27. The
Fertility
Diet

Ple
To r
or vi

rro

The
Fertility
Diet

How to Maximize Your Chances of Having a Baby at Any Age

SARAH DOBBYN

ON &
JSTER

First published in Great Britain by Simon & Schuster UK Ltd, 2008
A CBS COMPANY

1 3 5 7 9 10 8 6 4 2

Simon & Schuster UK Ltd
Africa House
64–78 Kingsway
London WC2B 6AH

www.simonsays.co.uk

Simon & Schuster Australia
Sydney

A CIP catalogue record for this book is available
from the British Library.

ISBN: 978-1-84737-200-0

Typeset by M Rules
Printed and bound in Italy by
L.E.G.O Spa

To my Mum, Judith Ann Dobbyn, who never needed a fertility diet

Contents

Foreword

by Dr John Simmons

As a doctor trained in both conventional and complementary medicine, with more than ten years' experience in general, family practice, I found *The Fertility Diet* a fascinating, well-written book and certainly a valuable resource that I would refer to when advising my patients. I would definitely recommend this book to anyone over thirty-five years old considering starting a family. It is well researched, clearly laid out and has an encouraging, step by step approach to changing your diet and lifestyle to maximize fertility (and indeed, overall well-being).

From my own research and practice, I observe that only 30 per cent of most disease conditions relevant to the western world are caused by genetic susceptibility and the remaining 70 per cent by environmental factors, showing that the overwhelming part of the healing outcome is totally changeable if you are prepared to commit to the process. We are always trying to empower our patients to take control of their health situations but they still need support in making the necessary changes – to have their hand held at times. The positive, motivational approach of *The Fertility Diet* will inspire readers to take charge of their diet and lifestyle and to do what it takes to lure the stork to their door.

Male infertility is a very common issue with semen analysis often identifying oligozoospermia (low sperm count). I had previously been at a loss as to how to advise these men to help themselves. Now I can refer them to the relevant chapter in *The Fertility Diet* and suggest they follow its guidelines: to increase their intake of organic produce and to ensure adequate daily consumption of anti-oxidants, in particular vitamin C , as well as the mineral zinc by eating plenty of fresh organic fruit and raw nuts and seeds every day.

With more and more women choosing to start their families later, *The Fertility Diet* offers a wonderful way to increase the chances of conception whether by assisted means or naturally. The latest in assisted conception technology (IVF, ICI, etc.) has helped thousands of couples who would never otherwise have had children. However, as Sarah Dobbyn points out, until very recently nothing was ever taught about nutrition or complementary and alternative medicine at medical schools. *The Fertility Diet* now allows men and women who are experiencing fertility issues to have the best of both worlds: complete information about what lifestyle choices, diet, herbs and supplements can do to help them conceive naturally, and, if they should subsequently need all the amazing technology allopathic medicine has to offer, greatly improved prospects of such assisted conception techniques succeeding. My approach to medicine is that it is about working together to achieve the best outcomes for our patients.

Often I have found that the healthiest diets are time-consuming and bland, but the recipe section in *The Fertility Diet* has some great ideas for preparing tasty, nutritious food in very little time. There is a lot of really useful information on healthy eating in general, some of which I intend to adopt myself!

When presented with a review copy of the book, I must confess I expected only to skim through it; instead I found myself completely engrossed and turning pages compulsively. I thoroughly enjoyed the book, finding it equally readable, entertaining and educational. I am sure it will prove a favourite addition to the library of anyone interested in fertility.

Dr John Simmons, GP, East Sussex

Acknowledgements

The gestation, development and safe delivery of this book into the world would not have been possible without the support, advice and inspiration of a number of people.

First, I must thank the good fairy behind the scenes who seems to have cast a lucky spell on the whole book project: my friend Stephanie Van Den Bergh, who introduced me both to my brilliant agent as well as to Dr Wendy Denning.

I have never looked back since being represented by Julia Churchill at the literary agents Darley Anderson. Julia's insight and editorial advice led to a vastly improved manuscript and her endless patience in dealing with all the naïve suggestions/queries inevitably made by a first-time author was remarkable.

The editor, Kerri Sharp, and her team at Simon & Schuster UK have been a pleasure to work with as *The Fertility Diet* evolved through various drafts into the exceptionally well-produced book you are holding in your hands.

Enormous thanks to Dr John Simmons and to Dr Wendy Denning – both for their vision in pioneering an integrated approach to medicine in which diet and nutrition play a key role, as well as for taking the time out of their unbelievably busy schedules to review *The Fertility Diet* and write the foreword/an endorsement respectively.

Astrologers tell me it is a 'Jupiter in the eleventh house' blessing but, for whatever reason, I have always had excellent friendship karma and must acknowledge all my wonderful friends – far too many to list individually – in the UK, Cayman Islands, Greece, USA, British Virgin Islands and around the world for your love, support and encouragement and for never betraying anything but total conviction that I could live my dream life as a writer.

My sincere appreciation to Dr Gabriel Cousens and all the talented staff at the College of Living Arts/Tree of Life Rejuvenation Center Patagonia, Arizona, USA, for creating a unique and amazing Masters Degree in Nutrition programme and for launching me on my new life path as a nutritional writer.

Thanks to my amazing family: to my wonderful mum who was always interested in good food and nutrition; to my brother, Johnny; his partner, Margaret; my sisters, Abigail and Judith, and their respective husbands, Alex and James, and to my darling nephews and nieces: Jack, Alice, Zoë, William, Henry and George, who are the sweetest reasons I know for wanting to write this book.

Most of all I suppose I must thank my soul mate, life partner and future father of my babies wherever he may be, for not being in my life yet. Had I met you before, this book would never have been written. P.S. you can show up now!

Part I:
The Ingredients for Baby Making

Introduction

Infertility and sub-fertility have now reached epidemic proportions, affecting one in every four couples of childbearing age in the USA and approximately one in six in Europe. One in every two couples in their forties are usually infertile. Women over thirty-five are told they have a better chance of being struck by lightning than of conceiving naturally. Research shows that the average sperm count in Europe dropped by 3.1 per cent each year from 1971 to 1990.[1] In the USA it dropped by a staggering 50 per cent in the period 1982 to 1992 alone.[2] An increasing number of abnormalities in sperm quality, motility and development are apparent.[3]

It is now not unusual for a couple with no evident fertility problems to take up to three years to conceive. Some 30 per cent of couples seeking medical assistance are told they have 'unexplained fertility' for which there is no treatment.

The medical establishment offers an array of assisted reproductive technologies such as in vitro fertilizations (IVF) and gamete intraFallopian transfer (GIFT). The prospects of success for such procedures are in the range of 15–20 per cent. For couples undergoing such assisted conception techniques, the experience is usually invasive, humiliating, very expensive and sadly, for the vast majority, ultimately disappointing.

Despite the huge amount of scientific research on the link between diet, proper nutrition and almost every other medical condition under the sun, the one thing on which doctors rarely advise adequately is the impact of nutrition on fertility. Huge amounts of money are being spent on assisted conception techniques by hopeful couples who do not know that alcoholic and caffeinated beverages are liquid contraceptives, that aspartame prevents ovulation, and that seemingly innocent 'health' foods such as peas, rhubarb and soya all inhibit conception.

There is no 'gold standard', double-blind and placebo-controlled, long-term medical study on a complete diet for fertility. However, there are hundreds of individual papers considering certain foods, drinks, micronutrients, and their direct impact on fertility, hormone levels and libido. In *The Fertility Diet* I have distilled this research into a comprehensive diet protocol. At the end of each chapter you will find a Fertility Action Plan that sets out suggestions for immediate steps you can take today to maximize your fertility and to bring the dream of having your own baby a lot closer.

Men and women who have been stigmatized as 'infertile' and women who have been told they are 'too old' to have a baby feel betrayed by their own bodies. Suddenly the most natural act in the world, the most primal human function of reproducing, is in the hands of people in white coats, with nasty syringes, unpleasant drugs, test tubes and Petri dishes. Of course it does not feel 'right', of course it is not 'natural'. How annoyed would you be to find out that some simple dietary changes could have spared you all this suffering and expense? Ultimately, *The Fertility Diet* aims to empower you to put your own fertility back where it belongs – in your own bedroom (OK, and your own kitchen!).

This book will be helpful to couples who wish to conceive naturally in the shortest possible time, and for men and women who wish to preserve their fertility at its optimum until the timing for starting a family is right.

The Fertility Diet will also help those who are already in the process of seeking medical treatment such as IVF, since it is vital for all assisted conception techniques that the egg and the sperm be as healthy as possible. Compelling evidence comes from a 1995 study[4], conducted by the University of Surrey on behalf of an organization promoting pre-conception nutrition called Foresight. During 1990–93 the progress of 367 couples trying to have a baby was followed. The women were aged between twenty-two and forty-five, and the men from twenty-five to fifty-nine. Thirty-seven per cent of the couples had a history of infertility and 38 per cent had had between one and five miscarriages. (Others had had other problems such as stillbirths, babies with birth defects and low birthweight babies.) All of the couples followed a healthy diet very similar to the principles of *The Fertility Diet*. They eliminated smoking and alcohol, bought organic food, ate more fruit and vegetables, cut down on caffeine, non-organic meat and dairy products and received individually tailored mineral and vitamin supplementation. By the end of the three-year trial, 89 per cent of the couples (327) had given birth; 81 per cent of the couples who had had a history of infertility had conceived and had babies; 83 per cent of those who had previously miscarried had a baby without experiencing a further miscarriage. None of the 327 babies born as part of the study was premature, the lightest one weighed 5 lb 2 oz (2.368 kg) and none needed to be admitted to a special care baby unit. Even more strikingly, there were no miscarriages, perinatal deaths or birth defects. On average statistics alone there should have been approximately 80 miscarriages (one in four) instead of none! And 65 per cent of the couples who had previously had IVF treatments conceived on this program without a further IVF cycle.

The work of the Reproductive Healthcare Clinic in St

John's Wood, London, shows that a highly nutritious diet such as that set out in *The Fertility Diet* will maximize your chances of having a baby even if you decide to undergo assisted conception techniques as well. At this London clinic women between thirty-two and forty-three years old who underwent assisted conception achieved a successful pregnancy rate of 50 per cent – an amazing statistic compared with the national standard of 15 per cent. The couples received both conventional and complementary medicine, including a full nutritional analysis and supplements.

Research from the University of Leeds, led by Dr Sara Matthews, on 215 women undergoing IVF treatment, found that the simple step of taking a daily multivitamin pill could boost a woman's fertility and double her chances of getting pregnant.

I am writing this book because I want this information on a diet that enhances fertility to become better known; I want to emphasize that the success rates of these incredibly expensive and interventionist assisted conception treatments can be doubled or tripled by something as simple as a simultaneous nutritional protocol.

The purpose of *The Fertility Diet* is to ensure that, for anyone trying to have a baby now or hoping to conceive in the future, a simple nutritional deficiency will not prevent you from having a successful pregnancy as soon as you want one.

The many well-intentioned doctors who sincerely wish to help couples trying to have a baby are never taught nutrition at medical school.

Fertility Action Plan

- Before making any changes to your diet to improve fertility, start to monitor what you actually do eat and drink right now by keeping a food diary for one week. List everything that you consume each day.

- Find out if you have any vitamin or mineral deficiencies by means of a blood test or hair-strand analysis. These can be arranged through your doctor, homeopath or naturopathic doctor.

Chapter 1
Parenthood at Any Age?

I have always had an inherent hatred of restraint. Being told that I cannot do something or even that some goal is objectively impossible inspires me more than any encouragement. My contrary spirit has been inflamed in recent years by the medical establishment presuming to tell me that, as a woman over 35, my chances of having a baby are dwindling with every passing year. They even have disparaging terms for me: I am now of 'advanced geriatric status'; were I pregnant I would be 'senile gravida'; and, since this would be my first baby, I would be 'elderly prima gravida'. Society's own prejudices about the appropriate time to conceive a child (until the mid-thirties) are equally pervasive: 'It's not natural to have a baby in your forties' and 'Who would even want to be a mother aged fifty or older?' are comments I have heard frequently.

With a twinkle in my eye, yet no sign of Mr Right on the immediate horizon, I have had no choice but to defy this wall of prejudice and pessimism and seek my own answers. After more than ten years' part-time study of health and nutrition, I knew that food was by far my best medicine. A book called *The Fertility Diet* or similar was nowhere to be found so I had to become a nutrition detective. I collected a few scraps here and there, from books, scientific journals and studies on natural medicine, anti-ageing, longevity, menopause, on fertility treatments, herbalism, minerals, amino acids, enzymes and, of course, nutrition and endocrinology generally.

A light beamed into the darkness one day as I read a book on anti-ageing and human growth hormone. The normally staid scientists at the Gerontological Society of America, when meeting in Washington DC a few years ago, had been thrown into uproar by the presentation of Dr Angelo Tarturro, who asserted that everything we call 'ageing' was no more than a collection of diseases and pathologies.

'Menopause,' he declared, is only caused by 'pathological changes in the hormonal balance that terminated a woman's fertile period. Fix this and motherhood could occur at any age.'

Yes! I knew it! Find a way to fix the hormonal imbalances that bring fertility to an end and *motherhood could occur at any age*! It is hard to describe the impact of these words upon me. My destiny as a future mother was within my own control if I could find out what to eat and, more importantly, what not to eat to keep my hormones balanced and at optimum levels for fertility.

It seems logical to me that eggs and sperm are only as healthy as the woman and the man producing them – no matter how old or, indeed, how young they are. Fertility at all ages is a condition of good health. Dr Christiane Northrup, a well-known endocrinologist, writes: 'A great disservice is done when "science" undermines the confidence of an entire group of women (everyone over thirty-five) concerning their fertility . . . If you're worried that you won't be able to have children because of your age, please know that this may not be the case at all.'

If you are under the age of thirty trying for a baby, you have youth and high hormone levels on your side, but this is no reason to become complacent. The advantages of being in your twenties can be undermined by unhealthy lifestyle and diet choices. I was interested to read that Dr Northrup would prefer to be the physician for a forty year old in excellent health who is planning a pregnancy than for a woman of twenty-five who smokes, drinks and eats junk food to excess.[1]

Post-menopausal women who have babies following egg donation and implantation prove that women's uteruses are fully capable of sustaining a baby into their sixties. So why is it that the ovaries, which of course supply many of the key reproductive hormones for women, normally age at a faster rate? One aspect of the fertility diet, as you shall see, is about creating optimal hormonal balance in the body in your twenties, thirties, forties and even fifties through healthy, plant-based, organic wholefoods and natural supplementation, to ensure that the ovaries also remain fully functioning as long as possible.

This is not just a pipe dream: there are reports of babies born to much older mothers living close to nature on a pure diet without any modern technology or medical intervention. The Huichol Indian women, who live in a remote part of Mexico, are said routinely to have babies in their fifties and even sixties.[3] On the Greek island of Paros, where I live some of the year, it is not a rare occurrence for a woman to have a baby in her late forties and early fifties, thanks to the local pure diet of home-grown herbs, fruits and vegetables, and, in particular, plenty of wild mountain greens (wild dandelion, chicory and amaranth).

In any case, all the doom and gloom one hears about 'old eggs' may be misguided. At least, that's what researchers at the University of Southern California School of Medicine think. Dr J. Lane Wong and his associates found that high-quality eggs for donor procedures are just as likely to be found in women between the ages of thirty-one and thirty-nine as in those from ages twenty-one to thirty. He reports: 'The pregnancy rate was 40 per cent among the women who received oocytes [eggs] from younger women and 41 per cent among those who received oocytes from older women.

Statistics from the American Center for Disease Control and Prevention show that, in 2004, there were 1,512 first-time mothers between the ages of forty-five and fifty-four.

'Menopause [is only caused by] pathological changes in the hormonal balance that terminates a woman's fertile period. Fix this and motherhood could occur at any age.' Dr Angelo Tarturro[2]

Take-home baby rates were also similar: 26 per cent among those who received oocytes from younger women and 30 per cent among women who received oocytes from older women.'[4]

Dr Monica Jarrett from the University of Washington has good news for older women who have been on the contraceptive pill a number of years: by inhibiting the release of an egg each month she thinks that they may actually have benefited by conserving their eggs.[5]

An even more intriguing theory was put to me in a private conversation by Dr Astley McLoughlin, former Professor of Biochemistry at the University of Indiana. Dr McLoughlin states that, since men manufacture sperm every ninety days, their sperm are made out of genetic material as old as the chronological age of the man at the time. In contrast, women are born as baby girls with, on average, 400,000 to 1,000,000 eggs already in place. So eggs are made out of genetic material that is zero months old – yes, the youngest, purest genetic material. Every other cell of a woman's body may be as old as she really is, but her eggs are as young as the day she was born. What a great hypothesis!

Besides, age norms have shifted significantly over the past fifty years: middle age now seems to begin at sixty and 'old' age at about eighty. The glamorous celebrities, movie stars, models and health gurus who have taken scrupulous care of their bodies for many years present a new yardstick for what a 'typical' forty, fifty and sixty-plus year old could be like and act like. They can inspire us to hold new beliefs about ageing. The actress Jane Seymour had twins, naturally, aged forty-five. Cherie Booth, wife of Tony Blair, gave birth to a healthy baby, Leo, when she was forty-six.

Britain's oldest mum, Dawn Brooke, was an astonishing fifty-nine when she and her then sixty-four-year-old husband, Raymond, naturaly conceived their son, a totally healthy, highly intelligent boy, now eleven years old.

Deepak Chopra, MD believes age is as much a state of mind as a bodily condition: 'Our cells are constantly eavesdropping on our thoughts and being changed by them . . . Because the mind influences every cell in the body, human ageing is fluid and changeable, it can speed up, slow down, stop for a time and even reverse itself. Hundreds of research findings from the last three decades have verified that ageing is much more dependent on the individual than was ever dreamed of in the past . . . In reality, the field of human life is open and unbounded. At its deepest level, our body is ageless, your mind timeless.'[6]

The elixir to fertility at all ages is one of health, the foundation to which begins with a good, pure diet of plant-based foods.

Fertility Action Plan

- Think some inspiring, baby-making thoughts for your cells to eavesdrop on!

- Women aged thirty-five-plus – create small notices reminding yourself MOTHERHOOD CAN OCCUR AT ANY AGE and MY EGGS ARE AS YOUNG AS THE DAY I WAS BORN. Post them somewhere you will see them daily, such as the fridge door or bathroom mirror.

- Men and women under thirty-five – make an honest assessment of any unhealthy lifestyle, eating and drinking habits, which may be depriving you of the fertility advantages of being young. Take some action today to improve your health.

Chapter 2

Pushing Snooze on the Biological Clock

In the drama of reproduction, age is always the villain. A villain who is also sexist, it seems. This chapter is therefore directed primarily at women who would like to stamp on the mythical biological clock and throw it out of the window, or at least hit the snooze button. Society as a whole is indoctrinated with the belief that, after thirty-five, women may be getting too old to have a baby. It's a bit like the four-minute-mile syndrome. Until 5 May 1954, it was universally accepted that it was impossible for any human to run a mile in under four minutes. Roger Bannister did just this on 6 May 1954. Once he had created this possibility, thirty-seven other runners matched his accomplishment the same year. In 1955 more than 300 other athletes achieved the 'impossible' feat, and now it is commonplace. The human body

It is all too easy to eat rubbish, drink rubbish, smoke, take dubious substances, lose sleep, maximize stress and forget exercise, and when your body finally fails to cooperate and give you a baby after all the years of abuse, to say, 'Oh well, I'm getting older, what could I expect? I need IVF.'

did not go through an evolutionary jump in 1954; it underwent a mental leap, a huge paradigm shift. So here is the new fertility paradigm, which I will capitalize to break through the hypnosis of the age thirty-five-barrier fertility programming:

ANY WOMAN WHO HAS NOT REACHED MENOPAUSE IS FERTILE AND ABLE TO HAVE A HEALTHY BABY!

And menopause can be delayed.

It is sometimes hard to trust the amazing regenerative and reproductive powers of your body at all ages. It takes courage to resist the thought programming all around us.

There is an important reason why the first part of this book, unlike other books on fertility presently available, focuses on anti-ageing. It is because ageing well is the key to enhanced fertility and libido, yet ageing is under your control to a significant degree. Your biological age and chronological age do not necessarily coincide. If your body believes you are young and healthy enough to have a baby, no matter how old you are, you will be able to conceive a child – and easily.

Immortality Syndrome

'Immortality syndrome', as I call it, can have a big impact on how well you are ageing. What on earth am I talking about? Everyone knows they are not immortal – right? Oddly enough, many people do not. At least not until their body reminds them of this unpalatable truth, often around the age of forty and most certainly by fifty. I observe teenagers and my friends in their twenties, still blissfully delusional that somehow they are going to look and feel forever as they look and feel now. They take little care of their health, they are almost contemptuous of their body in terms of the junk that goes into it because, hey, that one little cocktail/cigarette/doughnut is not going to make them old or infertile, is it?

Time is often blamed for the damage, which, in large measure, we in fact do to ourselves. The younger you are when you begin to treat your body with respect, nourishing it with mainly healthy foods and drinks and obtaining enough sleep and relaxation, the younger you will stay.

Knowing that how rapidly you age is largely within your control is liberating: you get to choose just how young and fertile you want to continue to be. It is never too late to begin this process. Look at yourself in the mirror – whether you look good, bad or average for your present age, now imagine you are ten years older and looking exactly the same or slightly younger. That is your goal for yourself – not necessarily to turn the clock back, but to slow it down or to get it to stand still. In this chapter and the next, I am going to explain everything I know about staying eternally young, and of course, fertile.

Genes Are Not Destiny

In my research I wanted to know all about women having babies naturally in their forties and fifties. I came across some interesting data suggesting that some women are born with a genetic advantage. Dr Neri Laufer of the Hadassah University Hospital, Jerusalem, Israel, and his team studied the genetic profile of 250 women, who 'conceived spontaneously' (meaning through good old-fashioned sex) aged over forty-five. Yes, forty-five! Dr Laufer noted, 'These women appear to differ from the normal population due to a genetic predisposition that protects them from the DNA damage and cellular ageing that helps age the ovary. What we do not yet know is whether this reproductive success is linked with potential longevity.'[1]

The women in the Israeli study were all Ashkenazi Jews, but the good news is that Dr Laufer's team believes that the same gene profile is seen in other ethnic and, thus, genetic groups. He already has preliminary results showing a very similar profile in Bedouin women who have also had children later in life.

But if there is one message I would like to get across in this book, it is that your genes are not your destiny. A 1996 study on 2,872 Danish identical twins showed, for example,

'Only about 35 per cent of the ageing process is genetic. That means 65 per cent is in your hands literally. Anti-ageing is possible, because metabolism can be changed.' Biochemist and anti-ageing expert Stephen Cherniske in *The Metabolic Anti-Ageing Plan* [3]

that genetic factors made up only 25 per cent of the variation of life span, with 75 per cent of ageing/longevity being caused by 'unknown environmental factors'.[2]

So what can you do with your major part of the equation to achieve the same reproductive potential as these super-fertile women?

You see, whether your genes are helpful or not, all ageing in the body – yes, every wrinkle you see – begins at the cellular level. When the 100 trillion cells in your body replicate there are three alternatives: the so-called daughter cells can be of better quality; they can be exactly the same condition; or they can be of an inferior standard, showing damage and wear and tear. It is nothing short of miraculous that the body makes the equivalent of 300 billion copies of your DNA every single day.

The Biochemistry of Ageing

Your DNA looks a bit like a twisted or spiralled ladder. During cell division, the DNA molecule comes apart and the bases (i.e. the 'rungs' of the ladder) must be duplicated perfectly in order to create a flawless copy for the new cell. During cell division, however, DNA is exposed to a number of potentially damaging conditions.

1. The presence of free radicals, which most people know are the vandal molecules inevitably produced during normal cell functioning, as a form of waste product or cell exhaust. In a non-smoker it is estimated each cell receives 10,000 free radical hits every day.
2. Toxins from food or the environment, which also increase the number of free radicals.
3. UVA radiation from the sun.

The cell has elaborate quality control systems. When DNA is damaged, a team of special enzymes fix the problem. But, with 100 trillion cells replicating a billion DNA strands (do the maths, that's a lot of zeros), inevitably errors creep in. If an error is not detected or repaired in time and certain internal cell functions go awry, a second level of control kicks in. Either the cell commits suicide, sacrificing itself for the good of the whole, or it is killed off by neighbouring cells – like a kind of cellular neighbourhood watch combined with a vigilante group!

It is folic acid, zinc, magnesium, B vitamins and other key nutrients which support critical enzymatic actions in the cells. Eating the right stuff means that your cells have what they need to make each new cell copy as perfect as the first one. Exposing your cells to toxins from your diet or from the environment or high levels of stress hormones will inevitably cause cell damage or even death.

Folic acid and zinc are key for repairing DNA strands in all cells – they are important anti-ageing and fertility nutrients.

Eternally Youthful Cells

This entire book is full of information on how to keep your cells young and happy through diet but here, in summary, are the key components:

- **Avoid cell damage by increasing your intake of antioxidants.** These are the friendly compounds that hook up with the vandal molecules, free radicals, giving them companionship and thus keeping them out of trouble. Antioxidants come from organic fruits and vegetables, as well as supplements of vitamin E, selenium and alpha-lipoic acid – men should add vitamin C supplements too. (I do not recommend vitamin A in supplement form because of its potential toxicity, nor vitamin C supplements for women, which have been found to interfere with fertile cervical mucus.) The fertility diet includes fruit and vegetables with an abundant supply of antioxidants. Your body also produces its own master antioxidant called glutathione (pronounced 'gloota-thigh-own') inside each cell. You can take certain nutrients in supplement form to increase your own glutathione levels, including: NAC (n-acetyl glutathione); milk thistle (silymarin) – a herb particularly helpful in repairing cellular damage caused by alcohol consumption; the amino acid gluta-mine – which can also kill cravings for sugar; and B vitamins, which are co-factors in the internal manufacture of glutathione.

- **Protect your cells from toxins.** Pesticides, heavy metals (including the mercury in the fillings in your teeth), smoking, alcohol, caffeine, artificial sweeteners, recreational drugs and junk food additives all contribute to cell damage and, not coincidentally, all cause infertility. The fertility diet emphasizes a pure diet of organic foods and drinks to reduce the toxic load on your body and remove these powerful contraceptive toxins from your life.

- **Help stabilize your DNA.** Certain compounds found in plants when they are under stress turn on their anti-ageing genes called sirtuins. Organically grown plants with no herbicides or pesticides to help them fight their life battles have higher amounts of these anti-ageing molecules than mollycoddled commercially grown crops. These anti-ageing compounds, which have been found by Harvard scientists to stabilize DNA, are then passed on to the humans who consume them. The fertility diet recommends the consumption of as much fresh, organic produce as you can obtain, and, of course, afford. Even better, grow your own fruit, vegetables and herbs.

- **Optimize your cells' quality control procedures:**
  a) Take a folic acid supplement every single day and each folate-rich foods such as leafy greens and spinach. This is a simple, but highly effective, anti-ageing strategy.
  b) Quit the caffeine. I know this is tough, but caffeine interferes with the normal cell replication cycle. Basically, instead of allowing the cell its usual pauses to check quality control, the presence of caffeine encourages the cell to 'skip on by' quickly, possibly overlooking cell errors. By the time you have read about the contraceptive qualities of coffee and tea in Chapter 5, your favourite cuppa may not look so appealing anyway.
  c) Make sure there is adequate zinc in your diet by eating nuts, seeds, parsley, spinach and asparagus – alternatively take a supplement of maximum 10 mg per day.

- **Help your cells communicate properly.** Water plays a critical role in cell communication; some biochemists now believe that the core of the double helix of your DNA is a column of organized water through which information is transmitted at lightning speeds.[4] MRI technology has now proven that dehydration results in cellular damage – i.e. rapid ageing. Water really is the elixir of youth. When calculating your water intake do not count tea, coffee, sodas or any other caffeinated beverage, which are all diuretic. So, from a daily goal of a minimum of two, preferably three, litres, always deduct 250 ml from your total of water consumed for each caffeinated or high-sugar beverage you drink.

The other key component in cell communication is glyconutrients – forms of sugar. Now, you may never have heard of glyconutrients before – indeed, their vital role in cell communication was unknown until 1996 – but, as of 2008, they are at the cutting edge of research in anti-ageing nutrition and nutrition for the cure of cancer, diabetes and heart disease. In fact, they may be an almost universal panacea because of their responsibility for intelligent interaction between cells.[5]

There are eight of these miracle sugars in total. The first two of them you are probably eating every day: glucose – yes, the usual form of sugar – and galactose, from dairy products. However, you are likely to be deficient in six of them.

1. Fucose: it sounds almost rude! It is found in medicinal mushrooms such as cordyceps (dubbed the 'fungal Viagra', without the side effects), resihi and shiitake mushrooms.
2. Mannose: not just for men, but women too! Aloe vera is an abundant source of mannose.
3. Xylose: the main source is my all-time favourite sweetener xylitol. Derived from fruit and birch tree bark, this low-glycaemic, low-calorie sugar looks and tastes like regular sugar, except it does not trigger an insulin release and is anti-bacterial.
4. n-acetyl glucosamine: which everyone with stiff joints loves.
5. n-acetylgalactosamine.
6. n-acetylneuraminic acid.

These last three glyconutrients can be found in supplements like echinacea, astralgus and brewer's yeast. While not yet commonly available in health-food stores, complete compounds of all eight glyconutrients can be found online.

Taking food or supplements which contain the miracle sugars called glyconutrients will keep you young and fertile.

The fertility diet will show you how to implement this cellular youthing plan into your diet and lifestyle. In the next chapter, we will look at how hormones are sending instructions to your cells all the time – either to degenerate and halt your reproductive potential, or to regenerate and keep you young and fertile.

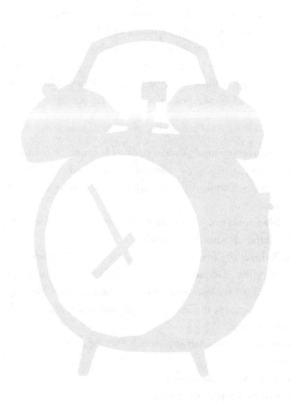

Fertility Action Plan

- Consider how you may have been harming your health and fertility through immortality syndrome behaviour. Resolve *now* to nurture your body, so you age very slowly.

- Take folic acid and antioxidant supplements including vitamin E and selenium, and those which boost glutathione levels, every day.

- Check out glyconutrients online and order yourself some of these anti-ageing miracle sugars as soon as possible.

Chapter 3

Growth Hormone and Insulin – the Master Hormones

Hormones are the communication internet, fax, phone, mail, courier and even the news-reporting media of the body all rolled into one – chemical messengers that enable the 100 trillion-plus cells of the body to function together as a unit and to keep the 'mission-control centre' part of the brain (the hypothalamus) informed on the state of affairs. They move continuously through the bloodstream to different cells; once at their destination they latch on to the surface of their target cell at sites called receptors (like a key going into a lock), where they trigger a specific reaction. Fertility lies in far more than sex hormones. For perfect reproductive health all the major endocrine glands – the pituitary, thyroid, thymus, adrenals, pancreas and ovaries/testes – have to be functioning well and producing appropriate levels of hormones.

The pituitary releases many hormones – growth hormone (the youth and regeneration hormone) being the most abundant one. Growth hormone is at the centre of much anti-ageing research since it has been found that it declines with age in every animal species that has been tested. In humans, after the age of thirty-one, levels of growth hormone usually fall about 14 per cent every ten years. At twenty years old we produce 500 mcg, at forty this has usually dropped to 400 mcg and by eighty it has often dwindled to a paltry 25 mcg.[1] Studies have shown that the decline of growth hormone from the pituitary seems to trigger a cascading decrease in all the hormones necessary for fertility and libido. However, if growth-hormone levels are boosted, the sex hormones are correspondingly elevated. The male authors of a number of books I read on human growth hormone and anti-ageing can barely contain their boyish delight at the testimonials of women taking growth-hormone supplements who have a return of libido, and, in particular, at men who are cured of impotency and low sex drive. Men as old as eighty start reporting a return to sexual vigour and activity at levels similar to when they were twenty-five! In fact, Vincent Giampapa, MD, an anti-ageing specialist, encourages couples who want growth-hormone treatment to start supplements together, saying that, otherwise, the relationship may run into trouble: 'We find that men start looking at young girls again, so we have to treat the wives also,' he observes.[2]

What I find particularly interesting is the fact that, as we age, the pituitary does not stop producing growth hormone, it just releases less of it into the bloodstream. Read that last sentence again. Isn't that remarkable? If you want to remain as young and fertile as possible, no matter how many candles are crammed on to your birthday cake, you have to do everything possible to keep the levels of growth hormone being released as naturally high as they are as in young adults. I am not recommending paying vast sums of money for monthly injections – growth hormone can be

'Growth hormone plays a role in both male and female fertility, improving the effect of the reproductive hormones and in the production of sperm and eggs.' Karlis Ullis, MD[3]

boosted naturally by diet, supplements, sound sleep and exercise.

How to Stimulate Production of Growth Hormone

1. Fasting. It has been discovered that fasting is one of the most potent inducers of growth hormone. It is safe for anyone in good health to carry out a three-day juice fast at home. But, if you have never fasted before, I recommend attending a health farm or fasting clinic to undertake a fast of up to seven days on fresh, organic fruit and vegetable juices. Fasting only on water (no juices) causes the highest elevation in growth hormone. However, water fasting can be challenging and is really only suitable for those who are already familiar with juice fasting and are not under-weight. (See Chapter 18 for more about the fertility benefits of fasting.)

2. Appropriate body fat levels. Body fat itself appears to be the biggest, reversible, obstacle to growth-hormone release. There is an exact correlation between both fertility and body mass index (BMI) as well as between growth hormone and BMI. With an average weight and a BMI of between twenty and twenty-five you will have normal fertility. A 1991 study by Dr A Iranmanesh and his colleagues estimated that growth hormone fell 6 per cent for each unit increase in body mass index. Two factors reduced the rate of twenty-four-hour production of growth hormone: going from twenty-one to forty-five years old or increasing BMI from twenty-one to twenty-eight. Think about that – supposing you were a 5-foot 6-inch woman weighing 12 stone 7 lbs (80 kg), with a BMI of twenty-eight. If you lost weight to 10 stone 10 lbs (68 kg) and a BMI of twenty-four, you would, by this alone, boost your daily growth-hormone release by 24 per cent and give all your sex hormones quite a zap! There is a lot of anecdotal evidence concerning women who have gone on diets, lost a lot of weight, then suddenly got pregnant. This can not only be attributed to improved self-esteem and libido from feeling more attractive in a slimmer body (leading to more hanky panky with the significant other), but also to a sudden surge in growth-hormone levels as the BMI decreases.

3. Exercise. Yes, I am sorry, this would not be a diet book without some mention of exercise. Exercise sends a wake-up call to the pituitary to start pumping out more growth hormone. There is also plenty of anecdotal evidence of men and women conceiving having started a fitness programme. I attribute this to the boost in growth hormone and, thus, a corresponding rise in gonadal hormones. But beware of overexercising – if exercise causes a woman's body fat levels to fall too low (below 17 per cent), this will cause infertility, so don't overdo it!

4. Supplements. Taking the amino acids L-arginine, L-ornithine, L-lysine, L-glutamine and L-glycine, together with niacin and GABA (gamma-amino butyric acid) just before bedtime can lead to growth-hormone levels being raised by 20 per cent while you sleep – completely naturally! Other helpful amino acids are leucine, valine, carnitine and tryptophan. The amino acid tyrosine helps too, but do not take this at bedtime, since it is a stimulant – first thing in the morning is better. (See Chapter 17 on amino acids and Chapter 9 for more details on fertility boosting nutrients.)

5. Sleep. Adequate sleep is very important in maximizing growth hormone. The strongest bursts or pulses of growth hormone from the anterior pituitary occur about one or two hours after we fall asleep and achieve a deep sleep state. If sleep is fitful or broken, a vicious circle occurs: the lack of deep sleep causes less growth hormone to be released, and lower growth-hormone levels can in turn actually cause poor sleep or insomnia. Research carried out at the University of Chicago by Dr Eve Van Cauter suggests that, if deep sleep can be restored, the ageing process can be slowed thanks to higher levels of growth hormone. There is also a school of thought that any sleep before midnight is of a better quality than sleep after midnight, that one hour before midnight is equal to two after.

If you are overweight, the level of growth hormone released in the body can be increased quite naturally by losing body fat.

A diet high in sugar, alcohol and refined carbohydrates causes insulin levels to soar and, in turn, shuts off the release of growth hormone, which can, therefore, cause impaired fertility.

The Growth Hormone – Insulin Connection

Insulin has a vital life-serving role; it regulates blood glucose levels in the body. However, I think of it as the hyper-ageing hormone.

1. Insulin inhibits growth hormone. Growth hormone is a fat-burning hormone, whereas insulin promotes fat storage. A vicious ageing circle ensues if your growth-hormone levels fall, you get fatter, then, because you are fatter, growth-hormone release declines, which means your growth-hormone levels are going to be even lower in proportion to your insulin levels.

2. Insulin accelerates cell turnover. This is not a good thing. You want your cells to replicate themselves as slowly as possible since it appears all your cells can divide only a maximum of fifty times before they (and thus, ultimately, you) die. You do not want your cells whirring at top speed though their finite divisions, like your electricity meter does when running every appliance in the house. You want your cells to be languid, positively snail-like in their division activities. It is no accident that the *only* thing researchers have ever been able to find that centenarians all have in common is low insulin levels.

3. Another reason insulin is the number one age-accelerating hormone is because it **stimulates the release of cortisol from the adrenals**. Cortisol competes with the master steroid hormone DHEA(dehydroepiandrosterone), which is one of the most powerful regenerative and procreative hormones in the body, converting into both testosterone and oestrogen. High insulin means high cortisol and thus low DHEA and, correspondingly, lower sex hormones. DHEA is abundant in young people and begins to decline from the age of thirty onwards. Trust me, you want to keep your DHEA levels as high as possible for as long as possible.

Instead of asking yourself the boring old question, 'Why do I eat this chocolate bar – why don't I just apply it directly to my hips?', you can enquire of yourself instead, 'Why eat this chocolate bar? Why don't I just bash myself around the eyes with it and give myself more crow's feet?' Because that is the truth of it.

Eating any high sugar and refined carbohydrate foods frequently enough will spike your insulin levels, decelerate growth hormone, accelerate ageing, and ultimately lower your sex hormones. The good news is that insulin can be controlled by eating foods low on the glycaemic index. This is a measure of how fast a carbohydrate enters the bloodstream and raises the blood-sugar level. Glucose (pure sugar) scores 100 on this index; most vegetables (apart from cooked carrots, sweetcorn and potatoes) are low on the glycaemic index, as is most fruit (apart from tropical fruit such as mango, banana, papaya and pineapple).

The fertility diet is a low glycaemic diet with a heavy emphasis on raw fruit and vegetables, with protein from organic free-range eggs, nuts, seeds, fish from pure sources and sea vegetables – so nothing even remotely like the Atkins diet. This diet ensures insulin levels will remain low and stable and thereby allows growth-hormone levels to remain proportionally higher.

The more fibre a food contains, the lower its glycaemic index, so raw fruit and vegetables are automatically lower on the glycaemic index than their cooked counterparts because their fibre has not been broken down in the cooking process. Fibre itself has a role to play in fertility since it reduces excess oestrogen levels by clearing out old hormone residues and preventing oestrogens that have been excreted in the bile from the gall bladder from being reabsorbed into the blood. Studies have shown that women who eat a vegetarian diet excrete three times more 'old' detoxified oestrogens than women who also eat meat. Carnivores reabsorb more oestrogens, so a low glycaemic, high-fibre diet will help to balance hormone levels.

Insulin and Women's Fertility

Researchers have found that there is a clear correlation between women's sensitivity to insulin and the phase of the menstrual cycle. During the first half of the cycle leading up to ovulation, when the hormone oestrogen is more dominant, you are more sensitive to insulin and glucose is more effectively metabolized in the body. From ovulation leading up to menstruation, when progesterone levels rise, women become increasingly resistant to insulin. This is why women experience a heartier appetite and more food cravings before their periods. Your body is laying down fat ready for any pregnancy and your cells will be 'deaf' to insulin, so the pancreas will be pumping out far more than normal.

Never start any kind of sliming diet in days fourteen to twenty-eight of your cycle. With progesterone and insulin surging, you are far more likely to fall off the wagon than if you started it earlier in your cycle, just as your period is ending.

Maintaining moderate levels of insulin may be key for fertility for yet another reason: insulin controls your cholesterol levels in the blood. Sex hormones, like all steroid hormones, are manufactured from cholesterol, which must be maintained at healthy levels.

Most importantly for women's fertility, researchers have found insulin receptors in the ovaries. Insulin acts with these so the enzymes in the ovaries make more androgens (male sex hormones such as testosterone) rather than the normal oestrogen balance. According to Dr Elizabeth Lee Vliet, these androgens feed back on glucose-regulating hormones and cause even more insulin production.[4] The higher the insulin levels, the more androgens are made by the ovaries – leading to another vicious infertility circle of weight gain and hormonal imbalances. On top of this, excess androgens stop the ovaries releasing an egg, causing irregular or non-existent periods. This syndrome is particularly seen in women suffering from Polycystic Ovary Syndrome (PCOS). (See Chapter 27 on PCOS.)

To enhance fertility, particularly for women, insulin must be kept under control. The answer is to follow a low-glycaemic, high-fibre diet, like the Fertility Diet.

Insulin and Men's Fertility

Men, do not be reaching for your high-sugar foods just yet, elevated insulin levels can lead to Type II diabetes, which is known to cause infertility and impotency! You will be at your most fertile and healthiest sticking to low-glycaemic, high-fibre foods as well.

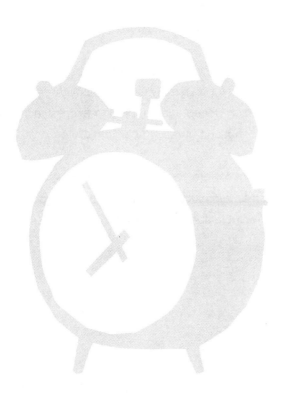

Fertility Action Plan

- Review the growth-hormone-stimulating protocol and decide which steps you can begin today to zap your youth and fertility hormones. Going to a health farm for a juice fast? Losing any excess weight? Increasing exercise? Taking amino acid supplements? Improved sleep?

- Immediately cut down (or preferably cut out) the high-glycaemic foods that cause high-speed ageing through excessive insulin release: sugar, alcohol and unrefined carbohydrates.

- Increase the amount of fibre you eat: choose wholegrain bread and rice, and high-fibre breakfast cereals, eat flax seeds, or take a supplement of soluble fibre like psyllium husks.

Part II:
The Fertility Blockers

Chapter 4
Infertility Foods

By now, we should all have got the message that we are what we eat. We understand that our health is affected by diet, so it will come as no surprise that processed/junk foods and saturated fats – the foods that are commonly known to lead to ill-health and disease – are also damaging to fertility. However, what you might not have realized is that some foods which are considered 'healthy' like soya or peas, whilst conferring certain nutritional benefits, have substances in them that act as a contraceptive and should be avoided when you are trying for a baby. In this section, foods both 'good' and 'bad' that hinder your chances of conceiving are described.

Aspartame

Consider all diet drinks and low sugar food containing aspartame to have a skull and crossbones on them. Aspartame is a so-called excito-toxin – a substance that was once listed by the Pentagon as a biological warfare agent! Every time you ingest it, a residue of wood formaldehyde is left behind – forever. The liver has no natural enzymes or detox pathway to get rid of this evil stuff out of your body, so aspartame assiduously accumulates in your nerve endings and neurons, just waiting to give you a terrifying list of ill-nesses: arthritis, fibromyalgia, lupus, multiple sclerosis, diabetes and Alzheimer's[1] – even a tiny amount of excito-toxic chemicals cause the brain cells to become so overexcited that they burn themselves out and die.

Since 2004, the National Justice League group has filed a number of lawsuits in the USA against the manufacturers of aspartame, which the claimants describe as 'a deadly neuro-toxin unfit for human consumption'. Imagine what eating this is doing to your fertility . . .

Mother Nature is not keen on reproducing a species chock-full of wood formaldehyde so she causes aspartame to stimulate the pituitary gland to secrete the hormone prolactin, which inhibits ovulation – thus ensuring you will not have a baby. Even if you do somehow conceive, this is not the kind of poison you want to be giving a developing baby, since it can penetrate the placental barrier and cause birth defects.

Aspartame is found in more than 5,000 foods so it is important to be vigilant. Check all food labels carefully, especially those on diet drinks and diet foods, many types of frozen desserts, diet sugars, sugar-free gum and some forms of gelatine. If they contain aspartame, chuck them straight into the rubbish bin.

Animal Fats

Fat is key in terms of reproductive health and has a signifi-cant impact on hormonal levels. Whereas consumption of uncooked essential fatty acids (EFAs) from plant sources boosts fertility and hormone levels, fats from animal sources and cooked fats interfere with the functioning of cell mem-branes and can also cause oestrogen levels to rise excessively.

A number of studies show that when both pre- and post-menopausal women cut back on their animal and cooked fat intake from 40 per cent of calories to 20 per cent, oestrogen circulating in the blood was significantly lowered.

Besides improving fertility, a diet low in animal and cooked fats has been found to prevent breast and other hormone-related cancers, which need excess oestrogen to thrive.

For men, several studies have indicated that eating fatty meals may lower sex drive and sex hormones, since they cause testosterone to plunge. Fatty meals mean a high risk of weight gain, and obesity also causes higher oestrogen and lower testosterone levels. Furthermore, a high-fat diet could interfere with having and maintaining an erection: eating animal fat clogs the arteries that also transport blood to the penis for an erection, in the same way that it clogs the arteries to the heart. Arterial blockages are a significant cause of impotence in men. Indeed, problems with maintaining an erection could be one of the warnings from the body that your cardiovascular system needs immediate attention.

Fish from Mercury-contaminated Waters

Mercury causes infertility in both men and women, and mercury toxicity causes both miscarriages and birth defects. The fish with the highest mercury levels are the bigger predatory fish – shark, tilefish and king mackerel. Under no circumstances should any woman wanting to have children eat these fish. Tuna, red snapper and mahi mahi have lower, but still significant, levels of mercury. Herring, like all smaller fish, has the lowest amounts. If you are a fish lover then I recommend you cut down to fish once per week, and choose a smaller, less toxic fish, if possible from pure waters – definitely not the Atlantic Ocean or North Sea region.

The mercury leaching into your body from amalgam dental fillings is more of a widespread cause of infertility than mercury from fish; mercury from fish is, nevertheless, a serious problem.

Fried Foods, Trans-fats and Commercial Oils

Your body will flourish on raw, plant fats. Organic cold-pressed nut and seed oils like olive oil support fertility and libido. The moment you heat any oil to a high temperature, however, it twists fat from their natural 'cis' shape to an unhealthy 'trans' shape. Trans-fats, found in all fried foods and most margarines, are alien substances to your fat-sensitive cell membranes and reproductive organs. A study in Nigeria found that, when rats were fed palm oil that had been heated to very high temperatures, their pregnancy rates were reduced by up to 55 per cent. The most heat-stable oils are coconut and canola, which can be used in small amounts to stir fry your fertility vegetables, if you wish. Ideally, do not fry any food or eat heated oils.

Genetically Modified (GM) Foods – the Frankenstein Foods

The more I read about GM foods, the more I am terrified and disturbed. Let me tell you a few more details about these Frankenstein foods. The biotechnology industry is taking plants – our food – and messing with their DNA; they are turning genes permanently on, permanently off, moving them, scrambling them, deleting some, and reversing others. To insert a GM gene into a plant and switch it on, they also have to attach an altered virus gene called a promoter which, whoops, they now find can set off other genes it is not supposed to.[2] It also turns out that the inserted genes are often unstable and can mutate in unpredictable ways (double whoops), creating proteins that were never intended or tested.[3]

It is already known that GM food can reduce the fertility of animals and insects feeding on them. Ladybirds who ate greenfly, which had been feeding on GM potatoes, had a drastic reduction in fertility and produced far fewer eggs. The fertility of the petunia plant has been shown to be significantly reduced by the introduction of a gene to increase redness in the flower.

More worryingly, experiments conducted by Irina Ermakova, a leading scientist at the Institute of Higher Nervous Activity and Neurophysiology of the Russian Academy of Sciences, showed that when rats were fed GM soya at the pre-conception stage and while pregnant, they gave birth to smaller offspring, of whom 55.6 per cent were dead within three weeks. This was compared with 6.8 per cent of infant deaths in the control group.[4]

At the moment we do not know the full price to be paid in terms of human health by eating these Frankenstein foods, but, instinctively, I feel this tampering with nature cannot be right and that eating unnatural produce is not going to assist my health and my fertility. The British Medical Association shares my concerns. In a report entitled *The Impact of Genetic Modification on Agriculture, Food and Health*, the BMA has called for research into these Frankenstein foods to see if they will damage the immune system and fertility, as well as a moratorium on GM foods altogether.

Genetically modified foods are now meant to be labelled, so check carefully. However, you can be sure that food from organic sources will not be genetically modified. Avoid commercially grown produce and choose the best organic food available, finances permitting.

Herbs to Avoid

Heavy use of the herbal supplements echinacea (to boost immunity); ginkgo biloba (to enhance circulation and memory); and St John's Wort (a natural antidepressant) may cause infertility in men and should be avoided. According to a study carried out at Loma Linda University School of Medicine in California, these herbs reduce the sperm's ability to penetrate the egg, lower sperm viability and damage sperm DNA – not exactly what a man who wants to be a father is looking for.

A number of herbs promote uterine contractions and should definitely be avoided in the first trimester of pregnancy (though they are great if you want to speed up labour). These are blue cohosh, raspberry leaf, burdock, chamomile, fennel, sage and thyme. Parsley, though a tremendous fertility food when it comes to conceiving, should be avoided in high doses in the first trimester too. Steering clear of high doses of these herbs will eliminate any small risk of miscarrying at the embryo implantation stage as well, when you might not yet know you are pregnant.

Junk Foods

It is estimated that some 80 per cent of foods found on our supermarket shelves (with 3,000 artificial additives) have only been created in the last twenty years. A diet of edible items (I think 'food' is too generous a description) from cardboard packages nuked in the microwave will certainly not help your fertility. A study on mice that were fed food colourings found they ended up with abnormal testicular function and reproductive performance. Their sperm count, motility and morphology were all affected. It seems the law of evolution makes junk lovers the losers in the survival of the fittest.

Meat

Non-organic meat should be eliminated from the diet completely. Increasingly, commercially raised cows, sheep, pigs and poultry are given hormones to stimulate growth. When the flesh of such animals is eaten, these hormones enter the human bloodstream, wreaking havoc with our own delicate endocrine balance.

Another reason to avoid all meat, even organic meat, is that it is loaded with saturated fat, which is the hardest of all foods for the body to break down and digest. The excess body fat caused by eating saturated animal fats can lead to elevated oestrogen levels, since one form of oestrogen, estrone, is manufactured by fat cells in the body. Obesity can cause infertility in women, as explained in Chapter 9.

Thirdly, even organically raised animals are likely to feed on pasture that is subject to air pollution – in particular dioxins, by-products of many manufacturing processes. These toxic chemicals do not dissolve in water so are only found in minuscule amounts in plants, but they are fat soluble, so tend to accumulate in the body fat of animals. Research shows that between 80 and 90 per cent of the average human intake of dioxins comes from milk and meat. Any person living in an industrialized country who has eaten animal fats or animal fat by-products will have dioxins in his or her body. Dioxins are linked to low sperm count and abnormal sperm in men and anovulation (failure to ovulate), endometriosis and miscarriage in women.

The regular consumption of the common pea is reported to be responsible for the low birth rate in Tibet![5]

Women's fertility is affected even at trace amounts. Thus, the only effective way to cut out dioxins is to avoid eating all meat and dairy products when trying to conceive. If giving up meat is unthinkable to you, then please choose only the best organic meats and trim off every ounce of fat.

Besides affecting fertility, dioxins at high concentrations can cause organ disease, an increased risk of cancer and heart disease, a suppressed immune system, diabetes and disfiguring facial cysts known as chloracne.

Monosodium Glutamate

If you love Chinese and Japanese takeaways be aware that monosodium glutamate has been shown to cause infertility in test animals according to a study published in *Neurobehavioral Toxicology*.

Peas

Peas, which seem so innocent a vegetable and have a number of health-giving vitamins and minerals, have been linked to infertility. They contain a natural contraceptive with the unpronounceable name m-xylohydroquinone, which interferes with both oestrogen and progesterone. To obtain the full contraceptive effect you do have to eat a lot: rats who were fed a diet of which 20 per cent consisted of peas had reduced litter sizes; 30 per cent of the rats failed to reproduce. To be on the safe side, however, peas are best avoided when you are trying to have a baby – opt instead for wonderful fertility-enhancing vegetables: broccoli, cabbage, carrots, spinach and other leafy greens and sweet potatoes.

Red Clover

For all the reasons set out below concerning soya, it is crucial to avoid supplements of the herb red clover, which is very high in isoflavones. This supplement can boost immunity and liver function and purify the bloodstream. However, wait until you have had all your babies and then consider taking it for these reasons – or as a natural contraceptive!

Rhubarb

The British love their traditional summer dessert rhubarb crumble. Unfortunately, rhubarb has been linked to infertility and so should be off the menu when you are trying to conceive.

Soya

Of all the foods I researched for *The Fertility Diet*, soya initially confused me the most. I had read so much hype about the innumerable health benefits of soya that I confidently expected it to be a fertility power food. I was in for a big shock. I found research suggesting that the isoflavones in soya can render you infertile. Yes, you read correctly. The soya industry's PR has done fine work with the media in convincing us into believing that soya is a health super-food. Well, whatever its many claims in relation to cardiovascular health as well as its cancer-protective effects, unfortunately, for fertility and libido, soya is definitely very bad news – indeed, it is one of the foods most likely to cause infertility in women.

Studies show that when high levels of isoflavones from soya are ingested they can compete with the body's own oestrogen at cellular receptors and thereby interfere with or block your body's own oestrogen production. A landmark UK study involving pre-menopausal women found that a daily intake of just 45 mg of soya for one month (about one cup of soya milk) could alter the length of the menstrual cycle and continue to disrupt the cycle for three months after the soya supplement was stopped.[6] Disturbed menstruation in young vegetarians has also been attributed to soya consumption.[7]

Soya can cause infertility in men too. Research carried out by Professor Neil McClure, a fertility specialist at the Belfast Royal Infirmary, found that the sperm of twenty-four men whose partners had been having difficulty in conceiving had significantly higher levels of genistein – one of the phytoestrogens found in soya – leading him to conclude that soya impairs sperm function.[8] Studies also show that a diet high in soya will cause men to lose testosterone as their oestrogen levels rise too high or fall too low.[9]

I was further dismayed to find out that soya inhibits healthy thyroid function, which, in turn, reduces fertility. Dr Larrian Gillespie, author of *The Menopause Diet*, experimented on herself. 'I did it in two different ways. I tried the (isoflavone) supplement (at 40 mg), where I went into flagrant hypothyroidism within seventy-two hours, and I did the "eat lots of tofu category", and it did the same thing, but it took me five days with that. I knew what I was doing but it still took me another seven to ten days to come out of it.' There is a well-established connection between hypothyroidism and infertility, so eating any substance that interferes with optimal thyroid function could never be recommended for any woman trying to become pregnant.

In addition to the harm soya can cause to fertility, 90 per cent of the US soya crops – which also end up in Europe – are said to be genetically modified, so fall into the Frankenstein foods category.

I now only eat soya in the form of minimal amounts of organic soya sauce and an occasional organic miso soup. My advice to anyone seeking to have a baby or with a low thyroid problem is not to touch any soya products with a bargepole with a condom on the end.

Sugar – Sweets, Biscuits and Cakes

I hope the pep talk in Chapter 3 on the dangers of too much insulin has curbed your sweet tooth and turned it into a xylitol tooth instead. Sugar and white flour products will rob your body of valuable fertility-enhancing minerals, accelerate cell turnover, cause insulin to soar and growth hormone to plummet. You are sending your body and sexual organs the message to age as fast as possible. Apart from inhibiting growth-hormone release, sugar interferes with enzyme actions in the body. Remember, refined sugar has no nutrients and only wreaks biochemical havoc in the body. It is the consumption of sugar that leads to more sugar cravings. To help your willpower in cutting it out, take supplements of the amino acid l-glutamine, which helps curb cravings for sugar and sweet treats while at the same time supporting your fertility.

Wheat/Gluten

Sometimes a severe gluten intolerance or allergy can interfere with fertility. In extreme cases, this allergy to gluten (which is also found in other cereals such as rye, barley and oats) leads to a medical condition known as coeliac disease. Research has confirmed that women with coeliac disease are sub-fertile and have an increased risk of stillbirths and perinatal deaths.[10]

Even if you do not suffer from coeliac disease, wheat is still a very common allergen and generates an ongoing immune system response, using up precious enzymes. One client of mine was having two periods a year when she was eating wheat at breakfast (in cereal and toast), lunch (in sandwiches) and often dinner (as pasta) as well. When she cut out wheat she had normal menstrual cycles for the first time in her life. It is recommended to avoid wheat as much as possible. There are many delicious wheat-free wholegrain breads and pastas available.

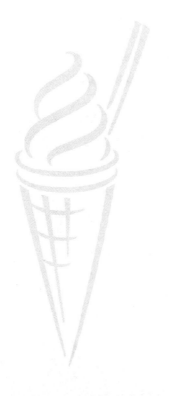

Fertility Action Plan

- Identify how many of these fertility blocking foods you eat regularly – refer back to the food diary you made following Chapter 1's action plan.

- Decide what you are going to do to cut these fertility blockers out of your life, and what foods you can eat as substitutes.

- Become a meticulous label reader – do not inadvertently consume foods that are contraceptive.

- Research the hormonal disrupting effects of soya for yourself online to satisfy yourself whether you should still be eating it.

Chapter 5

Barren Beverages

Even the healthiest organic diet is not going to help your chances of having a baby if you are washing your food down with drinks that have contraceptive properties. Since the most commonly consumed beverages like tea, coffee, beer and wine can reduce fertility by as much as 50 per cent, just eliminating alcohol and caffeine (as well as the other barren beverages described in this chapter) might be enough for you to hear the patter of tiny feet in nine months, even without any of the other recommended changes to your food diet.

'Alcohol provoketh
the desire but
taketh away the
performance.'
Macbeth, William
Shakespeare

Alcohol

'Alcohol is an aphrodisiac, surely?' queried all my young, socialite friends, fascinated by this one area of my research. Well, you may lose your inhibitions, your sense of discrimination and be feeling pretty randy after a few drinks, but you are not likely to be producing babies from any drunken frolics.

When it comes to men who drink, if the liver is burdened with dealing with alcohol and producing alcohol-digesting enzymes, its role in getting rid of excess hormones will be impaired, and men who drink alcohol can begin to accumulate residues of oestrogen, i.e. the female hormone, which men have in small amounts. Apart from giving men who drink heavily a lower libido and the unsexy appearance of having breasts, this hormone imbalance is then exacerbated by the fact that booze interferes with the synthesis and secretion of testosterone.[1] This means lower sperm count and reduced sperm potency and production.

As if this were not bad enough, alcohol blocks the absorption of the superstar fertility mineral zinc. Zinc is found in high concentrations in sperm and is essential for the manufacture of healthy sperm by the testes. Research has shown that, if zinc is reduced in the diet, the sperm count goes down.

Alcohol is also well known to cause cell mutations. Research has demonstrated that giving male mice alcohol damaged their sperm and increased the number of stillborn and miscarried offspring by 300 per cent. As any sperm produced while alcohol is being consumed will be less healthy and effective,[2] and since it takes three months for sperm to mature, alcohol should ideally be avoided by men for at least this amount of time prior to planned conception.

Perhaps the most telling evidence comes from research that shows that 80 per cent of chronic alcoholic men are sterile and that alcohol is a common cause of impotence.[3] Quite a sobering thought.

For women who like a drink, the picture is equally gloomy. Research has shown that women who are heavy drinkers may stop ovulating or having their periods and may take longer to conceive. Even very moderate drinking, such as one or two drinks a week, can raise levels of the hormone prolactin, which inhibits ovulation. In fact, a study on 430 women showed that as little as five units per week – equivalent to five glasses of wine or five small bottles of beer – could act as a contraceptive and prevent conception. (Great when you're a student, not so fab when you want a baby.) The study found that women in the survey who drank less than five units of alcohol a week were twice as likely to get pregnant within six months compared to those who drank more.

Drinking any alcohol at all can reduce a woman's fertility by 50 per cent and her chances of conceiving decrease in direct proportion to the amount she drinks.[4]

Most women are aware of the disastrous consequences of drinking alcohol while pregnant: Foetal Alcohol Syndrome (FAS) is a very serious condition, which leads to the baby being born with birth defects; it is the third major cause of mental retardation and neurological problems in babies (after Down's Syndrome and spina bifida). Children born to mothers who drank alcohol when pregnant have been found to have an IQ seven points below the average of children born to women who abstained in the critical pre-conception stage and pregnancy.[5]

The most critical period during which alcohol should be avoided is the first six weeks of pregnancy, when the foetus is developing the fastest. Since you could already be at least two weeks' pregnant before you even find out you are expecting, you could already have caused irreparable harm to your baby if you have been out partying in this crucial period.

Nature is so clever: when it realizes the foetus is not viable, it will naturally terminate the pregnancy – this is why women who drink every day have a much higher risk of miscarriage than non-drinkers (two-and-a-half times more). You could even have conceived but miscarried within two weeks, and just assume your period is a little heavier than normal. The same research found that, if a woman smokes as well as drinks, her chances of miscarriage are four times higher.[6]

Men only have to remain teetotal for the three months prior to their partner conceiving, then they can go back on the beers, or preferably the red wine, to celebrate (not that

I endorse anything other than very moderate drinking). However, women must remain on the wagon throughout pregnancy, and, ideally, while breast feeding too, in order to have the best chance of a healthy baby.

Caffeine

If you are a Java junkie I have more bad news for you: drinking as little as one cup of coffee a day decreases your fertility and cuts your chance of conceiving in half! Research has also clearly demonstrated that caffeine (from coffee, tea, colas and some painkillers) delays conception. Sorry, men, you do not escape. The more coffee you drink, the more you are likely to have a low sperm count and problems with sperm motility or abnormality.[7] Researchers have noted an increase in miscarriages, stillbirths and premature births among the babies of men who drank caffeine even when their female partner didn't; they attributed this to caffeine's negative affect on the production of sperm.[8] So, I'm afraid, guys, it really will matter if you drink caffeine in the three months prior to trying to conceive, when you will be manufacturing sperm.

Women who drink coffee will find it three times as difficult to conceive within a one-year period compared with women who do not drink coffee.[9]

Tea (especially green tea) contains antioxidants and bioflavonoids, which do support health, and certainly black and green teas contain less caffeine than coffee – only 50 mg a mug compared to 260 mg in a mug of coffee, so tea does seem to be relatively better for fertility than coffee. A study at the Kaiser Permanente Medical Care Program of Northern California found that tea drinkers were twice as likely to conceive as coffee drinkers. But neither tea nor coffee are helpful for fertility.

The downside of black tea, apart from the caffeine, is that the tannins in tea bind with important minerals and prevent their absorption in the intestines. If you drink tea with or after meals, a very common habit in the UK and Ireland particularly at breakfast, then all those excellent vitamins, minerals and micronutrients you are eating could be swept up by the tannins and pass through you unabsorbed – what a waste. Green tea has a further serious defect: drinking large amounts of green tea may decrease the effectiveness of folic acid, which is critical for perfect cell replication and avoiding defects. Research has shown that women who drink a lot of green tea around the time of conception and early pregnancy experience an increased risk of having a child with a neural tube disorder[10] – it is not worth the risk.

As a former tea addict myself, it came as a huge shock to discover that drinking any caffeinated drink significantly accelerates ageing (and thus reduces fertility). Here's why:

1. Caffeine decreases absorption of key minerals. Coffee in particular, is so acidic that minerals are leached from the bones to maintain a proper alkaline balance in the body.[11]

2. Caffeine has a diuretic effect. Vital nutrients and minerals such as zinc and calcium needed for conception and producing healthy sperm and ova, are thus peed away down the toilet in higher quantities. Dehydration is also likely to result, and MRI technology has now proven that dehydration results in cellular damage, i.e. rapid ageing. Water is lost in significant amounts every time you drink coffee or tea.

3. Caffeine lowers the production of the master steroid hormone DHEA (dehydroepiandrosterone), produced by the adrenal glands.[12] This hormone is a key component in the manufacture of testosterone and oestrogen and generally protects the body against ageing and degeneration. Levels of DHEA peak between the ages of twenty-five and thirty and decline thereafter. Producing adequate DHEA is key for preserving youthful hormonal balance and libido.

4. Caffeine elevates the stress hormones cortisol, epinephrine (a.k.a. adrenalin) and norepinephrine for hours after it has been consumed,[13] and thus upsets the delicate endocrine balance in the body as a whole. The long-term effect of stress hormones in general is rapid ageing. Further, excess cortisol stimulates appetite, cravings for fats and sugars and leads to abdominal obesity. Unfortunately, excess weight is a common cause of infertility. Despite its zero calories, your coffee could be making you too fat to have a baby.

5. Caffeine alters DNA repair and metabolism. Caffeine interferes with the quality control systems in normal cell turnover, preventing proper DNA repair and increasing the likelihood of cell damage and deterioration, the hallmarks of ageing.[14]

The answer to all of this is to cut out tea and coffee while you are trying to conceive – or even beyond, if you want to remain young! Try weaning yourself off caffeine by switching to an ever-increasing percentage of decaffeinated beverages – preferably those that have been decaffeinated using a water or other natural method (you do not want to start adding other exotic toxins used in some decaffeinating processes to your system). I have found some excellent herbal and decaffeinated black teas and a very palatable caffeine-free organic grain 'coffee'. Try all kinds of brands from your supermarket or health-food store until you find the ones you particularly like.

Diet Drinks

Diet drinks can cause infertility in women by causing levels of the hormone prolactin to rise, inhibiting ovulation (see the section on aspartame in Chapter 4).

Milk

Now, I am going to get a bit controversial: drinking this calcium-loaded supposed health drink may be stopping you from conceiving a baby. There is a vast body of research showing a negative correlation between milk consumption and fertility in women. The leading study, conducted by the Harvard Medical School in 1994, found that, in countries where milk consumption is at its highest, there was a corresponding increase in age-related infertility in women. This eight-year study involved 18,555 women between the ages of twenty-four and forty-two with no history of infertility, of whom 438 became infertile by the end of the research period. The Harvard researchers found that eating two or more low-fat dairy products a day increased a woman's chance of infertility by 85 per cent.

An age-related decline in fertility associated with drinking milk has been found in women who were just twenty years old.

Beyond childhood we do not have the necessary lactase enzymes, which break down the sugar molecules in milk. Thus, the main sugar in milk, galactose, cannot normally be properly digested. Galactose is toxic to unfertilized eggs, and so women with the highest concentrations of galactose in their blood stream are infertile. Even worse, galactose is linked to ovarian cancer as well as infertility – women who consume dairy products on a regular basis have triple the risk of ovarian cancer than other women.[15] This finding was echoed by a study that found that poor absorption of lactose could double the risk of ovarian cancer.[16] Lactose malabsorption has also been linked to pre-menstrual syndrome and depression.[17]

The prolonged use of enzyme-free pasteurized milk has been shown to be a contributing factor in infertility. It is implicated as one of the main causes for the infertility epidemic sweeping the USA, in particular. Unless you are drinking organic milk, you should also be aware that many commercially reared cows are given hormones such as bovine growth hormone and antibiotics to speed up their growth and massively increase their milk yield. The situation is far worse if you are drinking American milk compared with European milk, which is more tightly regulated under EU law.

Even more frightening is that milk can contain high amounts of dioxins, the same as meat products, since this poisonous substance (170,000 times more deadly than cyanide) is fat soluble and thus ends up secreted into milk from the body fat of cows exposed to dioxins. As mentioned previously, even organically farmed cows cannot avoid dioxin exposure, since this is an airborne toxin created as the by-product of industrial manufacturing processes.

All pasteurized milk is almost certain to have been homogenized. This is the process by which milk is passed through a fine filter at pressures equal to 4,000 pounds per square inch. Homogenization makes the fat molecules in milk very small, so small in fact that they can bypass the usual digestion by which proteins and fat are broken down in the intestines or stomach. Instead these fat globules in milk can pass directly into the bloodstream and, if non-organic, can deliver their poisonous load of hormones, pesticides and steroids directly into the body. This means that milk, especially non-organic milk, is full of fertility-damaging compounds and that, thanks to homogenization, your body is absorbing them effortlessly, with none of the usual digestive defence mechanisms to protect you.

Milk also interferes with the absorption of magnesium, and a deficiency in magnesium has been implicated in infertility, PMS and miscarriage.

Non-organic milk is a poisonous stew that can upset your body's finely balanced hormones, not the healthy drink the glossy advertisements of well-known people with white moustaches would have us believe.

I know it is hard to swallow but cow's milk of any kind is *not* good for your fertility. If you are sceptical, like I was initially, check out the website www.notmilk.com for a wealth of information and data. You will need to know this information once you have had your baby to find out about the well-established link between many childhood diseases and milk consumption in babies and children. There is even an increased risk of the terrifying Sudden Infant Death Syndrome (cot death) for babies fed a cow's milk formula. Dr Benjamin Spock, perhaps the most famous paediatrician of all time, was quoted as saying, 'Cow's milk in the past has been oversold as the perfect food, but we are now seeing that it is not the perfect food at all and the government really shouldn't be behind any efforts to promote it as such.'[18] Another paediatrician, Dr Frank Oski, has also written a book called *Don't Drink Your Milk*.

Switch to oat, rice, almond (my favourite) or other nut milks, which are all readily available, but please avoid soya milk for the reasons previously explained. Drinking soya milk can cause infertility and thyroid problems in both women and men. Switch to grain or nut milks instead.

Replace butter with organic nut butters or dairy-free margarines from organic sources, which consist of cold-pressed oils that have not been hydrogenated so are labelled 'free of trans-fatty acids'. You will notice the improvement in your overall health, particularly in how few colds, flu and ear infections you get.

Tonic Water

Having thrown out the gin, you will not miss your tonic water (or your bitter lemon). The key ingredient in tonic water is quinine, which has been linked to birth defects and may be implicated in miscarriages. Sorry, stick to fruit juices and mineral water if you want to have a healthy baby.

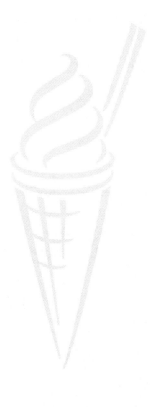

Fertility Action Plan

- Put down this book. Go to your fridge or kitchen cupboard and pull out all the barren beverages.

- Throw all the drinks in the bin that are going to prevent you from having a baby, or give them away to a friend who wants liquid contraceptives. Start with the diet drinks immediately and move on to any alcohol.

Chapter 6
Smoking and Recreational Drugs

When preparing to get pregnant, it is important to pay attention not just to what you might be eating and drinking, but your exposure to other toxic compounds as well. Unlike toxins from the environment, to which we are often exposed involuntarily (see the chapter which follows), you can very significantly increase your chances of pregnancy by avoiding the toxins in cigarettes and recreational drugs, which are ingested voluntarily. No 'high' could surely compare to the high of having a longed-for healthy baby?

Smoking
can cause
premature
menopause

Smoking

If you want to have a baby, smoking is very bad news; in the struggle for survival of the fittest, nature, unsurprisingly, seems to frown upon those habitually introducing 4,000 toxic compounds into their bodies every day. To make babies, your cells do not want or need carbon monoxide, radioactive polonium, benzopyrene, oxide of nitrogen, ammonia, aromatic hydrocarbons, hydrogen cyanide, vinyl chloride, nicotine, lead and tar.

Couples who smoke also have very high amounts of cadmium – a heavy toxic metal that stops the utilization of zinc, the fertility mineral needed by both men and women in order to conceive. The trouble is, cadmium does not just vanish from the system once you stop smoking; you have to take active steps to remove it by increasing the intake of antioxidants in the diet, both by eating more raw fruit and vegetables but also by supplements of zeolite, vitamin C, vitamin E, alpha-lipoic acid and selenium. More worryingly, the cadmium already present in the body, even from passive smoking can concentrate in the placenta once you are pregnant,[1] so testing for toxic metals such as cadmium and mercury before you try to get pregnant is very important. A midwife told me that, at one delivery, the placenta from a chain-smoking mother was grey and heavily pitted from smoke. So do not deceive yourself that the smoke will not be affecting your baby.

For men, studies on smoking show that chemicals in tobacco smoke can damage the DNA in sperm and deplete the antioxidant vitamins C and E, which help to protect the sperm from free radical damage. Sorry to scare you even more, but ponder the following: the constriction of blood vessels caused by smoking applies equally to those blood vessels supplying the penis with the blood needed for an erection. I gather that, in Canada, you can find cigarette packets with a graphic warning from the Health Authorities: a picture of a flaccid cigarette phallus, with suggestively drooping ash. Guys, you need to think about whether you enjoy smoking more than you enjoy sex. What's more, there is clear evidence that men who smoke, if they are able to father children despite the reduction in their fertility and potency from smoking, have children who are more likely to develop cancer in childhood such as leukaemia and brain tumours. According to Oxford University, if the father smoked between ten to twenty cigarettes a day, the increased risk for cancer for his child is a massive 31 per cent, rising to 42 per cent if more than twenty cigarettes are smoked.[2] Basically, the more a man smokes, the more damaged his sperm will be – so, if you are finding it hard to quit for your own health, then do so to increase your chances of fathering a child by a very significant degree, and for the sake of your unborn children.

Women, do not suffer any delusions: there is a direct link between smoking and female infertility.[3] Older women should also be aware that smoking can accelerate the age of menopause by up to six years.[4] So, if you are in your forties or early fifties and trying to conceive, cigarettes are right up there with alcohol and caffeine in what you should jettison out of your life first. If you intend to give up once pregnant, remember that your baby (should you be able to conceive, with your reduced chances by smoking) could have had two weeks' or more exposure to this cocktail of toxic rubbish before you even know it. For you to be part of the happy statistics the cigarettes and booze have got to go. You will also be doing your unborn baby a huge favour in guarding his or her health and normal development. The further good news is that by following the fertility diet, a diet rich in antioxidants, the damaging effects of smoking and alcohol can be reversed in a relatively short space of time (depending on your previous levels of addiction, of course).

Recreational Drugs

All recreational drugs have a detrimental effect on fertility in men and women. It is Mother Nature at work again; she does not want to propagate a species off its box, tripping on dubious substances. If you are one of those people who think a little spliff of marijuana is harmless and relaxes you, think again: in men, marijuana can lower follicle-stimulating hormones and luteinizing hormones, both needed to make sperm. It lowers sperm count and can also lower libido.[5] In women, the same studies show marijuana can lead to menstrual irregularities, reduced fertility and

Nicotine is said to be even more addictive than heroin, so use everything it takes to give up smoking before you try to conceive: acupuncture, hypnotherapy, nicotine patches and gum – just stop!

can cause ovulation to stop. Cocaine causes men to have a lower sperm count, sperm with poor motility and a high rate of abnormal sperm.[6] Heroin can cause a decrease in testosterone levels in men, and, when taken together with cocaine by a woman, make it harder to conceive, increase the risk of miscarriage, stillbirth or a baby born with birth defects.[7]

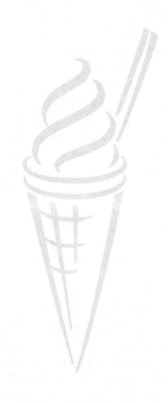

Fertility Action Plan

- Face up to the bitter truth that your addiction is likely to prevent you from having a baby.

- Please get all the help, therapy and support you need to quit smoking or taking recreational drugs.

Chapter 7
Environmental Factors

Today, chemical contamination pervades our air, water, country-side, homes, workplaces, food supply and, inevitably, our bodies. There are many excellent books and articles written on the topic of reproductive damage caused by environmental contaminants, so I want to focus on solutions – what you can do to protect yourself and your fertility (short of moving into a cave in the Himalayas).

Toxins in the Kitchen

1. Choose organic foods. Some fifty different types of pesticide and many other oestrogen-mimicking substances (commonly found in plastics) are known to cause serious reproductive damage – even sterility. So avoid these pesticides that are stopping you conceiving. The worst non-organic fruit and vegetables in terms of pesticide levels are strawberries, bell peppers, spinach, cherries, peaches, cantaloupe melon, celery, apples, apricots, green beans, grapes and cucumbers. If you cannot find or afford the organic equivalent, please do not eat these foods. The crops that have fewest pesticides are avocados, bananas, corn, onions and spring onions, sweet potatoes, cauliflower, Brussels sprouts, plums, watermelon and broccoli. If you do buy non-organic produce, at least peel it, and then soak it in filtered water to which apple cider vinegar has been added, then rinse. This will remove some pesticide residue.

2. Filter your water. This is a critical step if you are to avoid chemicals, heavy metals and hormone residues that are common in municipal water supplies. At the very least use a charcoal filter jug (and change the filter each month) to filter all the water you use in cooking and hot drinks. Ideally install an under-the-counter filter system, so you have a spigot on the kitchen sink for purified water. Another option, finances permitting, is to invest in a water steam distiller. These will save you a fortune in mineral water too. You will then be drinking and cooking with the absolute purest water available.

3. Replace cleaning products. The chemicals and solvents stored in the kitchen could be impairing your chances of having a baby – especially if you are inhaling the fumes as you clean, and not wearing rubber gloves, so the toxic compounds can enter your skin. Give your liver a break. There are many brands of non-toxic cleaning materials, washing-up liquids and laundry detergents. Do invest in these.

4. Avoid plastics – choose glass. The most powerful hormone-disrupting compounds – fake oestrogens – leach from plastic into food and drink. The softer the plastic, the more likely that it will be leaching these contraceptive chemicals. If you microwave food in plastic containers you will consume high doses of them. Use glass containers to store food. And if you must kill off all nutrients in your organic food by heating it in a microwave, then please at least use something like Pyrex cookware. Buy water in glass bottles (or, better still, with your own water distiller, store your purified water in glass bottles).

5. Avoid non-stick/Teflon frying pans and bakeware. The toxic chemicals in the non-stick surfaces break down at high temperatures and contaminate the food you eat (this is why newborn babies are being found with Teflon in their blood). Fried foods are not recommended on the fertility diet anyhow. If you want to roast vegetables, use glass, clay or ceramic casserole dishes and grease with olive oil.

Toxins in the Bathroom

1. Filter your water. Ideally, the water supply to your house should be filtered and purified at the point it enters your home, so that all the water you use is free of heavy metals and contaminants. If not, filters that attach to shower heads are relatively inexpensive and very easy to install. If you prefer baths to showers, just fill up the bath using the shower head. Unless water is filtered, your skin and then your liver and kidneys will be left to do the filtering – so do help them out.

2. Upgrade bath and beauty products. Any artificial chemicals and fragrances you put on your skin *will* be entering your bloodstream and potentially disrupting your hormone balance. Replace junky cosmetics, gels, lotions and potions, with their organic natural equivalent. I never buy anything for my skin until I have checked from the label that I could eat every ingredient if I wanted to. I often put food on my skin: aloe vera, blue-green algae, avocado, olive oil, coconut oil. You get the idea. Use your skin as another way to get the fertility nutrients you need into your system, not as another burden on the liver and kidneys.

Toxins in the Garden

1. Forget the pesticides and herbicides. It is annoying when pests eat your prize geraniums or well-tended vegetables; it is irritating to have to pull out weeds. These bothers do not compare to the annoyance and irritation of not conceiving the healthy baby for which you long. Give up the weed suppressants (such as Roundup) and any pesticides. Clear this stuff out of your shed, basement and garden as soon as possible.

2. Avoid exposure to agricultural chemicals. If your home borders commercial farmland, you need to be extra vigilant when the crops are sprayed. Close all windows and doors and stay inside or away from home if possible when the pesticide vapour is in the air. If it has not rained since the spraying, hose down the walls of your house and garden furniture and as much of your property is feasible to lessen the concentration of toxins.

Other Toxins in the Home

1. Decorate using eco-paints. The chemicals found in non-eco-friendly paints and solvents are particularly harmful for fertility and the health of an unborn child. Ideally, repaint your home only in the spring or summer, when you can leave doors and windows open to allow the toxic paint fumes to 'out gas'.

2. Choose second-hand or antique furniture. Most modern furniture/upholstery fabric is manufactured with chemicals, which will not be helping you with your baby plans until they have 'out gassed' – which can take some time. Try to find second-hand or antique furniture, where this will not be an issue.

3. Fertility clothes. Of course, the best clothes for fertility are no clothes! Since wearing just your birthday suit is not always possible or, indeed, legal, always wash new clothes (in non-toxic detergent) before you wear them for the first time. Dry them out on the line to further help remove the chemicals used on cotton crops and in fabric manufacture. The solvent used in dry-cleaning is a disaster for fertility. Studies has shown that even living near a dry-cleaning shop can harm your chances of conceiving. Try hand washing dry-clean only clothes, and just avoid any dry-cleaned clothes when attempting to conceive.

Avoid Toxins in the Workplace

1. Pest control? Find out if your workplace is sprayed to control pests. The law firm I used to work at in the Cayman Islands used to be sprayed once per month with pesticides, which, on investigation, I found were banned in the USA because of the health and reproductive damage they caused. I used to barricade my office from the sprayers and advised my female colleagues who wanted babies to do the same. When I sent concerned emails to the six partners on this issue, they could not have been more uninterested (apart from one who had four daughters) – in fact, they were annoyed that I should be such a troublemaker. So, I left that toxic law firm. If your office or work environment is being sprayed (which is very common in schools and – horror! – hospitals) find out from the pest-control people what pesticide they are using. Then conduct an online search into this toxin and start to write your own memos to the powers that be to get this fertility-harming process stopped. Make every reasonable effort to avoid chemical exposure at work.

Electromagnetism and Fertility

Compared even with twenty years ago, we are bombarded by more electromagnetic fields than ever before: mobile phones, computers, TVs, microwave ovens, other electronic appliances. We tend to forget that our bodies are electrical and that wavelengths that disrupt our own electromagnetic field have serious consequences both for health and fertility. The more men use mobile phones, the poorer their sperm, both in quantity and quality (see Chapter 31 for further details). The longer women spend in front of computer terminals, the higher their chances of not conceiving, endometriosis or of miscarriage – which I look at in Chapters 26 and 28.

To protect yourself from infertility caused by electromagnetic stress take the following steps.

1. Avoid using a mobile phone, even with a headset. If you are holding the phone near your body your fertility will be adversely affected, especially if you are a man. Use landlines as much as possible for calls.

2. Try to limit time at the computer or in front of the TV. Twenty hours per week is the maximum amount of exposure before fertility is damaged. If not using the computer or TV, turn it off – at least the monitor – and move away from it. Do not sleep with a TV in the bedroom.

3. Remove as many electrical appliances from the bedroom as possible. Certainly remove heated mattress pads, electric blankets and TVs. This will allow your own magnetic field to recover overnight.

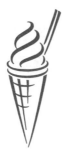

Fertility Action Plan

- If your budget permits: take a large garbage bag and, wearing rubber gloves, go around your home removing all toxic chemical products – especially garden pesticides, herbicides and old tins of paint/solvents. Replace kitchen and bathroom items with safe, eco-friendly, fertility-friendly equivalents.

- If your bank manager would disapprove of the radical course of action suggested above, replace your cleaning products, cosmetics, etc. with fertility-friendly products on a piecemeal basis as each runs out.

- Decide what recommendations in this chapter you are going to implement immediately to protect your fertility – and take action.

- Stop using your mobile phone to make unnecessary calls. Wait until you are on a landline.

Chapter 8
The Sterility of Stress

The adverse effects of stress on fertility can be seen from the beleaguered efforts of the captive breeding programmes of zoo animals and endangered species. The testes of many captive gorillas actually shrivel up; elephants in zoos lose their mojo[1] and they often fail to sustain any interest in sex even with a frisky new mate; maned wolves may breed but most of their offspring die soon after birth. For years, I watched BBC news coverage of London Zoo's attempts to get their giant pandas to mate. At first it was thought that these gorgeous animals, a gift from the government of China, just did not fancy each other since they showed no sign of wanting hanky panky, but even IVF failed. If you thought any assisted conception techniques for humans were a bit sordid and messy, let's all take a moment to pity the poor person who had to collect sperm from a giant panda without the help of any panda porn!

While some zoologists like Cindy Engel also attribute the lack of critical phytonutrients in the diet – namely the many unidentified plant secondary compounds available in 'the wild' – as having a role in the reproductive difficulties of animals in captivity,[2] there can be no doubt that the stress of confinement is a major cause. A panda can spot the difference between a bamboo forest and a concrete enclosure, it would seem.

A whole medical science of psycho-immunology has grown up around the incontrovertible evidence that long-term stress undermines the immune system and, thus, health.

There is clear evidence that stress has a detrimental effect on the reproduction of both men and women.

Men under Pressure

Research has shown that stressed-out men have a lower sperm count and far more abnormal sperm with decreased motility.[3] In one study involving 150 men, stress caused by a death in the family, separation or divorce slowed their sperm enough to affect their ability to conceive.[4] Dr Marilyn Glenville, in her book *Natural Solutions to Infertility*, cites the example of a patient who suddenly produced an abnormal sperm sample at the time he had to attend his mother's funeral, but a few weeks later his sperm sample was fine.[5]

Stress has also been found to affect a man's hormonal balance, lowering his levels of testosterone and luteinizing hormone.[6] Men on death row – surely the most stressful of all possible life experiences – have been found to have sperm counts close to zero.

Women and Stress

In February 1996 I thought I was pregnant. For the first time ever, my twenty-eight-day period – regular as clockwork; you could set the moon by me – was late. Really late, like six or seven days. At the time, I was a student at the University of Bonn in Germany completing a Masters Degree in Comparative Law, and in a state of great agitation and stress with the final deadline for my thesis looming. In the six months it took me to write my ninety-page thesis *in German* on a particular decision of the European Court of Justice on cross-border services and right of establishment under European law (about as dull and as difficult as it sounds), I did nothing apart from read EU law reports and have sex about three times a day with my Greek boyfriend, also a student, and also understimulated by his studies. So, despite the meticulous use of condoms, it did seem as if fate was about to punish me for my wanton frolics. The pregnancy test was negative, but still my period did not arrive. I went to see a gynaecologist in case the test was wrong. I remember a horrid, aggressive woman prodding and poking me, shrieking at me for using only condoms as a contraceptive instead of the pill. She took one test – it was negative. She scowled at me, then repeated the test – it was still negative. She never took the time to ask me if I had been under stress or to explain to me (as all endocrinologists and gynaecologists know, or should know) that women going through a bereavement, severe stress or some other trauma can stop menstruating all together.[7] My period arrived two days later. As this gynaecologist was German, I am surprised she was not aware of research from the women's hospital of Berlin Charlottenburg in the late eighties, which found that, out of 2,000 couples experiencing infertility, stress was the cause in 25 per cent of all cases.[8]

If you are under severe stress your system will pump out adrenalin – the fight or flight hormone. This has an adverse impact on your libido, fertility and general hormone balance; it has been found to block the body's utilization of progesterone, which is critical both for a normal corpus luteum to form and to avoid miscarriage. The lower levels of progesterone can also lead to an overall reduction in oestrogen levels, as the body tries to balance out the sex hormones.

Stress can upset the pituitary gland, triggering increased levels of follicle-stimulating hormone (FSH), with correspondingly lower fertility. It also inhibits the release of gonadotrophin-releasing hormone (GnRH) from the hypo-thalamus, which in turn reduces the levels of luteinizing hormone (LH) from the pituitary necessary for ovulation and conception.

The hormone prolactin is also released by the pituitary gland surge during stressful experiences (or by overstrenuous exercise when the body is under physical stress). This hormone inhibits ovulation and thus conception in women, and in men may cause impotence.

Apart from adrenalin, the other main hormone released under stress is cortisol. This is an anti-inflammatory hormone. I think of it as the 'grit your teeth and endure – let's not punch anyone today' hormone. Its effect is different to the heart-pounding, hyped-up feeling of adrenalin, but it keeps the body in a state of readiness for action (even if you are just sitting in daily traffic or coping with an aggravating boss or co-worker); it suppresses sleep, growth, reproduction and libido in the body. It reduces the release of GnRH and LH from the pituitary, and estradiol and testosterone from the gonads.

Symptoms of endometriosis, fibroids, Polycystic Ovary Syndrome (PCOS) and premenstrual syndrome are all made worse under stress due to the general destabilizing effect on hormones. Further, since stress upsets hormonal balance, it leads to the production of malformed eggs and sperm, and thus increases the risk of miscarriage.[9]

Addressing Stress

I can imagine how galling it is to have unhelpful people telling you 'just relax and it will happen' when you are trying to have a baby, but, all the more annoying, I am sorry to say they are right. Two studies have shown that, when women become completely obsessed with getting pregnant, they may release eggs that are not mature enough to be fertilized.[10] Stress has also been shown to send the Fallopian tubes into spasm, causing them to repel incoming sperm.

We all know stories of the couples who gave up trying to have a child, decided to adopt and then conceived almost immediately. One of the best ways to conceive is to go on a relaxing holiday in the sun (see also Chapter 21 on sunlight).

At times of stress it is important to get nutritional support since many nutrients, which are critical to fertility, are depleted by the adrenal glands going into overdrive when we are under pressure. First vitamin C, then vitamin E, B6, vitamin A and all the B vitamins (called nature's tranquillizers) are used up in huge amounts. Levels of zinc, calcium, magnesium, phosphorous and potassium also fall.[11]

By taking vitamins B, C, and E and minerals in supplement form (copper is only recommended in very small amounts since it can be toxic) or, preferably, from food sources, you will help safeguard your fertility (not to mention your immune system and health in general) during the most difficult of times.

Stress reduction is vital in normalizing hormone levels. The relaxation response is mediated by the hypothalamus – hormonal mission control – which also regulates all aspects of reproduction. It is logical that relaxation will enhance fertility. Of course, trying to tell someone not to be stressed is like telling them not to think about the colour blue: it's then the first thing they will think of. Try to practise any technique of relaxation, stress management or meditation that works for you, such as massage, yoga, mindfulness, body scan, progressive muscle relaxation and autogenic training.

I strongly recommend aromatherapy massage and aromatherapy oils for relaxation as aromatherapy oils are able to aid fertility by affecting the nervous system on very deep levels, overriding the anxious mind.

Another tip is to take natural flower remedies such as Bach flower remedies, which are widely available. These belong to a system of so called vibrational healing. I have had excellent results using such remedies.

Acupuncture and reflexology are both excellent tools for enhancing fertility and can also help you cope with the pressure of home, work and infertility itself. They are definitely worth looking into.

Sometimes the solution to stress is on an even more mundane, practical level – hiring a cleaning lady, a part-time gardener, or finding extra child support (if you have a child already). Can you delegate any of your workload in your job? Can you ask your boss to recruit extra staff if your responsibilities are just too much for one person? Explore solutions that will give you the extra time you need to relax.

Any steps you take to relieve stress and relax will yield fantastic dividends in terms of enhanced fertility. In a series of amazing studies conducted by Dr Alice Domar and her team at the Harvard Medical School, 34 per cent of one group of 'infertile' women and 32 per cent of another group became pregnant within six months of participating in a stress management mind–body programme. In a third group of women who had been struggling with infertility on average for more than three years, 43.7 per cent were pregnant within six months of completing ten weeks' of stress management sessions and 38 per cent went on to give birth.[12]

In a later study funded by the National Institute of Mental Health, the Harvard medical team divided infertile women into three groups: one received cognitive emotional therapy, one joined a support group and the third, a control group, received no psychological intervention. Within twelve months of entering the study, 55 per cent of the women in the cognitive behaviour group and 54 per cent of the women in the support group were pregnant and went on to have healthy babies. In the control group only 20 per cent ended up having viable pregnancies.

In this chapter I have only looked at the effect of everyday pressure and stress on fertility; I have not dealt here with the bigger issues of anxiety, depression and infertility, and the general question of the interface between emotions and hormones. This is covered in Chapter 25.

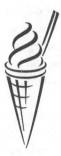

Fertility Action Plan

- Explore ways to reduce some of the everyday stresses in your life.

- Seek help at home or at work to reduce your load and create extra time.

- Schedule time to relax, meditate or pamper yourself every day.

- Find some kind of guided relaxation CD to listen to daily.

Chapter 9
Weight and Infertility

Sometimes the solution to infertility is the most simple, inexpensive and obvious one. For women, maintaining an optimum, healthy weight is vital for peak fertility and a successful pregnancy. Losing or gaining weight, as appropriate, might be the only change necessary to conceive. The impact of appropriate weight for men's fertility is less important and will be addressed at the end of the chapter.

Body fat is not just lifeless blubber that accumulates on your thighs or belly to distress you: it is a metabolically active substance. Yes, your fat cells communicate with your body on a daily basis, via the hormones leptin and insulin, letting the brain know how much is in storage, capable of supplying nutrients to sustain a pregnancy and breastfeed a baby thereafter in case a famine should strike. The stomach also communicates with the brain, through the hormone ghrelin, which is secreted in the cells in the stomach lining (and later by the placenta too), that triggers growth-hormone release and stimulates hunger.

These are interesting times in the nutrition of weight control. Scientists are eager to unravel the mysteries of leptin, ghrelin and body fat set point (the weight to which your body seems to automatically revert) because the 'fat code' is a puzzle science has not yet fully cracked. All we do know is that the body itself closely monitors your weight and, unless there is enough fat for a feasible pregnancy (but not too much), you will not conceive.

Whether your body weight is within optimum levels for fertility can easily be checked by reference your body mass index (BMI). This is calculated by dividing your weight in kilograms by the square of your height in metres. If this sounds like scary maths, just search under BMI on any online search engine and it will take you to a number of websites that will do the computation for you and tell you if you are underweight, the perfect weight or overweight. For absolute peak fertility you should aim for a BMI between twenty and twenty-four. Women with a BMI of 25, 26 and 27 (slightly chunky) are also very fertile, but could increase their fertility even more by losing just a little weight. Skinny women with a BMI of between 17 and 19 are likely to be sub-fertile if their periods are irregular or absent and could increase their chances of conceiving significantly by aiming for a BMI of 20, which may involve a weight gain of just a few pounds. Women who are thin to the point of emaciation, with a BMI below 17, are unlikely to be menstruating and may well be infertile. In the opposite direction, overweight women with a BMI of between 28 to 30 have a significantly increased risk of infertility, and obese women (BMI over 30) are also likely to be infertile. Very obese women with a BMI of 40 are highly likely to be infertile. The good news is that bringing your weight up to a minimum BMI of 20 or down to a maximum BMI of 27 (a BMI of 24 is even better) helps creates the perfect hormonal environment in which to conceive.

Leptin, Weight and Fertility

The hormone leptin mentioned above, which controls appetite, body weight, metabolism, and signals the brain when enough fat has been eaten, is a significant regulator of reproductive function. Leptin is produced in the body, predominantly in the fat cells, with small amounts also being secreted by the lining of the stomach (and in the placenta when pregnant). There are leptin receptors in the brain, in the centres that control feeding behaviour, hunger, body temperature, energy expenditure and that help the body to regulate and monitor how much fat is being carried. Leptin is therefore the chemical messenger responsible for reporting back to the brain that there are sufficient reserves of body fat to make having a baby viable. The ovaries appear to respond directly to levels of both leptin and insulin (see Chapter 3 on insulin).

This is why women who are significantly overweight as well as those who are significantly underweight are more likely to be infertile or sub-fertile – their leptin levels will not be in the optimal range to signal the release of the hormones needed for ovulation. Having enough vitamin D from sunshine (see Chapter 21 on sunlight) will also help make sure you have optimum levels of leptin to maximize the release of hormones needed for conception.

Gaining Weight for Fertility

In our diet-conscious society, with most actresses and models having a body mass index of approximately 17 ('normal', healthy weight is a BMI of between 20 and 24.9), there is extreme pressure to be underweight since thinness is now associated with beauty. One aspect of this drive to maintain thinness at the expense of good health is the complete avoidance of fat in the diet, even the 'good' plant-based fats from nuts, seeds and avocados. However, ovarian and adrenal steroid hormones responsible for fertility actually require a certain level of dietary fat for normal functioning. The liver converts dietary fat into cholesterol – the essential raw material of estradiol, progesterone, testosterone, DHEA, cortisol and aldosterone. A lack of fat in the diet upsets the production of all these hormones as well as the absorption of key fat soluble vitamins such as A, D, E and K.

It is imperative to eat sufficient calories on a daily basis if you wish to preserve your fertility. A very troubling study from 1985 concerning women aged 20–29 found that dieting for just six weeks on approximately 800–1,000 calories a day caused estradiol to fall to *menopausal* levels during the final two weeks of the diet. Some two thirds of the women had disrupted menstrual cycles, which did not return to normal for three to six months after dieting ended. The authors of the study concluded that even mild dieting interferes with hormone production and disrupts the menstrual cycle.[2]

Consult a BMI chart or calculate your own BMI and note the weight range for a BMI of 20–21 and make this your initial goal weight. This is still a very slim weight. Do not let vanity prevent you from having a baby. When your family is complete (and your babies are breastfed) you can restore your weight to whatever low level feels good and healthy to you.

If you need to gain weight to achieve a fertile BMI it is important to do so in a healthy manner. Bingeing on sweets or junk food is not the way to go about it. If you exercise more than one hour a day, you need to cut down – to an average of approximately seven hours a week at most (Chapter 23 deals with optimal amounts of exercise for fertility). One option is to exercise on alternate days or to train with less intensity in whatever sport you do. Snacking on nuts and seeds throughout the day is an excellent and healthy way to gain weight. Nut milk smoothies are also perfect – healthy, high calorie and easy to consume (see recipes section for ideas). Many health stores also sell excellent fruit and superfood smoothies – often with algae, spirulina and other super greens. These are a good choice to

If you are underweight, sometimes gaining as little as five or six pounds extra is all that is needed to go from infertile to fertile.

drink between, or with, meals to add additional, healthy, calories; even better, make your own fresh smoothies. Wholegrains such as brown rice, millet, quinoa and buckwheat, and wholegrain breads and pastas should also be consumed every day.

Losing Weight for Fertility

Women with a BMI higher than 27 are three times more likely to be infertile than women in the normal BMI range because of problems with ovulation.[3] Very obese women (BMI over 35) seeking assisted conception treatment are 60 per cent less likely to conceive with IVF than women with a BMI of 20–24.9.

If you are overweight, even a modest reduction in weight can boost fertility: in one study carried out by the University of Adelaide, Australia, eleven out of twelve formerly overweight women conceived naturally after a six-month programme of diet and exercise.[4] Italian research found similar results – in a study involving thirty-three overweight women (also with Polycystic Ovary Syndrome), a weight loss of only 5 per cent (that's 10 lb for a 200 lb woman) led to ten pregnancies; fifteen resumed ovulation spontaneously and eighteen returned to regular menstrual cycles.[5]

If you are overweight, the chances are you have read and tried every diet book under the sun, and that there is nothing new I can tell you. You know a celery stick is less fattening than a Mars bar. Let the dream of a baby inspire you now to reclaim your most radiant good health and to optimize your weight. Following the recommendations of the fertility diet, in particular cutting out alcohol and caffeine and eating plant-based, organic foods, will automatically decrease your weight. I will however give you a few of the top tips I have learned in my own battle to rid myself of my unwanted 20 lb.

1. Kick start your metabolism: a) eat breakfast; b) aim to eat five times a day, rather than just three large meals (my own pattern is 8 a.m.: fruit smoothie breakfast; 10.30 a.m.:

main breakfast; 1.30 p.m. large lunch; 4 p.m. 'tea' i.e. a small snack; 7 p.m. – sometimes later if I am going out – light dinner); c) if you suspect your thyroid is sluggish take supplements of iodine and tyrosine and/or find a good thyroid-supporting supplement containing these.

2. Cut out all the obvious junk, candy and processed food. You know what this is – it is no good for your waistline or your fertility.

3. Cut out alcohol. Apart from being a contraceptive, alcohol contains a lot of calories; far worse, it also actually prevents the body from burning fat. The compounds acetaldehyde and acetate (produced when the liver breaks down alcohol) signal the body to stop burning fat, and another compound – acetyl CoA – triggers the body to store fat.

4. Take omega 3 fatty acids – either soaked flax seeds, or capsules with flax seed oil or borage oil, or fish oil capsules – three times a day. These essential fats help burn body fat and lower cortisol, which stimulates insulin, the fat-storing hormone.

5. Get into coconut. Coconut oil, milk and fresh coconut itself all stimulate the thyroid and help break down body fat.

6. Drink masses of water, a minimum of three litres a day. Fat can only break down if you are properly hydrated. Water will also fill you up. Sometimes we eat when in fact we are thirsty.

7. Get moving any way you can – a few extra steps across the parking lot, at work, in the shopping mall. Aim for thirty minutes exercise per day – walking is excellent.

8. Finally, anytime you are tempted to overeat, or to eat something highly calorific and unhealthy, **ask yourself the following question:** 'Do I want this more than I want a baby?' Good luck.

Fertility and Weight in Men

Being overweight has been found to affect male fertility by reducing the quality and quantity of sperm count.[6] At the other end of the scale, men who are too thin also have decreased sperm function and lower sperm counts as a result of inadequate production of the male sex hormones.[7] Men who overexercise can find that this lowers sperm count (see Chapter 23 on healthful exercise for fertility). Of course, using steroids for bodybuilding will dramatically decrease your sperm count and fertility over all (this is dealt with in Chapter 11 on medicines; safe alternatives for steroids are included there).

All the evidence suggests that men too should strive to keep their weight in the BMI 20–24 range if they are to maintain peak hormone levels and high quality sperm for fertilization.

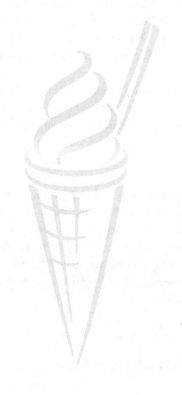

Fertility Action Plan

- Weigh yourself then check your BMI online.

- If your BMI is under 20 you need to gain weight to conceive easily.

- If your BMI is over 30 you need to lose weight to improve fertility.

- If your BMI is 25–27 losing a little weight will enhance your chances of conceiving.

- If your BMI is 20–24 strive to keep it there – you are in the optimum weight range to conceive a baby soon.

Chapter 10
Genito-Urinary Infections

A survey from a London infertility clinic found that 69 per cent of patients suffered from genito-urinary infections,[1] most commonly known by the more pejorative term sexually transmitted diseases (STDs). STDs are the leading cause of infertility among women in their twenties – the decade during which incidence of these infections is at its highest.[2] An unsuspected genito-urinary infection can, however, be the cause of infertility in men and women of all ages – and one that is easily treated. If you want a baby, please insist upon a blood test from your doctor to rule out the presence of STDs since you can be infected yet have no obvious symptoms (see below). In the book *It's my Ovaries, Stupid!*,[3] Dr Elizabeth Lee Vliet recounts a chilling story of a woman who was not diagnosed with chlamydia until she was 48, despite innumerable visits to top doctors starting in her late twenties and ultimately costing her twenty years of unnecessary, heartbreaking infertility. Do not let this be you, or your partner! A simple blood test will reveal if you have any infection.

Chlamydia and Infertility

The most common bacterial infection affecting fertility is chlamydia (*Chlamydia trachomatis*). In women, chlamydia spreads insidiously from an inflammation in the cervix (cervicitis), through the uterus (causing endometritis), to the ovaries also causing inflammation (oophritis) and premature loss of ovarian function, including a decline in ovarian hormones. If left untreated it can ascend to the Fallopian tubes, infecting them (acute salpingitis) and possibly permanently damaging them. And, finally, chlamydia is known to cause pelvic inflammatory disease (PID),[4] which can impair fertility. Your chances of being a future mother can be significantly compromised by chlamydia.

Damage to the Fallopian tubes caused by acute salpingitis and/or pelvic inflammatory disease from chlamydia is one of the most common causes of female infertility.[5]

In men, chlamydia can cause inflammation of the prostate (prostatitis), the epididymis (ducts at the rear of the testicles) and of the seminal vesicles, which lie behind the prostate gland and secrete fluids into the tube called the vas differens that runs from the testicles to the urethra, thus adversely affecting the fluids needed by sperm. If untreated, chlamydia in men can also cause inflammation of the testes resulting in infertility. A study of seventy-one infertile men carried out by the University of Tampere in Finland found chlamydia antibodies (indicating infection) in 51 per cent of them – compared with a finding of only 26 per cent of fertile men.[6]

Chlamydia has reached epidemic proportions – it is now probably the most common STD in the Western world.[7]

The mildest symptoms of a chlamydia in women are a slight vaginal discharge and occasional mild abdominal pain. More pronounced symptoms, which can appear within one to three weeks of sex with an infected partner, include genital inflammation, vaginal discharge, difficulty urinating and painful urination, painful intercourse and itching around the inflamed area. Men who are infected by chlamydia may notice a discharge from the penis (sometimes very copious amounts of pus), difficulty urinating and painful urination, and pain and swelling in the testicles. However, the most scary thing about chlamydia is that 50 per cent of men and 75 per cent of women experience no symptoms at all, so that it is possible to pass undetected for a very long time – hence the importance of having a blood test before trying to conceive to rule out the possibility of infection, not least since babies whose mothers have chlamydia may be born with pneumonia or conjunctivitis (an eye infection), unspecified viral diseases and, of course, the chlamydia infection itself.

Gonorrhoea

The second most common STD affecting fertility, gonorrhoea (*Neisseria gonorrhea*) is another bacteria that lives in the male and female reproductive tracts and is passed on through sex. In women, untreated gonorrhoea can lead to the more serious infection, pelvic inflammatory disease, which can cause infertility.

Half of all cases of gonorrhoea produce no symptoms – women normally experience no symptoms while men usually do. Of those which do manifest in women, the most common include increased vaginal discharge, lower abdominal/pelvic pain, pelvic inflammation, rectal itching, abnormal menstruation, and frequent urination with pain or burning. In men, classic symptoms of gonorrhoea include a yellow discharge of pus and mucus from the penis, and difficult, painful urination. The infection can scar the genital tract and prevent sperm from being ejaculated, and cause sterility and urethral stricture (blockage of the tube through which urine passes). Any symptoms appear within 2–21 days after sexual contact. Worryingly, since the infection can cause aches and inflamed joints it is sometimes misdiagnosed as arthritis. For men, in particular, it is important to test for gonorrhoea if you have had had unprotected sex.

Other STDs

STDs such as herpes, hepatitis B, cytomegalovirus, syphilis and HIV don't necessarily cause infertility. However, they can have very serious consequences for your baby in terms of birth defects, so they are a factor well worth eliminating at the pre-conception stage.

Treatment of Genito-urinary Infections

I am not a fan of antibiotics in general, and believe them to be often shockingly over-prescribed by doctors. Antibiotics also appear to suppress fertility while they are being taken. However, since STDs, especially chlamydia, can usually be totally successfully treated by a course of antibiotics, this is one instance when their use is entirely appropriate, beneficial and recommended. If you prefer to follow a completely natural approach, then the natural antibiotic, garlic, is my number one tip – take massive doses of capsule supplements for best results, and, of course, eat it in foods (with fresh parsley, to kill the smell on your breath). Honey has some antibiotic properties as well. The mineral zeolite (often sold under the brand name Natural Cellular Defence (NCD)) is also a potent antimicrobial and antiviral nutrient and will assist in eliminating bacterial infections and even alleviating some of the symptoms associated with HIV/AIDS. The above-mentioned nutrients can of course be taken in addition to any course of antibiotic medication and I am unaware of any adverse synergistic affects of the combination of these supplements with medicinal drugs.

At the same time as undergoing any course of antibiotics it is critical to replenish the 'friendly flora', i.e. good bacteria, in the gut, which will be wiped out by the medication. Look for supplemental acidophilus or bifidus, or eat organic, natural yogurt every day, which has live cultures of these friendly bacteria in them.

Bacterial infections also diminish the body of zinc, so supplementing this mineral – a fertility superstar mineral in any event, and which boosts immunity – is strongly recommended. The mineral silver – taken in liquid colloidal form – also supports the immune system and will help the body rid itself of any pathogens.

Fertility Action Plan

- Make an appointment to be tested for all STDs, especially chlamydia, which usually has no symptoms (there are outpatient clinics for these tests if you do not want to go to your own GP).

Chapter 11
Medicines

A number of common medicines can have an adverse affect on fertility.

Headache/Pain Medication

Avoid headache and pain medications that may cause levels of the hormone prolactin to rise, which will inhibit ovulation. Aspirin and other non-steroidal anti-inflammatory drugs (NSAIDS) such as Ibuprofen, Advil or Aleve may also interfere with ovulation and should be avoided. Aspirin has also been linked to male infertility.

Try the herb feverfew (short-term use) as a natural headache remedy without any adverse impact on your fertility. My nutritional advice to migraine sufferers is to take a liquid magnesium supplement daily (some 70 per cent of migraine sufferers are deficient in magnesium) together with a daily supplement of vitamins B2 (riboflavin) 400 mg daily, and B3 (niacin) 500 mg first thing in the morning and immediately a migraine begins.

Antihistamines/Decongestants

Fertile cervical fluid can thicken or, worse, dry up due to use of antihistamines and decongestants, leaving sperm high and dry with nowhere to go. However, if you have too much cervical mucus which might be acting as a barrier to conception, one old wives' tale says take cough syrup (orally) containing the active ingredient guaifenesin (such as Robitussin), since this is said to thin cervical mucus, helping sperm glide to their destination egg. There is anecdotal evidence of couples who have conceived with a swig of cough syrup, but no formal scientific studies exist to confirm this.

Antidepressants

Antidepressants such as Prozac can also impede ovulation. They appear to interfere with normal menstrual cycles and can increase the risk of birth defects. Monoamine oxidase inhibitors (MAOIs) such as phenelzine (Nardil) and tranylcypromine (Parnate) elevate the risk of foetal malformations when taken during the first three months of pregnancy; this could also increase the risk of miscarriage. In men, antidepressants can cause erectile dysfunction, a loss of libido and an inability to orgasm/ejaculate.

Anti-anxiety Drugs

These drugs, including the well-known Valium (diazepam) and Xanax (alprazolam), have been linked to birth defects and are best avoided if possible when trying to conceive. Natural tranquillizers include the supplement 5-HTP (5-hydroxytryptophan) as well as bananas. The amino acid GABA is a natural tranquillizer too.

Corticosteroids

Medicated ointments to treat skin conditions such as psoriasis and eczema can cause irregular menstrual periods in women and reduce sex drive in men. Try instead lotions containing MSM (naturally occurring sulphur), as well as MSM supplements.

High Blood Pressure Medications

Some medicines that are designed to lower blood pressure, such as potassium-sparing diuretics including spironolactone (Aldactone), can interefere with normal menstrual cycles and may lead to erectile dysfunction in men. Of greater concern is the fact that calcium channel blockers such as Procardia may impair the motility and viability of sperm. Alpha-blocker drugs such as Cardura can lead to retrograde ejaculation. Blood pressure can be lowered without medication by taking garlic capsules, magnesium supplements and by juice fasting. (See Chapter 18 for more details on fasting.)

Anabolic Steroids

If you are a man who takes or has taken anabolic steroids as a bodybuilder, you need to know that, in excessive amounts, these can cause infertility. In the book *The Perricone Weight-loss Diet*,[1] Dr Nicholas Perricone sets out the following shopping list of supplements that will naturally help burn fat and build muscle: carnitine, acetyl l-carnitine, alpha-lipoic acid, DMAE, conjugated linoleic acid (CLA), glutamine, chromium picolinate, gamma linoleic acid (GLA), co-enzyme Q10 and astaxanthin. All of these supplements have no adverse effect on fertility or virility; in fact they will help both.

Ulcer Medications

The ulcer medicines cimetidine (Tagamet) and ranitidine (Zantac) may decrease sperm count and even produce impotence.

Medications Known to Cause Erectile Dysfunction

Over-the-counter nose drops, which act by constricting small blood vessels in the nose, reducing swelling and thus improving breathing, can be absorbed in the bloodstream and go to the genitalia where you may want some swelling! A New York University Physician reported that the impotency in sixteen of his patients was caused by long-term use of nose drops![2]

Here's quite a list of other drugs that can lead to impotency in men (some have already been mentioned):

Aldomet, Aldactone, Catapres, Chlorpromazine, Dibenzyline, Furdantin, Haldol, Ismelin, Librium, Macrodantin, Meillar, Priscoline, Regitine, Serax, Tranxene, Trecator-SC, Valium.

Fertility Action Plan
(And Common-Sense Caution)

- Consult your doctor to find out if some prescription medicine you are taking may be interfering with your chances of conceiving, and explore if there are any alternative medicines, or if an alternative or dietary approach is available for controlling your symptoms.

- Please do *not* stop taking any medication you are on – even if it is listed here as having an adverse impact on fertility – without consulting your health-care practitioner first.

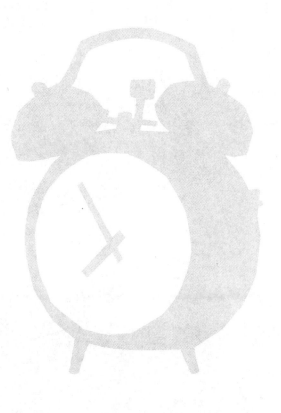

Part III:
The Fertility Diet

Chapter 12

Extraordinary Enzymes – the Power of Living Foods

In contrast to foods that are actually harmful to fertility, there are a number which greatly enhance your chances of having a baby. By no coincidence these are the foods that are themselves bursting with life – and in the case of nuts and seeds even the intrinsic potential for creating new life in the form of plants and trees. The fertility super-foods are all organic fruits, vegetables and seaweed; the fertility 'neutral' foods are free-range eggs and fish from pure sources. The more you can eliminate the food and drinks which hamper your chances of conceiving discussed in the previous chapters and focus on magical fertility foods, the faster you will conceive a healthy baby.

When a roasted almond is planted in the ground it will rot and decay. A fresh, raw almond, on the other hand, will sprout and grow into an almond tree. The difference between a cooked and a raw almond is enzymes, which carry the very spark of life within them.

One of the most compelling examples of the vital, life-giving role played by enzymes comes from studies carried out by Oxford University. Both raw (i.e. unpasteurized) and pasteurized milk have identical components: a very high calcium and protein content. However, in electromagnetism and crystalline structure, raw and pasteurized milk are found to be very different. A calf suckling on raw milk full of enzymes will flourish and grow into an adult cow; a calf fed its own mother's milk that has been pasteurized, thus destroying all the enzymes in the milk, will die within three weeks. In a nutshell, through heating, the milk is no longer alive.[1]

Microwaving your meals is a great way to eat food that is dead. In another English study a group of cats was kept in an artificially lit room and fed only food and water that had been heated in a microwave (and later cooled). Despite consuming a huge array of abundant foods – an entire feline gourmet buffet – all the cats died of starvation within one month.[2] The short-wave radiation of the microwave alters the molecular structure of the food. Biophysicists would say that no resonant, i.e. life energy, could be measured.

Where is that spark of life to be found? Enzymes. If you are in the habit of eating microwaved foods you need to be aware that this will only be giving you calories, i.e. fuel. It will not be supplying you with any micronutrients or the life-giving essence of enzymes so essential for both fertility and health in general.

The short-wave radiation of microwave ovens alters the molecular structure of food, depleting it of fertility-giving nutrients.

Every cellular action in our bodies depends on enzymes: they convert the food we eat into the raw materials of our bodies; every hormonal action and reaction is dependent upon enzymes.

Eating for Enzymes

It is a logical first step in eating for fertility to consume plenty of foods that are 'alive' and bursting with enzymes. This means eating foods (fruit, vegetables, nuts and seeds) in their raw state or only gently warmed to a temperature under 118°F/47.7°C (the point at which all enzymes are killed off). Raw meat, eggs and fish are not recommended, however, even if they do have more enzymes, because of the high risk of bacterial infection from the pathogens with which they are teeming.

To bring forth life, to tune into the reproductive capacity of nature itself, life-giving foods must be eaten in abundance. Seeds and nuts contain the reproductive elements of plants and trees. The role of fruit in nature is to contain all the vitamins, minerals and enzymes the seed will need in its fertile path from germination to seedling.

Eating more fresh fruit, nuts, seeds and uncooked vegetables therefore brings the entire cornucopia of nature's fertility into your body.

Herbalists, naturopaths and those practising natural medicine have known for thousands of years that there is an magical correlation between the healing and medicinal properties of plants in 'the wild' and the effect in a human body. For example cordyceps, a Chinese mushroom, was first discovered by yak herders who noticed that their yaks ate a lot of it at the start of the breeding season. When the herdsmen themselves tried eating it they found they became jolly, agile, strong and very frisky!

The mushroom cordyceps has been dubbed the 'fungal viagra' because of its ability to reverse the loss of sexual drive in humans.[3]

There is even a school of thought – 'the doctrine of signatures' – which states that every living thing has a 'signature' that tells us its use, function and role in the universal plan. The colour, shape of a fruit or vegetable and how and where it grows gives us a clue as to its properties. Thus, by amazing coincidence or design, kidney beans are good for the kidneys, beets nourish the blood and the cerebrum-shaped cauliflower is good for the brain! Based on this concept, men should go for the phallic shapes: celery, bananas, cucumbers, asparagus. Women should gravitate towards peaches, melons and apples.

The fresher and the better the quality of the fruit and vegetables, the more life force (i.e. reproductive force) they contain. If you are wondering whether organic food is worth the extra money, there can be no doubt that it is, unless you want to short-change your own fertility. Organically grown foods have significantly higher nutritional values than the same foods grown commercially in the same local soil. One major study at Rutgers University in the US found that organic produce has an average of 83 per cent more nutrients in it. This study, the Firman Bear Report, found that organically grown foods were much richer in minerals than the same commercially produced vegetables. For example, organic tomatoes had more than 5 times more calcium, 12 times more magnesium, 3 times more potassium, 600 per cent more organic sodium, 68 times more manganese and 1,900 times more iron. Organic spinach had more than double the calcium, 5.5 times the magnesium, more than 3 times the potassium, 70 times the sodium, 117 times as much magnesium and 83 times more iron. Organic lettuce had 3.5 times the calcium, 3 times the magnesium, 3 times the potassium, 33 times the sodium, 169 times the magnesium, and 157 times the iron.[4] The amazing fertility benefits of organic food are set out in greater detail in Chapter 6.

If you want 83 per cent more fertility power out of your foods, make buying organic produce a priority.

Raw Versus Cooked Food

As mentioned above, enzymes are involved in every cellular action including the production and use of hormones in the body. Enzymes that are present inside the body are called metabolic enzymes and can be likened to a team of highly skilled technicians with large tool bags, who work throughout the body to keep its trillions of cells running smoothly. When fruit and vegetables are eaten raw they come with their own integral enzymes: for instance, pineapple contains the enzyme bromelain; avocados, nuts and seeds contain the fat-digesting enzyme lipase. Such foods are effectively self-digesting in the body. However, when the same fruit and vegetables are cooked, and nuts and seeds are roasted, the enzymes are wiped out and the food cannot self-digest. Without enzymes coming from outside the body from raw foods, the body is forced to draw on its own precious source of metabolic enzymes to digest cooked foods. I imagine a picture of all my metabolic enzymes hard at work, clearing out rubbish in the body, making sure my cells are reproducing perfectly. Then, suddenly, the cry goes out from the stomach, 'Help! Cooked food on the way! Request emergency enzyme assistance to deal.' To which the enzyme chief obligingly responds, 'OK, lads, down tools here, forget about that hormone we were making, we're off to the intestines to deal with some fish and chips.'

While very oversimplified, the picture described above is borne out by the research of Dr Paul Kouchakoff, who found that every time cooked food is eaten a significant rise in white blood cells can be measured, a condition known as leukocytosis – namely, an immune system response.[5] This means the body reacts to cooked food as if it is under attack. Eight different amylase (starch digesting) enzymes are found in white blood cells, and other studies have shown that they also contain proteolytic and lipolytic (protein- and fat-digesting) enzymes too.[6] White blood cells clearly play a role as the means of transportation of the enzyme 'workers' to wherever they are needed in the body, whether to break down and digest cooked food or to destroy bacterial invaders. Dr Kouchakoff found that when raw foods were eaten there was no white blood cell response since no enzymes are needed. He also found that, when the balance of raw to cooked foods eaten at the same time was approximately 50–50, there was no immune response.

It is not unusual for people to eat a diet of 100 per cent cooked food, particularly in colder climates in the winter months. By cooked foods, I do not mean just 'hot' food. For example, most breakfast cereals have been cooked, even if you are eating them cold. This is the same for all processed foods; for example, ice cream is a cooked, processed food. The continual draw on the body's metabolic enzymes to deal with cooked and processed food and the constant need for the body to go into overdrive in the enzyme manufacturing glands such as the pancreas and the pituitary, are not without their consequences for your fertility.

Research by Dr Howell shows that eating foods devoid of enzymes because of cooking, microwaving or irradiation leads to an enlargement of the pancreas and associated endocrine glands such as the adrenals, pituitary, ovaries and testes. This is because the body uses up a great deal of energy in digestion, and to maintain the supply of necessary enzymes the pancreas becomes enlarged to keep up with output. Thereafter, as it is forced to draw on enzymes from other glands, they in turn are forced to overwork and enlarge – or 'hypertrophy' as the medical jargon puts it. After enlarging, the endocrine glands gradually become exhausted. So, for anyone wanting a baby, there is a tough choice to make. Do you want your adrenals, testes/ovaries and pituitary pumping out optimum levels of hormones for reproduction, or do you want them producing enzymes to the point of exhaustion in order to support the pancreas in digesting your cooked and processed food?

To maximize your chances of conceiving a baby or just to keep your hormonal levels high and balanced, I recommend that at least 50 per cent of your daily intake be raw fruit, vegetables, seeds and nuts. This can easily be accomplished by an entirely fruit breakfast and a salad with lunch or dinner and some nuts or seeds (especially raw sunflower seeds loaded with fertility boosting zinc and vitamin E) as a snack. If you can make 50 per cent of every meal raw by eating salads and uncooked vegetables, according to Dr Kouchakoff, you will not be burdening your immune system. If you are looking to lose weight to enhance fertility, eating a large salad (not drowned in an oily dressing) as a first course will help enormously. The volume of the fibre bulk of the salad will stretch your stomach and the sensitive stretch receptors will signal to the appestat centre in the brain that you are full much sooner than if you were eating only a calorie-dense, cooked food meal; this will lead to the consumption of fewer calories overall.

> A diet composed of 70 per cent raw plant foods (emphasizing the fertility power foods described in Chapter 13) will bring about the fastest results both in terms of general health and fertility.

Digestive Enzyme Supplements

While you work at increasing your intake of fresh fruit and salads, I can give you one tip on how to cheat a bit: whenever you eat cooked foods take a digestive enzyme supplement beforehand or at the same time. This will spare your own enzymes and thus your glands, allowing them to get on with their more important jobs of producing perfect levels of hormones. Friends of mine who have suffered frequent indigestion, acid reflux or wind are delighted to find these problems disappear with digestive enzyme supplementation too. Personally, I am a digestive enzyme junkie: I take them now with every meal, even if it is raw fruit or salad, but I take a higher dose if I am eating cooked foods. I want to preserve all my metabolic enzymes and endocrine glands for keeping me young and for baby making later on.

Fertility Action Plan

- Review what percentage of your diet is made up of cooked foods devoid of enzymes.

- Plan ways to introduce more organic raw fruit and vegetables into your diet until at least 50 per cent of everything you eat is bursting with fertility-enhancing enzymes.

- Buy some digesting enzyme supplements at a health-food shop and start to take them with every meal (note: supplements of acidophilus or bifidus, the friendly intestinal bacteria, are not the same as digestive enzymes).

Chapter 13
The Fertility Power Foods

In this chapter you will find out all the delicious things you can be eating/drinking from Nature's amazing treasure chest of fertility foods as well as aphrodisiacs to maximize your chances of having a baby – at any age.

Organic Farming

If you were to make only one change to your diet to improve your fertility, then buying organic foods instead of commercially grown, pesticide and artificial-chemical laden, non-organic produce would be my top recommendation. It is no coincidence that human fertility has been decreasing over the past 50 years, exactly the time span that intensive commercial agricultural methods have been widely used.

Organic farming prohibits the use of hormones, antibiotics and pesticides. Animals raised on organic farms are not only healthier, they are significantly more fertile than their reproductively challenged counterparts fed on fodder grown with chemical fertilizers and pesticides. According to the Organic Consumers Association,[1] when bulls are transferred from organic to non-organic fodder, the motility of their sperm declines, but bounces back to normal levels once they are fed organic fodder again. It was also found that organically fed rabbits produce far more eggs, have a higher pregnancy rate (100 per cent as opposed to a feeble 29 per cent and 26 per cent), more embryos, larger litters and are healthier than rabbits fed non-organic foodstuffs. The organic bunnies' offspring had a greater birthweight and about 50 per cent fewer deaths prior to weaning.[2]

Rabbits, the animals that symbolize prolific fertility and mating drive in our culture, can be rendered infertile in the course of three generations, just by being fed non-organic foods.

This phenomenon is not unique to cows and rabbits: organic hens produce more eggs with higher egg weights. One study found that, when chickens are fed organic grain, they lay twice as many fertile eggs, begin laying earlier and at faster rates; the eggs even keep better.[3] Do you know any women who would like their own eggs to keep better for longer? I do!

The few studies published exploring the link between the consumption of organic food and fertility show that human beings benefit as much as our furry friends from eating organically produced foods and from low exposure to pesticides. A

1994 study found that organic farmers had much higher sperm counts than other blue-collar workers; in fact, they were more than twice as high in organic farmers (363 million sperm per millilitre of semen) as in a control group of welders and printers (164 million per millilitre).[4] Interestingly, it has also been found that conventional farmers who do not eat organic foods (and would inevitably have higher exposure to pesticides) have a significantly lower proportion of normally shaped sperm.[5]

Men who eat organic foods have much more fertile sperm: they have higher sperm counts and better sperm quality than men eating normal, pesticide-laden food.

Can Organic Fruits and Vegetables Slow the Ageing Process?

In research carried out by David Sinclair, an associate professor of pathology at Harvard, together with Professor Leonard Guarente, it seems that plants under stress, such as organically grown plants (which have no herbicides or pesticides to help them fight their life battles), produce molecules that turn on the plants' defence genes (sirtuins). When consumed, these molecules – Sirtuin Activating Compounds or STACs – have been shown, on tests on yeasts, worms and flies, to turn on their anti-ageing genes – extending their lifespan significantly – and seemingly boosting fertility. Sinclair observed that the longer-lived flies 'were laying more eggs than usual'.[6] In comparison, mollycoddled, commercially grown plants do not produce anti-ageing STAC molecules in any significant amounts.

As mentioned in Chapter 2, STACs and the sirtuin genes can preserve our own youth by stabilizing the chromosomes in cells' DNA. The best known of the STACs derived from plants is called resveratrol; this has even been shown to be antiviral, to suppress the growth of implanted cancer tumours and to be effective in animals against heart disease, stroke and high cholesterol.

Eating organic and wild foods generally could extend your life and boost fertility.

Which Fertility Power Foods to Choose?

OK, so now you are standing by the organic produce section of your supermarket or at your local farmers' market, what should you buy?

Alfalfa

Alfalfa is a nutritional wonder food loaded with magnesium, iron and calcium. In fact, this little sprout is bursting with all the vitamins and minerals necessary for life, including new life. With four times the vitamin C of citrus fruits, it will boost the sperm count and sperm quality of infertile men and enhance fertility in women. It contains an array of natural digestive enzymes and even amino acids. Alfalfa is both cleansing and detoxifying and will help remove fertility-inhibiting toxins out of your body.

One reason I pick alfalfa as a top fertility food is because of its high magnesium content. Magnesium deficiency has been linked to miscarriage. It has been found that the magnesium content of the diets of many North American and British women is too low to sustain a pregnancy. If you load up with alfalfa and other sprouts you will not be part of this statistic any more. Alfalfa's mineral balance makes it very beneficial for sufferers of endometriosis.

Alfalfa leaf is said to have a regulating effect on oestrogen levels thanks to compounds called inflavones.[7] Alfalfa is also high in vitamin E, which is critical for fertility. Sprinkle the sprouts into your daily salads.

Algae (Blue-green)

This is my all-time favourite superfood, and one that I take in the form of capsule supplements every single day. You could literally live off this miracle seaweed – it is a perfectly balanced spectrum of all amino acids, minerals, live enzymes and almost every nutrient so far discovered. Its protein content is so easily assimilated it will literally fly into your cells – unlike meat, which is much harder for the body to break down and access. An unexpected side effect of blue-green algae is that it seems to make your hair and nails grow twice as fast. Algae is rich in vitamin B6 (as well as B2 and B12), one of the top fertility nutrients for women, especially women who have elevated prolactin levels (a hormone that prevents ovulation), such as is found in women who drink diet sodas, or take the artificial sweetener aspartame in any form. Algae also helps detoxify heavy metals from the body, including mercury and lead, toxins that prevent conception. And finally, the high level of antioxidants found in algae make it a top anti-ageing food.

If you do decide to take a blue-green algae supplement, build slowly up to six capsules a day. Taking too much initially could trigger a 'cleansing crisis' – you may become completely nauseous as your body rapidly dumps toxins out of your system.

Every aspect of fertility nutrition is enhanced by blue-green algae.

Almonds

Raw almonds are perhaps the best overall fertility nut. They are very high in vitamin E, which is important for reproduction in both sexes; it also contains the amino acid arginine, which has been shown to markedly increase sperm count and motility. Almonds also contain vitamin B2, which helps with hypothyroidism, a condition linked to infertility. Get munching on those raw almonds; roasted almonds will have only 10 per cent of the nutrients of raw almonds, so don't waste your money on them. Note that, in the USA, many almonds labelled as 'raw' have in fact been pasteurized and are useless for fertility so please check your sources carefully.

Aloe Vera

This powerful medicinal plant is another one of my all-time favourites – and one I take every day for its anti-ageing properties. An entire flowerbed in my garden is devoted to aloe plants. The gel inside when the spiky leaves are cut open contains eighteen amino acids, vitamins, minerals, enzymes and the anti-ageing glyconutrients I mentioned in Chapter 2 – especially mannose. In its natural form, it is a laxative, which helps detoxification and thus supports fertility. Many supplemental forms have had the laxative compound removed. See Chapter 19 to learn more about your intestines and fertility.

Apples

Good source of flavonoids, vitamins – especially vitamin C (the best one for male fertility) – and minerals including boron, a mineral that has been found to raise estradiol-oestrogen to optimum levels, higher than HRT in perimenopausal women. Apples contain anti-ageing antioxidants and are very high in fibre. An apple a day will keep the fertility doctors away!

Apricots

These luscious fruits are fertility foods because of their youthful antioxidant vitamin C content and the fact they are good sources of magnesium (an anti-miscarriage mineral), iron, copper, potassium and silicon.

Asparagus

Asparagus is a very well-known aphrodisiac – it even looks phallic. It contains aspartic acid, an amino acid that is said to neutralize toxic wastes in the bloodstream and eliminate them through the kidneys, so it is an excellent diuretic, which is also why it can make your urine smell very strong. It is also said to revitalize the reproductive organs, perhaps because it contains so many great nutrients: beta-carotene, vitamins B, C, and E (all fabulous for fertility), iodine, potassium and the mineral zinc – a fertility super-nutrient.

Avocados

A wonderful source of healthy plant fats, avocados will boost your fertility with the vitamins E and B, beta-carotenes, copper and potassium. Avocado has always been a traditional remedy for erectile dysfunction and some men report avocado boosts their libido in general.

Bananas

Bananas contain an enzyme that facilitates the production of sex hormones. According to Chinese medicine they increase the 'yin fluids', i.e. they will help in the production of fertile cervical mucus. This popular fruit contains the anti-ageing star vitamin, folic acid, as well as vitamins B6 (great for women's fertility) and potassium. They are also rich in tryptophan, a vital amino acid involved in nerve function and for boosting serotonin levels, making you feel happy and relaxed. Tryptophan is important for men and women since chronic deficiency in this nutrient causes infertility in both sexes.

Bee Pollen

Bee pollen is probably the ultimate fertility food. One teaspoon of bee pollen granules contains about 2.5 to 10 billion pollen grains. Each of these grains is the male semen, seed or germ cell of the plant kingdom, able to fertilize and create a life – a fruit, grain, vegetable, flower or tree.[8] It is bursting with the overwhelming reproductive force of nature, so imagine what it will do to you!

Loaded with amino acids, bee pollen is one of the most protein-rich foods available, in a form that is easily assimilated by the body. Bee pollen is a potent stimulator of sexual hormone production in both men and women and is thought to balance glandular activity. In one study, forty infertile men who were given bee pollen reported improved health in general, an increase in libido and improved sperm production.[9] In a further study involving women with menstrual irregularities, the group who took bee pollen showed either a significant improvement or the elimination of their menstrual complaints. In contrast, the control group saw no improvement.[10] The Hunzas from Pakistan and the Caucasus people of Russia – both of whom are well known for their longevity and good health – eat high amounts of bee products.

Bee pollen contains all the vitamins and minerals necessary for health and reproduction.

Bee pollen comes in granules that taste quite mild. The easiest way to eat them is mixed into fruit smoothies, but, if you like the taste, you can sprinkle them on your food. I know people who eat teaspoons of bee pollen straight from the jar.

However, please note that bee pollen may cause an allergic reaction in some people, so start with a very small amount and stop if you notice any adverse side effects. Anyone who is allergic to bee stings should not take bee pollen.

Beetroots and Juice

Beets contain B and C vitamins, and the fertility-enhancing mineral manganese. They are meant to be an aphrodisiac too.

Mixed with carrots and cucumber in a juice, beets are great for cleansing the reproductive glands and organs by boosting kidney function in the body. Remember not to be alarmed when, going to the bathroom after eating beets, you find your pee is bright red!

Berries

Blueberries, blackberries, cranberries and strawberries are loaded with vitamin C and other phytonutrients, they are powerful antioxidants and protect both sperm and eggs from cell damage. Vitamin C is the best overall tonic for sperm; it increases sperm count, motility, and protects against sperm clumping and genetic defects.

Broccoli

Broccoli has far too many health-enhancing nutrients for it to be left off any list of fertility power foods. Broccoli contains selenium, which is good for sperm count and motility. Its folic acid and boron content will also go a long way to helping you conceive a healthy baby. Just one cup of broccoli is sufficient to provide 24 per cent of your daily vitamins and 5 per cent of all minerals to sustain perfect health and fertility.

Carrots and Carrot Juice

Carrots are loaded with zinc. Domestic rabbits are thought to breed even more prolifically than wild rabbits because they are fed more carrots. Carrot juice is the best fertility drink, combining rich vitamin C with zinc, bioflavonoids and other phytonutrients. One 8 oz glass is equal to 5 lb (2.2 kg) of carrots, which would be very difficult to eat even in one day. A mixture of carrot, beetroot and cucumber juice is one of the best blends for cleaning and alkalinizing the kidneys, sexual organs and sexual glands which, according to principles of Chinese medicine, are influenced by kidney function and condition. Freshly prepared organic carrot juice would be my top tip as a fertility drink for men and women.

Cauliflower

This familiar vegetable has fertility vitamins folic acid, B6 and C as well as the mineral boron, which can raise oestrogen levels if they are falling. On the other hand, cauliflower appears to aid the body's excretion of excess oestrogen – keeping the balance just right! It is beneficial for fibroids. Like broccoli and cabbage, it is best eaten gently steamed, not raw, for anyone with a low thyroid, since a compound in raw cauliflower can suppress the thyroid.

Celery

It looks so innocuous. It tastes so bland (to many people). But do not underestimate the humble celery with all its folic acid, beta-carotene, vitamin C and array of fertility-enhancing minerals including magnesium. It contains a compound similar to the male hormone androsterone and is a powerful aphrodisiac, especially for men.

Coconut and Coconut Milk

Coconuts are a wonderful plant fat. Loaded with iodine, coconut improves fertility by optimizing thyroid function. Coconut water is a great source of easily absorbed minerals. It is also said to increase sperm production. Coconut – both the nut itself and the oil – has antifungal, antiviral and antibacterial properties. Use coconut to counteract any niggling health complaints that could be undermining your fertility.

Coconut can be taken internally or topically to treat any complaint that stems from a fungus, virus or bacteria.

(Other) Cruciferous Vegetables: Bok Choy, Brussels Sprouts, Cabbage, Collards, Kale

These vegetables are a good source of the mineral boron, which has been found to raise levels of estradiol, i.e. the metabolically active form of oestrogen, to a level higher even than HRT. They contain indoles, which have cancer-fighting properties, are loaded with vitamin C, a key fertility nutrient (especially in men – see the section on vitamin C below), and contain bioflavonoids, which are said to promote a healthy uterine lining.

Cucumber and Juice

An excellent alkalinizer, great mixed with beetroot and carrot juice for giving the reproductive organs a cleansing boost

Fennel

Fennel is a highly effective blood tonic and helps correct menstrual disorders. It is very good taken as a juice with beetroot and carrot juice.

Flax Seeds (Linseed)

Another one of my favourite superfoods. Flax seeds are one of the richest source of omega 3 essential fatty acids, of which most people do not get enough. The brain is 60 per cent fat, as are the nerves running throughout your body. Every single cell membrane is made of a layer of fat, so the quality of fat you eat plays a significant role in your general health and fertility. The reproductive organs seem to be especially affected by the quality of the dietary fat con-sumed. Infertility can sometimes be caused by essential fatty acid abnormalities and the consumption of bad fats, like dairy fats and trans-fats found in processed foods. Flax seeds, on the other hand, assist in hormone production as well as the health of the ovaries and testes.[11] I recommend flax seeds in particular to women who show any sign of an oestrogen dominance. When oestrogen levels are disproportionately higher than progesterone levels you typically you get excess body fat around the stomach, mild hypothyroid and a shorter menstrual cycle – under 26 days. The mild phytoestrogens in flax seed will gently help to balance out oestrogen by reducing the absorption of the hormone at the cells' receptor sites.

Garlic

Garlic is a powerful antibiotic and antifungal vegetable (as are onions, leeks, mustard green and radishes, all high in natural sulphur). It contributes to fertility in women by killing off bacteria that could affect the ovaries, causing hormonal imbalance and endometriosis, or chlamydia, for example, which can lead to inflammation of the Fallopian tubes, pelvic inflammatory disease and thus infertility. Garlic also prevents the overgrowth of the candida fungus, which also impairs fertility.

As a source of selenium, garlic is good for male fertility in that it leads to an increase in sperm count and an improvement in motility.

Grapefruit

With high levels of fertility-enhancing vitamin C, grapefruit is also rich in bioflavonoids, which are said to support good uterine lining. As a small additional benefit, fasting exclusively on grapefruit for three days is meant to cure cellulite. I have not had the willpower to be able find out if this claim is true. If you prove to yourself it is, please let me know!

Grapes (Red)

Grapes contain the mineral boron, which is the key in maintaining balanced oestrogen levels. Organic grapes, particularly red grapes, have very high levels of the compound resveratrol, recently found to turn on the body's anti-ageing genes – just what you need to stay young and frisky.

Hazelnuts (Filberts)

Rich in B vitamins, these nuts are a great source of amino acids and good for the prostate. By eating one cup of raw hazelnuts you would be treating your body to a huge 20.3 mg of vitamin E – the superstar fertility nutrient; that is 135 per cent of the minimum daily amount needed to stay healthy. With a further 41 per cent of your zinc requirements being met at the same time, what's not to love? They taste yummy too!

Hemp Seed Protein

I have never met, heard of, or seen a protein-deficient vegetarian. Indeed, I doubt such a person exists, what with broccoli containing eleven times more protein than steak (11 g of protein per 100 calories in broccoli, 1 g of protein in 100 calories of steak). Nevertheless, sooner or later, anyone not eating meat will hear the tedious, misconceived question, 'But where do you get your protein from?' as if the enquirer expects their fingernails to drop off at any moment. Well now, vegetarians everywhere need no longer quote the broccoli statistic, they can simply shrug and say 'hemp seed protein'.

Hemp seed is a nutritional wonder food – for general health, as well as for fertility. Hemp seed contains over 33 per cent digestible protein and is rich in iron, vitamin E and omega 3 essential fatty acid. Unlike most soya, hemp is not genetically modified. Hemp is mainly produced in Canada; its production is illegal in the United States because, if someone ate an entire field of this agricultural hemp, they might manage, after many weeks of chewing, to consume around one-tenth of the same amount of the psycho-active compound found in a marijuana joint. Sorry, folks, hemp seed will not cause you to become unnaturally high. You may, however, get a blissful buzz just from the fantastic nutrients. Hemp seed is usually found in powder form and is consumed, just as you would any other protein or whey powder, in a smoothie.

Himalayan Crystal Salt

Normal table salt, sodium chloride, is a white poison that will do nothing much for your health except raise your blood pressure. Crystal salt, mined from the East Karakoram range of the Himalayan Mountains in Pakistan, on the other hand, is white gold as far as nutrition for fertility is concerned. This moist, pink miracle salt contains all natural minerals and trace elements found in the human body.

By taking a half pint jar of water and spooning in the salt until it no longer dissolves fully (the pink salt crystals remain visible at the bottom of the jar), you have made a solution called sole (pronounced 'solay'). If you then add one or two teaspoons of this sole solution to an 8 oz glass of pure/mineral water and drink this first thing in the morning, you will be giving yourself a mineral infusion, replacing electrolytes and balancing your energy. The sole solution helps the body to get rid of heavy metals such as lead, mercury and arsenic that inhibit conception, since the crystal salt is able to break down their molecular structures. Our blood is saline, and the mineral composition of blood is remarkably similar to sea water.

The stunning health and fertility benefits of pure water with sole solution were demonstrated in a study carried out by the Institute for Biophysical Research and The Inter-University, Graz, Austria. The volunteer subjects were divided into four groups. In addition to their usual diets, one group drank tap water, the second group drank tap water with table salt dissolved in it, the third group drank Fiji (pure mineral water) and the fourth group drank Fiji water with sole, Himalayan Crystal salt solution. Of the four groups, those taking the sole solution with Fiji water had stunning health improvements on every parameter of the body's functioning. The female patients in the Fiji water and sole groups had less menstrual pain and emotional exhaustion. All the patients taking sole found an increase in libido. Best of all, one forty-seven-year-old woman, who had wanted to become pregnant her whole life, naturally conceived a healthy baby for the first time while participating in this study.[12] I strongly recommend drinking a glass of sole solution first thing every morning to mineralize the body and help flush out toxins.

Celtic sea salt (which is usually from Brittany and is moist and grey), like Himalayan crystal salt, contains 84 minerals and, when used as a condiment, is a great way to take a mineral supplement.

Supermarket-type, pure-white crystal 'sea salt' has usually been heated to terrifically high temperatures to remove impurities and does not have the same levels of trace minerals as crystal salt or Himalayan crystal salt or Celtic sea salt.

Many health-food stores are now selling Himalayan crystal salt. It is also widely available online.

Leafy Greens and Spinach

Spinach and leafy greens, particularly kale and mustard greens, are very supportive of your fertility. They are loaded with folic acid, which is needed for anti-ageing and to prevent birth defects, and are also high in vitamin K and iron, both of which help guard against miscarriage and foetal abnormalities. I add spinach to everything these days – soups, salads, curries, even tomato-vegetable type sauces for pasta – ever since I found out that one cup of spinach, at only 48 calories, provides 34 per cent of all vitamins I need on a daily basis and 20 per cent of all minerals. One cup of spinach is enough for 24 per cent of your daily calcium requirements, 36 per cent of your magnesium and a whopping 62 per cent of the necessary mineral manganese.

Lemons and Limes

Lemons, lemon juice and lime juice are some of the best foods for the female sexual organs and glands. Whole lemon contains bioflavonoids, which have an affinity for the uterus and the vagina; it dissolves vaginal mucus (not the same as helpful cervical fluid), restores an optimal pH balance necessary for conception and regulates the female reproductive system. Lemons are helpful in cleansing and alkalinizing the urogenital tract, prostate and sexual organs in men too. Drinking lemon in hot water first thing every morning is a great way to start the day. The warm water also flushes the bowels, clearing out accumulated waste and helping with detoxification, which is essential for good liver and hormonal function.

Maca

In case you were ever wondering why Peruvians have almost no fertility or libido issues, the answer lies in maca, a pleasant-tasting root, grown high up in the mountains. Rich in nutrients, it balances hormones in men and women, boosts fertility and immunity, increases strength and energy in and out of the bedroom – and is a very potent aphrodisiac as well. Maca is one of those foods that makes you feel so well, so bursting with life and full of the joys of spring that you just want to jump in and be part of the reproductive cycle.

Maca is the fertility secret of people in the Andes.

Some specialist health stores will have maca, usually in powder form, sometimes in capsules. It is widely available online. I like to add a couple of spoons of maca to my usual fruit and flax seed breakfast smoothies.

Mesquite Meal

Unless you are from Southern Arizona or Mexico, you may never have heard of mesquite meal. This is a traditional Native American food, which is produced by gathering ripened seed pods from the mesquite-cactus tree and grinding it into a fine powder. Traditionally, a valuable source of nutrition for desert dwellers, mesquite is high in absorbable protein, and loaded with fertility minerals calcium, magnesium, potassium, iron and zinc. It has high levels of the amino acid lycine which is not commonly found in plant foods, apart from quinoa. It has a sweet, slightly molasses-ish flavour. Whenever I make a smoothie based on a nut milk, I always add a tablespoon of both maca and mesquite. Mesquite also seems to add a dairylike creaminess and thickness to smoothies.

Mesquite meal may be found in specialist health-food shops and is also easily found online.

Pecans

Pecans, like walnuts, are the best dietary sources of vitamin B6, the nutrient dubbed the infertile woman's best friend. B6 balances oestrogen and progesterone and also lowers elevated prolactin levels, which prevent ovulation. B6 has been found to be as effective as the bromocriptine drugs in correcting infertility issues caused by elevated prolactin. If you are suffering from PMT, forget the chocolate and reach for your bag of raw walnuts or raw pecans.

Pumpkin Seeds

For men, pumpkin seeds are one of the best fertility foods, very rich in unsaturated essential fatty acids, organic iron and pangamic acid (vitamin B15) all of which are vital for a healthy prostate gland. They are rich in zinc, a deficiency in which is linked with low sperm count, decreased sperm motility and potency. Zinc is the aphrodisiac mineral, boosting libido in men and in women. With 10.3 mg of zinc in every cup, pumpkin seeds provide 129 per cent of the recommended daily amount of zinc. As a side benefit for men, zinc is the key mineral in protecting the prostate. For women, zinc and vitamin B6 is one of the best fertility-enhancing combinations and guards against miscarriage.

In general, one cup of pumpkin seeds will meet 20 per cent of your daily vitamin requirements and 59 per cent of your mineral needs. Sprinkle pumpkin, sunflower and sesame seeds on salads, in soups, in sandwiches, wherever you can – you'll soon be sowing your own seed.

Quinoa

Quinoa was a staple food of the Incas in Peru, and called 'the mother grain' – perhaps because it helps you to become a mother? Quinoa (pronounced 'keen-wah') is a grain prepared in the same way you would rice, that contains even more usable protein than meat and more calcium than milk. It includes all the fertility-enhancing essential amino acids – including lysine, which is missing from corn, wheat and rice. When sprouted, it contains vitamins A, B6, B12, C, D, E and K, biotin, folic acid, niacin, pantothenic acid, riboflavin and thiamine. It contains a number of minerals too, all great for your health and your fertility.

Quinoa is frequently recommended by doctors of Chinese

According to traditional Chinese medicine, quinoa is good for your sex life!

medicine for its 'kidney strengthening' qualities. According to traditional Chinese medicine, strong kidneys are the foundation and root of all bodily functions and vitality, and are key to fertility and libido.

Sea Vegetables, Spirulina and Kelp

Sea vegetables are chock-full of minerals, and the more mineralized your body is, the more fertile you will be. Since they contain iodine, sea vegetables also help boost thyroid and correct hypothyroidism, a common cause of infertility. There is also a link between endometriosis and hypothyroidism – one study found women with endometriosis had thyroid antibodies 20 per cent higher than the control group – so kelp and other seaweed sources should be taken on a daily basis by endometriosis and hypothyroid sufferers. Sea vegetables also contain B vitamins and vitamins D, E and K, all of which are great for fertility.

Kelp, spirulina and chlorella are available in tablet form, but dried seaweed can also be found in most health-food shops and in the Japanese sections of supermarkets. I often use dulse flakes instead of salt – it is particularly good in soups. In fact, adding strips of dried seaweed will give a great mineral and taste boost to most vegetable soups. Making your own vegan sushi at home is another way to bring the amazing sea vegetables into your life.

Sprouted Seeds and Grains

Sprouted seeds and grains have more enzymes, amino acids, minerals, vitamins and phytonutrients than any other food. The super sprouts are the one food source that can actually reverse ageing and regenerate the body. Baby sunflower and buckwheat sprouts are my favourite and make delicious salads. It is logical that at a time when you want to bring forth new life in the world you should be eating the most life-filled offering of the plant kingdom – sprouted seeds and grains. The Ann Wigmore Institute in Puerto Rico, which bases its diet entirely on sprouts and living foods has had miraculous results on this green regime in treating everything from AIDS to multiple sclerosis and terminal cancer, compared with which baby-making challenges ought to be a cinch!

Sprouted seeds and grains have to rank as the number one food for overall health and, thus, fertility enhancement.

Sunflower Seeds

Sunflower seeds are a nutritional feast. If you only lived on these seeds, one cup would be giving you 46 per cent of your daily vitamins and 62 per cent of your minerals. You would get 49.7 mg of vitamin E – the baby-making vitamin – which is 331 per cent of the daily dose you need! Added to this is 91 per cent of the zinc, 156 per cent of the selenium, 159 per cent of the magnesium and 162 per cent of the manganese, together with loads of B vitamins that you require on a daily basis, and you can see that these little seeds pack a huge fertility punch.

Like pumpkin seeds, sunflower seeds are one of the best fertility foods for men. They are also very rich in unsaturated essential fatty acids, organic iron and pangamic acid (vitamin B15), all of which are vital for a healthy prostate gland. The high zinc content counteracts any deficiency in this mineral, which is linked with low sperm count, decreased sperm motility and potency. Zinc is the aphrodisiac mineral, boosting libido in men and in women. For women, zinc with vitamins E and B6 is one of the best fertility-enhancing combinations and helps prevent miscarriage.

Sprinkle sunflower and sesame seeds all over your food, into your salads and in your fruit smoothies, or just keep a packet in the car or office drawer to have as a healthy snack. You'll be glad you did.

Sweet Potatoes

Sweet potatoes contain sixty minerals, compared with white potatoes that have only three. Being more fibrous, sweet potatoes are also lower on the glycaemic index and, therefore, carry all the health benefits of foods that trigger only a moderate glucose and insulin response. Every woman I know who has eaten sweet potatoes every day on my recommendation has either had a baby or is pregnant at the time of writing, having conceived within four months of being on the sweet potato-rich diet!

A further anecdote to contemplate: the birth rate soars in the USA in August, nine months after Thanksgiving. While I have no doubt that the holiday festivities and couples being relaxed and on vacation play a role, it is intriguing to note that sweet potato is the traditional Thanksgiving vegetable and it is the one time a year Americans *en masse* will be eating it. Just a coincidence?

Walnuts

Walnuts and pecans are the best dietary sources of vitamin B6. B6 balances oestrogen and progesterone and lowers elevated prolactin levels, which prevent ovulation. B6 has been found to be as effective as the bromocriptine drugs. If you are suffering from PMT avoid chocolate; reach for your bag of raw walnuts or raw pecans and you will soon be sublimely balanced.

Wheatgerm/Wheatgerm Oil

Wheatgerm oil is particularly rich in organic vitamin E, which is essential for the production of sperm and ova and for maintaining the health of the prostate. Wheatgerm, being high in vitamin E, selenium, vitamin B2 (riboflavin), B6, PABA and zinc – the whole army of fertility nutrients – will raise sperm count and motility, balance menstrual rhythms, prevent miscarriage and help with endometriosis. If you are not certain you will digest it well, then one option is to use wheatgerm oil on your face or as a massage oil, so it will absorb through the skin. Vitamin E is great for stopping wrinkles too, so even if you are going to be an older mum or dad, at least you will not look it!

If you are not wheat intolerant, wheatgerm is an excellent fertility food.

Xylitol

As I mentioned in Chapter 3, normal sugar releases the enemy – the rapid ageing hormone, insulin. Luckily, there is a completely natural sugar found in fibrous vegetables and fruit, corn cobs and hardwood trees like birch. Xylitol looks and tastes exactly like normal white sugar, but could not be more different. A potent anti-ageing glyconutrient (see Chapter 2), the best thing about xylitol is that it warrants a mere seven on the glycaemic index, meaning it provokes virtually no insulin response whatsoever. Normal sugar scores 100 on the glycaemic index and even something as savoury as an onion is 15! Yes, you can have your cake, and you can eat it – since you can bake with xylitol too. This healthy, all-natural sugar, which is also antibacterial and good for your teeth, will keep you young and fertile.

Yams

The yam now has legendary status in terms of fertility enhancement for women. A remarkable study was carried out by a professor at the University of Ibadan in Nigeria on the women of the native Yoruba tribe, which has one of the highest rates of fraternal twins in the world: one in every four pregnancies instead of one in every forty! That is a lot of twins – with no IVF involved. He found that their diet contained huge amounts of wild African yams. Yams contain the substance dioscin, a form of natural progesterone. Many women are advised to use wild yam cream topically on their abdominal area if they have low progesterone levels, as suggested by a cycle of only 21 days or less.

Perhaps more relevantly, yams, like flax seeds, contain weak phytoestrogens, which inhibit the bodies own oestrogen (where there is an excess or an imbalance), and are said to act much like the drug Clomid, in that this anti-oestrogen effect can stimulate the ovaries to release an egg. The research from Nigeria mentioned above found that the steroidlike compounds in yams also triggered the release of follicle stimulating hormone (FSH), which is what was thought to be responsible for stimulating the ovaries. Women in the Yoruba tribe had consistently high levels of FSH. Certainly the Nigerian women in the study must have been releasing multiple eggs each ovulation to have so many twins.

Yams are helpful for women with luteal phase defects, short menstrual cycles, endometriosis and poor cervical fluid, or indeed for anyone wanting twins! Since an excess of phytoestrogens is linked to a *decrease* in fertility, it is prudent not to go too overboard with yams. It is recommended to take them in the first fourteen days of the cycle only (in the same way the drug Clomid is taken).

Yams are not the same as sweet potatoes, although many supermarkets confuse the two. Wild yams from Africa, the Caribbean and Mexico, from the tuber family Discorea, are the ones responsible for stimulating FSH release and ovulation and increasing the chances of twins.

Yams and sweet potatoes are, however, two of the best fertility vegetables.

Conclusion

The fruit, vegetables, nuts and seeds mentioned in this chapter have been singled out for their exceptional ability to boost fertility in men and women and maximize your chances of having a baby. However, all organic, whole plant foods are great for your health, and just because I have not mentioned them here does not mean you should not eat them. The only ones to avoid, as you have seen in Chapter 4, are soya, peas and rhubarb, which have contraceptive compounds in them. Bon appetit!

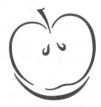

Fertility Action Plan

- All you Bridget Joneses out there should try to find out if there are any nice, single, organic farmers – the most fertile men on the planet – in your area.

- Decide what fertility power foods you are now going to eat on a regular basis and be sure to try some new ones.

- Replace all white sugar with xylitol and all white table salt with Himalayan Crystal Salt.

Chapter 14
Aphrodisiacs

If you are starting to think that your get up and procreate has got up and gone, then I have some good news for you. There really are foods that enhance mojo. While all the fertility foods discussed in Chapter 13 serve to improve your general energy levels significantly, there are certain foods that are particularly good for libido.

Artichokes

Artichokes have been used as an aphrodisiac since the 1700s in France, where street vendors would tout them under the promise that they heated the genitals! In fact, they contain a compound called cynarin that strengthens and helps to regenerate the liver. The liver is the organ which, in traditional Chinese medicine, is responsible for sexual vigour.

Asparagus

Asparagus has a long pedigree as an aphrodisiac, being cultivated by both ancient Arabs and Greeks for this purpose. The seventeenth-century English herbalist Nicholas Culpeper observed that asparagus 'stirreth up bodily lust in man and woman'.[1]

Bananas

Bananas not only contain enzymes that stimulate the production of sex hormones and thus libido, they can help to improve sexual stamina. In traditional Chinese medicine they are said to improve the 'yin fluids', which help things to . . . ahem . . . flow smoothly. Rich in potassium and B vitamins, and in particular the amino acid tryptophan, bananas stimulate the production of serotonin, the 'don't worry, be happy' brain chemical, so do eat bananas if, rather than wanting to go bananas, you would like to be aping around with a loved one.

Beans

According to herbalist Brigitte Mars, adzuki beans, garbanzo beans (chickpeas) and lentils are great for libido. I agree, assuming you are someone who digests beans well, otherwise passion-killing flatulence may not create the right atmosphere for your baby-making projects.

Beetroot

One has to wonder if there is a reason that, in French, the slang term for penis, *betterave*, is apparently the same word for beetroot. Beetroot are loaded with love-boosting nutrients:

beta-carotene, vitamins B and C, calcium, phosphorus and manganese. Brigitte Mars, in her excellent book *Sex, Love and Health*, even states that there is a folk tradition that two people who eat from the same beetroot are likely to fall in love. Single ladies, keep a good stock of beetroot in the fridge, just in case some likely life mate should cross your kitchen.

Cabbage

Cabbage is full of natural sulphur, which increases circulation to all areas of the body – yes, even those tiny capillaries to the male genitals. It is thought to be a warming nutritive sexual tonic.

Cacao (Chocolate)

Pure cacao, in the form of raw cacao beans which can be found in whole and powdered form, is loaded with the 'love chemical' phenylethylamine (PEA). Research shows that when we fall in love our PEA levels increase and are elevated whenever we are happy. Dark chocolate (with more than 70 per cent cocoa solids) also keeps PEA levels high, no matter what is going on in your love life. PEA, together with magnesium, helps to maintain high levels of the neurotransmitter dopamine, the brain chemical responsible for gusto, mojo and feelings of pleasure. Cacao's role in increasing PEA and dopamine is, no doubt, part of the answer as to why chocolate has long been known to be an aphrodisiac. It was dubbed 'the Aztec viagra' after the Emperor Montezuma was observed by the conquistadors to consume some 50 cups of a cacao drink before visiting his harem of over 300 women in 1528! And just in case you were wondering where the expression 'Montezuma's revenge' came from, it no doubt relates to the fact that cacao, in high amounts, is a laxative! There is another reason to be very moderate in your chocolate consumption (apart from not wanting to rush to the bathroom): cocoa contains caffeine, which, as you already know, is a contraceptive and accelerates ageing.

Celery

There is nothing about the innocent-looking celery with its mild taste that would lead one to guess that this is a love food for men or that it has a long history as a general aphrodisiac. Studies have shown that this vegetable contains chemicals that in a number of animals appear to stimulate sexual arousal in females because they elevate sex hormones, and to stimulate readiness to mate in males. So get munching – a mere two stalks of celery will also give you a good daily dose of potassium, magnesium, calcium, phosphorus, sodium, vitamins A and C, thiamine, riboflavin, B6, niacin, folic acid and iron.

Cucumber
Cucumbers are not just phallic in shape and aphrodisiac in nature; according to recent research these cool vegetables also stimulate women's olfactory senses.

Ginger
This spicy herb can spice up your love life. It is a powerful sexual stimulant and is supposed to increase the sensitivity of your erogenous zone.

Honey
Honey is a natural aphrodisiac thanks to its mineral and trace amino acid content. It also provides sustained energy, just what you need to be on an extended honeymoon.

Maca
Grown in the high mountains of Peru, this pleasant-tasting root, which is available in powder form, is one of the most potent aphrodisiacs around. Loaded with nutrients, maca is a sexual libido enhancer. Its amazing action is because of its effect on balancing hormones.

Onion and Garlic
Onions and garlic are among the oldest known edible aphrodisiacs. In fact, in some spiritual traditions such as the traditional yoga teachings, their consumption is strongly discouraged because they are so sexually stimulating.

Maca is sometimes called the Peruvian Viagra.

Other Fruits

Figs, grapes and berries are also great passion foods. Perhaps this is why libido has never been a problem for men in the Mediterranean region.

Peach

This sensual-looking fruit has been known by the Chinese for centuries to be as engaging to the sex drive as it is to the palate.

Pomegranate

The media health star of recent times, whose numerous nutritive and healing properties are only just coming to light, this delicious fruit has in fact been a symbol of fertility and sexuality since ancient times. It contains a compound called pelletierine, which is meant to raise states of consciousness. On a more mundane level, in traditional Chinese medicine it is said to assist in both kidney and liver function – key organs for good fertility and libido. The seeds also contain phytoestrogenic compounds, which may assist in optimizing oestrogen levels.

Shellfish and Seafood (from Pure Sources)

I hesitate to recommend shellfish and seafood because most contain traces of the mercury that now pollutes our seas and oceans (not to mention other contraceptive pollutants such as PCBs). This heavy metal makes both men and women sterile and massively increases the risk of miscarriage. However, the long history of shellfish and seafood as aphrodisiacs compels me to at least briefly mention them here. If you want to eat them, try to find shellfish and seafood caught in the cleanest waters possible.

Oysters: their suggestive appearance, combined with the fact they are loaded with zinc and iron, makes them perfect for virility.

Mussels: An even more effective sex aid than oysters – yes, these molluscs will really put you in the mood.

Other fishy love foods are scallops and anchovies. Caviar is reputed to have been the virility fix of choice for both Casanova and Rasputin.

Truffles

This underground black mushroom, traditionally snuffled out by pigs from the forest, always reminds me of Peter Mayle's book, *A Year in Provence*. In the South of France, it would seem from Mr Mayle's account, 'les truffles' are more precious than diamonds. Perhaps their long history as an aphrodisiac and the fact they are very high in minerals goes some way to explaining this. Or maybe it's just because they are so prohibitively expensive that the very fact that your partner could have bought these for you fills your heart with love (and passion).

Vanilla

This sweet spice is also a passion booster.

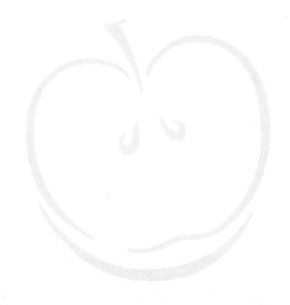

Fertility Action Plan

- Come on, people! You know that anything I could suggest after reading a chapter on aphrodisiacs is going to be indecent. Have fun!

Chapter 15
Fertility Drinks

Water

Pure water, uncontaminated by fluoride or other toxic chemicals, is by far the best drink for fertility and optimal health in general. Some 70 per cent of the body is composed of water – assuming you are one of the rare people who is properly hydrated. The regular consumption of dehydrating drinks like sodas and caffeinated teas and coffees means that most adults have only a 50–60 per cent hydration level. To maximize your chances of having a baby, you need the DNA of your egg cells or your sperm, respectively, as well as all the cells of your body in general, in tip-top, youthful shape. Some biochemists now think that the core of that double helix of the DNA in every single one of the trillion cells in your body is a column of organized water, which transmits information throughout your body. MRI technology has shown that dehydration leads to cell damage, which, in turn, leads to impaired fertility.

When you are dehydrated you will be on a fast-track ageing path and significantly reducing your fertility. This applies to both men and women.

Green 'Superfood' Powders

The next most fertility-enhancing drinks on the planet after water are green! Drinking some form of concentrated green juice, or 'superfoods' powder drink from wheatgrass, barley grass algae, spirulina, other seaweeds and chlorophyll from plants in general, is one of the most cleansing and mineralizing fluids you can put in your body. One teaspoon of any of the organic concentrated green superfood powders is the equivalent of eating fifteen plates of salad. Now, unless you are a gorilla, that is about thirteen more plates than most people can manage in a single day.

Wheatgrass and barley grass contain all the known minerals and trace elements, a whole spectrum of vitamins, hundreds of enzymes, and are loaded with amino acids. The best thing about wheatgrass and barley grass is that they have very high levels of the antioxidant superoxide dismutase (SOD), which protects the cells from damage and removes pollutants, radiation, heavy metals, toxic chemicals, foreign substances and other toxins from the body. By protecting the cells from damage, SOD is a key anti-ageing and fertility nutrient. Barley grass is usually only available in green-powder form. Wheatgrass is often available fresh at juice bars in the form of 'shots'.

A word of warning: do not overdose on these powerful, cleansing grasses/superfood powders. You are likely to become completely nauseous as your body dumps toxins out of the system, then be unable to face drinking them again for a long time.

Liquid Chlorophyll

Chlorophyll, the green pigment found in plants, has a number of health and detoxifying benefits. Although you are unlikely to be swigging it back as a drink all on its own, stirring a few teaspoons into a glass of fresh whole fruit smoothie (turning the concoction completely green) is a great way to take this. Chlorophyll is helpful in regularizing menstrual cycles and in the treatment of endometriosis. Most sources of liquid chlorophyll come from alfalfa plants and contain the same fertility benefits of alfalfa (see Chapters 13 and 14, above). It also helps protect the body against pollutants, radiation and toxins and in general strengthens the immune system by providing super high quality nourishment to the cells.

Organic Freshly Squeezed Vegetable Juices

All vegetable juices are fantastic for fertility, providing concentrated doses of nutrients, which can be absorbed immediately into the bloodstream, bypassing the digestive process. One 8 oz glass of carrot juice is the equivalent to 5 lb of carrots, which would be almost impossible to eat in one day. All non-starchy vegetables can be juiced. I particularly recommend beetroot, carrot, celery, chard, cucumber, dandelions (yes! very good for you, but a bit tricky to juice), kale, lettuces of all kinds and spinach. Tomatoes (strictly speaking a fruit, of course) are also great to juice. Since carrot and beetroot juice contains very high sugar, it is best to mix them with lower glycaemic green juices – celery and kale are a good mix. If you find pure green vegetable juices too bitter, the addition of a green apple will help make it a lot more palatable. (I do not recommend the packaged or tinned vegetable juices, which tend to be loaded with salt and have nothing like the nutritional quality of fresh squeezed juice.)

Whole fruit smoothies

Packaged or tinned fruit juices are little more than sugar water – and nutritionally not much better than sodas. They have always been pasteurized, so have no enzymes and are thus also likely to be nutritionally depleted. If you are used to having fruit juice in the morning, or like to take any supplements with a juice rather than pure water, then I recommend the whole fruit smoothie. This is a cinch to make. You put pieces of whole fruit – peeled, if you would usually peel it before eating – together with mineral water in a blender, and blend. Voila! The easiest imaginable 100 per cent pulp juice. The better your blender, the more you will have a real smoothie tasting beverage. I find this a lot less fuss than messing around with a juicer too – my blender jug is easy to clean.

My favourite fruit to blend is oranges, grapefruits, all types of berries, melon/watermelon and pineapple. Sometimes I mix a whole thick fruit 'shake' by adding in bananas, or other sweet fruits like plums and peaches. I usually add soaked flax seeds and maca too.

The advantage of eating fruit like this is that none of the fibre or nutrients of the whole fruit is lost. Thanks to the retained fibre, the fruit sugar, fructose, is not absorbed as rapidly as pure fruit juices and so does not cause an insulin spike (which you will recall from Chapter 3 is not good for those planning on ageing slowly and staying fertile as late as possible). Adding flax seeds slows down the rate at which the fruit sugar can be absorbed still further. For busy people, this is also a very quick way to eat a serving or two of fruit in the morning; to me it seems a lot less bothersome than taking the time to chew on a whole fruit. You can even pour your flax/fruit smoothie blend into a (glass) bottle and take it with you as a healthy meal to go. Just be careful of people in the office who start trying to steal your breakfast.

There are a number of delicious smoothies made with fruit and superfoods available in the refrigerated section of most health-food stores. While these will never be as nutritious as a fruit smoothie you have made fresh at home, they are a good choice if you are very hungry and want to avoid eating anything bad – sweets, or a tired old sandwich.

Coconut Water

One of the things I loved the most about living in the Caribbean was my access to abundant, fresh from the tree, coconut water. If you can get hold of this, even on vacations, then drink as much as you can. It is loaded with electrolytes and trace minerals, it is both a hydrating and a cooling drink that supports kidney function for both men and women. It is especially good for male fertility since it boosts male sexual fluids.

Rejuvelac and Kambucha

Rejuvelac and kambucha are both fermented beverages, which are loaded with B vitamins, friendly flora bacteria that populate the intestines (the first line of defence of the immune system), and vitamins E and K. They are also rich in enzymes and amino acids.

Kambucha is a form of fermented tea, originally from China. It tastes fizzy and I think it's delicious. It can be found in the refrigerator section of larger health stores, and, since I can find it in two shops on the small Greek island of Paros, I am sure you will be able to get it in your neighbourhood.

Rejuvelac is made from fermented wheat berries, rye or millet and sometimes even cabbage. It is not usually available to buy – since like all fermented foods there is a risk of it putrefying and becoming anything but healthy. You have to make this at home.

Herbal Teas

I recommend peppermint, spearmint, fenugreek, rosehip, nettle and all 'fruit' herbal teas. Of course, I strongly recommend you take any herbs prescribed by a qualified herbalist or doctor of oriental medicine for your particular reproductive state. The main teas to avoid for their contraceptive or abortive properties are red raspberry leaf (which is great to bring on labour), fennel, echinacea, sage and pennyroyal.

Fertility Action Plan

- Buy some superfood green powder and make up a health drink every morning, no excuses. Think of it as your fertility medicine.

- Start to carry a water bottle around with you everywhere and aim to drink three litres every day.

- Make a fresh whole fruit smoothie your usual breakfast.

Chapter 16
Fertility Supplements and Herbs

In much of the Western world, society has become lazy; we have become accustomed to 'fixing' anything wrong with us by popping a pill. It's a lot easier than having to make any effort, such as dietary or lifestyle changes. We pop a pill when we do not want to have a baby, so why not just take some pills in order to have one? The danger of this type of approach is that encourages you to think that you can carry on eating tasty but nutritionally depleted junk food and drinking any sugary, alcoholic and/or caffeinated beverages you like, and just rely on supplements to rectify the damage. Drug companies pander to this indulgence: a multibillion pound/euro/dollar supplement industry is now part of our nutritional landscape and consumers are lulled into a false sense of security by believing they are buying health.

'For those relying on supplements, beneficial and sustained diet change is postponed. The dangers of a Western diet cannot be overcome by consuming nutrient pills.' Dr T. Colin Campbell, *The China Study*[1]

Apart from vitamins and minerals, new so-called phyto-chemicals are being discovered in plants everyday. Scientists have only begun to scratch the surface of the role played by these compounds, and how they can support health when eaten as part of a whole fruit or vegetable. No supplement can ever match the exquisite genius of nature for packaging broad-based, fertility-enhancing nutrition. For example, you can take your zinc as a supplement or you can eat carrots instead, and get a wallop of vitamins A and C and carotenoids all at the same time.

Furthermore, supplements vary considerably in their quality and nutritional content. Read labels carefully – does it say 'all natural ingredients'? Or, even better, 'all organic ingredients'? Many supplements are full of binders and fillers that have no nutritional benefit. The cheaper, bulk-produced ones may also have been synthesized or made from foods grown with pesticides, in which case they will also include concentrations of pesticides which, even at very minute levels, are damaging to fertility and hormonal health in general.

The best supplements, like blue-green algae capsules, always come from natural food sources.

My own philosophy regarding taking supplements is that they should be used in moderation as 'nutritional insurance' only, an adjunct to a healthy, plant-based diet and not as a substitute for good wholefoods. This is why they are called 'supplements', not 'substitutes'. For instance, I would recommend *all* women hoping to conceive should take the B vitamin folic acid every day, even if you are eating plenty of folate-rich leafy green vegetables and fruit. This vitamin, thanks to its key role in protecting the DNA from damage during cellular replication (see Chapter 2), is critical for anti-ageing and for avoiding spinal-neural defects in a developing foetus. I take it every day, even while I'm not trying to conceive at present, as a general anti-ageing measure; I want all the 'daughter' cells in my body (including ovarian cells) to be perfect duplicates of their parent cells, with none of the degeneration or genetic damage that we call 'ageing'.

Another reason to take some good quality supplements, in accordance with your special fertility or health needs, is that, regrettably, thanks to destructive commercial farming practices, many fruit and vegetables contain now only a fraction of their previous levels of micronutrients. A recently reported study in *The Journal of the American College of Nutrition*, which looked at the nutritional composition of forty-three garden crops, shows new findings from University of Texas that levels of calcium, riboflavin, vitamin C, iron and potassium in vegetables and fruit have significantly declined since 1950.[2] There are a number of explanations as to why our fruit and vegetables no longer pack the same nutritional punch as 50 years ago.

First, commercial growers selectively breed vegetables for pith and water – so that the produce looks good, ships well and weighs a lot. It's called 'the dilution effect' – more pith and water but less vitamin content (and taste!). This is why most supermarket tomatoes, peppers and strawberries look great, but taste like juicy cardboard.

Secondly, nearly all commercial fruit is picked when it is green and not given a chance to ripen in the sun. Such fruit never has the chance to develop sunlight-related nutrients such as anthocyanins (plant sunscreens), which have been shown to provide protection against DNA damage (needed for anti-ageing, as you know from Chapter 2), brain-cell deterioration, cancer and other conditions.[3] A study from Spain shows that when cherries are picked when ripe (but not overripe) they have twice as much vitamin C compared cherries picked at a much earlier stage, when they are still green.[4] This phenomenon appears in many other fruits too – tomatoes have fewer carotenoids, less antioxidant activity and no folate (folic acid – critical for fertility) if they are picked unripe.[5]

Added to this gloomy picture comes the impact of commercial fertilizers, which are known to reduce vitamin C, antioxidants and enzymes in plants. Further, the composition of soil and erosion of topsoil, and, in particular, the increase in carbon dioxide levels, are known to significantly reduce trace minerals, such as zinc, which are essential to fertility and vibrant good health generally.[6]

In light of all this, supplements can help give a nutritional boost – especially if your diet has been poor and you are feeling run down and depleted.

Herbs

Many modern medicines are created out of compounds in plants. The problem is that medicines have side effects, because the isolated compounds do not contain the complete package of phytonutrients (many of which are still unidentified) that balance the active ingredient in the plant. Herbs, when used in the correct doses and with common sense, rarely have side effects. This chapter will introduce you to some of the best, easily available herbs for enhancing fertility and libido, but the information given here is no substitute for the advice of a qualified herbalist, who will be able to mix you up a potion tailor-made for your own particular health, fertility and libido challenges. Please exercise great caution, however. Do not underestimate the power of herbs and, in no circumstances, exceed the stated/recommended dose.

Astralgus

Astralgus has been found to stimulate sperm motility. It is a tonic for the kidneys, which, according to principles of Chinese medicine, support reproductive health and libido. It is an energizing herb that also supports the immune system. Note that this herb should not be taken if you have a fever since it stops you sweating.

Black Cohosh

This herb has been used extensively by Native Americans as a hormone-balancing herb to help both irregular and absent periods. It normalizes the reproductive system and is a powerful relaxant. Herbalists recommend that this herb should only be taken in small amounts, so, unless you are being treated by a herbalist and can be guided by them, do not otherwise exceed the stated dose on the label.

In the United States, a vegetable herbal compound containing black cohosh, sold from 1875 by medical manufacturer Lydia Pinkham, was credited with being responsible for one third of the American population! It was known as a 'baby in every bottle'.

Blue Cohosh

The best friend of all women going into labour, since it relaxes the uterus, making for a faster, less painful delivery – something to remember in the future. Meanwhile, blue cohosh regulates menstruation and helps start periods that have stopped. It relieves cramps and other symptoms of PMT. Of course, stop taking this herb immediately if you suspect you could be pregnant, since it could stimulate a miscarriage. So, just to spell it out once more: this herb is good for getting pregnant but bad for staying pregnant.

Cordyceps (*Cordyceps sinensis*, caterpillar fungus)

This mushroom is great for improving libido and is also rumoured to have anti-ageing properties. For many years cordyceps was hard to get hold of, but now it is cultivated commercially in China. It is available in most health-food shops.

Damiana

This herb, which grows in the desert of the southwest United States and Mexico is said to enhance sexual function in both sexes. A known sexual rejuvenator, herbalists use it for increasing fertility and libido. Its Latin name, *Turnera aphrodisiaca*, suggests its helpfulness! Mexican women use it for female reproductive complaints and it has been used to strengthen the ovaries. It is also used to treat impotence, since it appears to have a testosteronelike action.

Dong Quai

A well known Chinese herb, often called the Queen of the Female Herbs, dong quai has been used for thousands of years by Chinese women as a tonic for the female reproductive system. It balances hormones and enhances fertility in women; it is also said to tone a weak uterus, regulate irregular periods, alleviate menstrual cramps, reduce spotting and restart periods that have stopped.[7] In some women it has the side effect of making their boobs bigger – you may be happy about this or you may not!

Dong quai comes from the root of the *Angelica sinensis* plant, and the name means 'compelled to return', referring to a woman returning to her normal reproductive functions.

Dong quai is said to need about three months to work, so be patient. It is readily available in health-food shops and pharmacies. One caution: dong quai, like aspirin, thins blood, so, if you are on medication to lower blood pressure or if this might otherwise be an issue for you, please consult a qualified herbalist or health-care professional before taking this herb.

False Unicorn Root (*Chamaelirium luteum*)

This herb from North America is said to balance hormones, and regularize delayed and non-existent periods. It is a good general tonic for women as it strengthens the reproductive system. Many herbalists recommend it for ovarian pain and dysfunction of the ovaries. Typically, it is given to women who have had miscarriages or uterine infections, as it can be used to prevent a threatened miscarriage. While no scientific studies on this herb exist, it has a very strong reputation among herbalists for promoting fertility and preventing miscarriage.

Green Oat/Oatstraw (*Avena sativa*)

If the reason for infertility in a man is the inability to maintain an erection, this is one of the best herbs to take, although it is not widely available.

Horny Goat Weed (*Acertanthus sagittatum* or *Epimedium sagittatum*)

This is a male aphrodisiac that also increases both sperm count and density. According to Chinese folklore, this herb was discovered in China by a goatherd who noticed his male goats became sexually aroused after eating this plant. In Chinese medicine this is regarded as the best herb for enhancing male potency.

Also known by the Chinese name Yin-Yang-Huo, Horny Goat Weed is the superstar of fertility herbs for men.

Liquorice Root

Liquorice is a useful fertility herb for women since it normalizes ovulation – particularly in women with irregular periods. Do not take liquorice if you have high blood pressure, however, since it can elevate it.

Maca

Maca is a root that grows in the high mountains of Peru – it is the strength and fertility superfood of the Andes. Maca is a natural hormonal balancer which enhances fertility in both men and women. It enhances sexual libido and is recommended for fertility problems, sterility and other sexual disorders. Maca is reputed to act on the endocrine glands, especially the ovaries and testes.

Parsley

Just adding about 1 cup of raw parsley a day to your food (in soups and salads, divided up into different meals) could be the one step needed to increase your intake of vitamins and minerals to outstanding levels. It benefits the liver, kidneys, adrenal glands and, most importantly, the uterus. However, while it is great for getting pregnant, stop taking parsley (more than an occasional sprig) once you become pregnant, since, in high levels, it can cause miscarriage. To avoid any chance of this risk, you could stick to only taking parsley in high amounts during the first half of your menstrual cycle.

Rosemary

Who would have guessed that this familiar, pleasant-smelling garden herb is great for women's fertility? It stimulates menstrual flow, eases cramps and regulates the menstrual cycle. Rosemary contains more than 240 medicinally and nutritionally active compounds and is thought to be a powerful antioxidant – even more effective than vitamin E. Start to drink fresh rosemary tea (which has quite a nice taste) by pouring boiling water over fresh sprigs of rosemary. Include the herb in many vegetable soups for a nutrient lift.

Sage

Sage has antibacterial, antifungal and antiviral effects. Sage tea is very easy to make by adding fresh sage to boiling water. Sage, of course, is a common kitchen herbal addition to soups and sauces. Like parsley, stop taking any sage the moment you know you are pregnant; it is another herb that can cause miscarriage since it is so stimulating to the uterus. To be on the safe side, drink it only during days 1–14 of your cycle.

Sage has been used as a cure for infertility since the time of the ancient Egyptians.

Sarsaparilla

Several studies have found that sarsaparilla, a herb found in Central and South America, is good for reproductive function in both men and women.

Saw Palmetto

This herb, from Texas and Florida, is also meant to enhance sexual function in men and is an excellent herb for the male reproductive system. It is a good tonic, male aphrodisiac and is traditionally used to treat impotency and prostate problems.

For women who have been told they have high levels of androgens (male hormones) or who suffer from PCOS, saw palmetto can help with acne and excess hair. Like dong quai, saw palmetto is sometimes known to increase the size of women's breasts (in case this side effect matters to you, one way or the other). While its active ingredient is still a mystery, European studies have shown that it seems to be able to counteract the effect of excess testosterone in women.

Wild Chasteberry (*Agnus castus*)

This Mediterranean herb is one of the best for women's fertility. It stimulates the function of the pituitary gland and helps in the formation and balancing of our hormones.

According to Dr Marilyn Glenville, author of *Natural Solutions to Infertility*, chasteberry regulates heavy periods, restarts periods that have stopped, controls heavy bleeding, helps with too-frequent periods, relieves painful periods, and increases the ratio of oestrogen to progesterone by balancing excess oestrogen. Dr Glenville also used this herb with older women with high levels of follicle stimulating hormone (normally a sign of approaching menopause), which meant they were not suitable for IVF treatment. Chasteberry lowered the FSH levels so the women could have IVF.[8]

The fertility of women suffering from Polycystic Ovary Syndrome will benefit greatly from taking chasteberry.

Chasteberry is a powerful herb which will probably work better than wild yam cream when used by women with a shortened menstrual cycle. One study of forty-eight infertile women who took chasteberry for three months led to seven of them becoming pregnant and a further twenty-five showing balanced normal progesterone levels, necessary for pregnancy.[9]

One disadvantage of chasteberry is that it can take three months before its beneficial effects are felt. So do not expect any dramatic or overnight changes with this herb.

One more thing: keep this herb away from your man! It puts a complete downer, literally, on male sex drive. The herb's name derives from the fact that it was taken by monks as an anti-aphrodisiac, to keep their libido under control, when their thoughts were meant to be directed towards more spiritual things. In fact some herbalists call this herb by its traditional name 'monk's pepper'.

Yohimbine/yohimbe

Yohimbine, extracted from the bark of the African yohimbe tree, is good for enhancing fertility in men. The herb has long been used in Africa as a treatment for impotency. Eighty per cent of men who have tried it for this purpose in clinical tests have found it worked for them.[10] As a hormonal stimulant, it has been found to increase testosterone levels and is thus a powerful libido enhancer in both men and women, but is best for men. Women with polycystic ovaries or any other symptoms of excess testosterone should of course NOT take yohimbine.

Minerals

Minerals are the magic ingredient in health and fertility. Tragically, as commercial farming practices deplete the soil of its minerals, nearly everyone is mineral-deficient to some degree. Arable farmers know that adding minerals to barren soil brings it back to life, and ground-up stone dust (free from most quarries) is a great soil mineralizer. Animals, too, show huge increases in fertility when they are fed minerals. In the book *Overcoming Infertility Naturally*, Karen Bradstreet describes the wonderful fertility experiments of a man called Rollin J. Anderson from Utah. First an infertile bull, whose sterility was about to cost him his life (now *that's* pressure), was saved by Anderson adding minerals to his feed; he sired a number of healthy calves. The same result occurred for a fourteen-year-old racing mare, who went on to produce several foals.

My favourite story is of Anderson taking sixteen elderly ewes from a herd about to be slaughtered because they were too old to breed, then he purchased an old 'infertile' ram. The sceptics around him wagered that they would produce at most six lambs, if any. Andersen mineralized the animals' pasture, gave the ram extra mineral supplements and sent him off to frolic and gambol with the female sheep. The following spring, these supposedly infertile animals produced thirty-one baby lambs![11]

Cute as these stories are, the main point to grasp is that there is a mountain of scientific evidence that minerals, especially the mineral zinc, will do for you what they have done for cows, horses and sheep – with no side effects and at very little expense.

Boron

Boron is an essential mineral in absorbing calcium from food and utilizing it to build bones, but it has in fact also been found to boost levels of estradiol, the metabolically active form of oestrogen. Dr Forrest Nielsen of the US Department of Agriculture believes this is caused by the boron boosting steroid hormones in the blood. Boron also assists in retaining magnesium in the body, a key mineral for achieving a successful pregnancy (see section on magnesium below).

Studies from the Human Research Center in Grand Forks, North Dakota, found that the level of oestrogen in the blood of perimenopausal and menopausal women given sufficient amounts of boron more than doubled, removing the need for HRT.

Boron is also found in fresh fruit and vegetables, especially apples, grapes, honey, nuts – particularly almonds and hazelnuts, raisins, peaches, pears, and cabbage and other leafy vegetables, which are also good sources of calcium.

Calcium

Calcium (which the mineral boron helps to be absorbed by the body) plays a role in balancing oestrogen and progesterone levels. A study conducted by Dr James Penland at the US Department of Agriculture, gave women with normal menstrual cycles either 6,000 mg or 13,000 mg of calcium a day for six months. He found that those on the lower dose had significantly more PMS symptoms – including greater mood swings, irritability, depression and anxiety – most obviously in the week before menstruation. They also had more headaches, backaches and muscle stiffness. Calcium is known to be a natural sedative.

Contrary to what the milk marketing people want you to believe, dairy products are a poor source of calcium. The best, by far, with the highest levels of absorbable calcium are sesame seeds, which taste great and can simply be sprinkled on your food like a condiment. Spinach is also great – one cup supplies a quarter of your daily calcium needs. Calcium is found in the following fertility enhancing foods: alfalfa, almonds, asparagus, brewer's yeast, broccoli, cabbage, dandelion greens, dulse, figs, flax seed, kale, kelp, leafy greens, maca, mustard greens, oats, parsley, prunes and shepherd's purse.

Chromium

Chromium plays a key role in metabolizing glucose and in stabilizing proteins in the body. Research has found that a diet low in chromium leads to a lower sperm count and decreased fertility.[12] Mothers of premature babies have been found to have low chromium levels compared with women who carry their babies to term. Research has shown chromium is needed by the developing foetus; it is also important to take enough of this mineral at the pre-conception stage.

It is estimated that 90 per cent of the population of the USA are chromium deficient. Europeans are also mostly deficient. Since chromium helps regulate insulin, a diet high in sugar and refined foods causes chromium to be lost from the body in large quantities. Fertility food sources of chromium include beans, brewer's yeast (one tablespoon gives you 380 per cent of the recommended daily amount), brown rice, corn, dulse, mushrooms, molasses and whole-grains. Chromium is also widely available as a supplement in the form of chromium picolinate.

Iron

Iron is vital for the formation of red blood cells and the transportation of oxygen around the system. Interestingly, taking iron has been shown to be helpful in boosting fertility in women. In one study, iron taken with vitamin C (which aids in the absorption of iron) helped a number of previously infertile women become pregnant, including one lady who had undergone nine years of unsuccessful fertility treatment![13] Iron also guards against miscarriage and birth defects.

Please note: an excess of iron is not a good thing, however, so do not take iron supplements unless you know you are deficient. Signs of deficiency, for instance, are because you have heavy periods, your hair has been shedding (falling out in higher amounts but re-growing) and you typically drink tea with your meals (the tannins in tea bind with a number of minerals and prevent them from being absorbed).

Fertility food sources of iron include: alfalfa, almonds, apricots avocados, beetroot, blue-green algae, brewer's yeast, chickpeas, dandelion, dulse, kidney beans, leafy greens, lentils, lima beans, parsley, peaches, pears, prunes, pumpkins, raisins and rice.

Magnesium

This is one of the minerals in which most people in Western Europe and the USA are deficient. Magnesium is involved in over 3,000 enzymatic actions in the body and is essential for optimum fertility. I call it the anti-miscarriage mineral. Without sufficient mineral levels, a pregnancy cannot be sustained. Research has also found that taking magnesium supplements while pregnant leads to a huge decrease in birth defects – a 70–90 per cent reduction.

A magnesium supplement should be taken by anyone wanting to improve their fertility.

Fertility food sources of magnesium include: alfalfa, apples, apricots, avocados, bananas, brewer's yeast, brown rice, cacoa (high cacoa content chocolate), cantaloupe, dulse, figs, garlic, grapefruit, kelp, leafy green vegetables, lemons, lima beans, nuts, parsley, peaches, sage, sesame seeds, watercress and wholegrains.

Manganese

Manganese helps in maintaining sex hormone production in men and women. A deficiency in manganese leads to defective ovulation and testicular degeneration. In cases of acute deficiency (which is rare), it causes sterility.

Manganese also appears to have an effect on menstrual flow. In a study conducted by the US Department of Agriculture, Dr Phyllis Johnson discovered that women with a diet deficient in manganese had a 50 per cent increase in volume of menstrual flow. The additional blood loss caused consequential losses of 50–100 per cent more iron, copper, zinc and manganese, all important minerals for fertility. Manganese is also an essential mineral for the healthy development of your future baby in the uterus. There is research indicating that women with low manganese levels are more likely to have a baby with birth defects.[14]

Fertility foods rich in manganese include: alfalfa, avocado, fruit (especially blueberries and pineapple), leafy green vegetables, nuts and seeds, parsley, seaweed, spinach (one cup of which will give you most of your daily requirement) and wholegrains.

MSM

MSM is a naturally occurring form of sulphur that comes from rainwater. We would normally obtain it from the residue left on fruit and vegetables that have been rained on. Clever cats and dogs go and lick dew off the grass in the morning to get their fix of MSM. Regrettably, even organically produced food is irrigated and grown in greenhouses these days and also often washed, meaning that no MSM remains. I have read that virtually 100 per cent of the population in the USA and Europe is now deficient in this mineral.

I add MSM powder (1 teaspoon per 1.5 litres) to all my water. I have been a fan of MSM since I learnt that, together with vitamin C, it makes collagen in the skin and, with sufficient quantities, you never wrinkle or scar. Vanity reasons aside, MSM is a component in the cell membranes of all your 100 trillion cells, which you need to look after in order to stay young. Having sufficient MSM will boost your health and thus your fertility on almost every level.

Apart from drinking rainwater (or licking dew in the morning!), MSM can be found in powdered form and in capsules at many health-food stores – it is usually sold as a supplement for arthritis or joint health (as it flexes up all your cell membranes, it helps these conditions too). A note: MSM in pure powder form tastes foul! When added in dilute amounts to water (max 1 teaspoon per litre), its taste cannot be detected at all; if you add too much, the water tastes very bitter.

Selenium

The mineral selenium is a key antioxidant that plays a central role in anti-ageing generally and in fertility by guarding against miscarriage and birth defects through DNA damage to sperm, ova and the developing embryo. Selenium is also essential both for sperm formation and for optimum testosterone production; one study found that a selenium supplementation programme raised fertility from 1.5 per cent to 35.1 per cent in sub-fertile men.[15] In another study sperm donors with low sperm counts were also found to have correspondingly low selenium levels.[16]

If you are a smoker, have smoked in the past, or live in an area of heavy traffic, then selenium will assist in detoxifying these toxic metals, which have been known to interfere with the development of sperm.

People living where there is a selenium-rich soil have higher birth rates than areas of lower selenium. Since our intake of selenium is, on average, 50 per cent lower than 25 years ago because of the depletion of selenium from soil, supplementation is important for both men and women to improve fertility.

Selenium can be found in fertility foods: alfalfa, avocados, brazil nuts, brewer's yeast, broccoli, brown rice, dulse, garlic, kelp, parsley, sesame seeds, spinach, sunflower seeds and wholegrains, together with any vegetables grown on selenium-rich soil.

Zinc

Zinc is the superstar of all the minerals for fertility. Domestic rabbits breed more prolifically than rabbits in the wild because they are fed more carrots, which are loaded with zinc! Zinc is important for the functioning of the reproductive organs.

For men, zinc is essential for the manufacture of healthy sperm by the testes.[17] Men lose around 9 per cent of their daily zinc intake with each ejaculation, so it is important that men have adequate zinc; supplementation is the best way to ensure this. Studies show that the low sperm count and low testosterone levels caused by a lack of zinc can be reversed when sufficient amounts of the mineral are taken.

For women, zinc is necessary to form and maintain the reproductive hormones oestrogen and progesterone.[18]

There are a number of studies that also show zinc is vital for both men and women, because it is an essential component of genetic material and a zinc deficiency can cause chromosome changes, leading to miscarriage. Without zinc, the cell division at conception cannot take place properly. For couples undergoing IVF, the fertilized egg can only be reimplanted once there has been adequate cell division, which will dependent on both the sperm and ova having adequate levels of zinc.

Zinc also assists in the absorption of folic acid, one of the most important anti-ageing vitamins in ensuring perfect cell replication in the body, and key for a developing foetus in the early stages. It is not surprising, therefore, that a deficiency in zinc means that, if one is able to conceive, there is a higher risk of miscarriage, and also of the baby being born with birth defects and poor development in the brain and nervous system.[19]

Good fertility food sources of zinc include: alfalfa, almonds, brewer's yeast, carrots, dulse, leafy greens, mushrooms, oats, pecans and pumpkin seeds. Other sources include eggs and shellfish, especially oysters (maybe this is why they are meant to be an aphrodisiac?), and sea vegetables.

Vitamins

Alpha-lipoic Acid

Alpha-lipoic acid (ALA) is one of the few antioxidants that is both fat and water soluble, meaning it can move to all parts of the cell; it even helps recycle the other antioxidants, vitamins C and E. ALA, particularly when taken with l-carnitine and co-enzyme Q10, is one of the most anti-ageing nutrients you can take. ALA is found in small amounts in spinach and broccoli and is best taken in the form of a supplement.

Vitamin A and the Carotenoids

Vitamin A and the carotenoids play an important role in reproductive gland function and are also excellent antioxidants and protective of DNA. Vegetable sources of vitamin A such as sweet potatoes, carrots and broccoli do not lead to birth defects even if consumed in high amounts, unlike vitamin A from synthetic sources found in supplements. Over 10,000 iu per day is the threshold over which the chances of birth defects might increase, so be careful! Do not exceed the dose given on the label of any supplement bottle – vitamin A can be toxic in high doses.

Fertility food sources of vitamin A and carotenoids include: alfalfa, apricots, asparagus, beet greens, broccoli, cabbage, cantaloupe, carrots, collards, dandelions, garlic, kale, papayas, peaches, pumpkin/pumpkin seeds, red peppers, spinach, spirulina, sweet potatoes, tomatoes, turnip and watercress.

B Vitamins

The B vitamins in general are important for the functioning of reproductive glands, maintaining levels of sex hormones and in supporting the nervous system in times of stress. The B vitamins seem to work best when taken together. A good B vitamin complex supplement – or, even better, a brewer's yeast supplement – is part of the fertility diet protocol. All B vitamins are water soluble and they are lost when urinating; it is, therefore, important to take B vitamins on a daily basis.

Folic Acid

You may remember from Chapter 2 that folic acid is the star nutrient when it comes to guarding quality control in your cells (i.e. keeping them young and perfect). Folic acid thus ensures the proper genetic formation of ova and sperm.

It is also now common knowledge that folic acid helps prevent neural tube defects in babies. It is critical to get enough folic acid before you get pregnant, since most defects occur in the first twenty-eight days after conception, i.e. before many women realize they are pregnant. Ideally, folic acid must have been in the body for at least a month before conception, as well as during the first three months of pregnancy.

Folic acid is essential for the production of the genetic materials DNA and RNA and works best when taken with vitamin B12.

Fertility foods containing folate/folic acid are: asparagus, barley, bran, brewer's yeast, brown rice, dates, leafy green vegetables (in particular spinach – just one cup of which gives you 50 per cent of the daily amount of folic acid), legumes, lentils, mushrooms, oranges and wholegrains.

Vitamin B12

B12 maintains fertility by working in combination with folic acid to build DNA and RNA (molecules involved in the transfer of information from DNA), and ensures cells reproduce perfectly – this is important for producing healthy sperm and ova, and for anti-ageing generally. Research has shown that vitamin B12 is very important in increasing male fertility: Men with low sperm counts who were given B12 each day showed significant increases in sperm count: 25 per cent of the men improved their sperm count by 500 per cent.

B12 is found in fertility foods: alfalfa and seaweeds such as dulse, kelp, kombu and nori. Blue-green algae is loaded with B12. Other sources of B12 are eggs and seafood.

Vitamin B6

There is now a huge amount of research proving vitamin B6 is great for healing all sorts of female fertility problems. In one study, women who had no periods because they had hormone imbalances were given the vitamin for three to four months, and some of them started to have a regular period again.[20] An even more amazing study showed that twelve out of fourteen women who had unexplained infertility and who were given B6 supplementation from 100 to 800 mcg daily for six months became pregnant – some of them had been trying for up to seven years! Progesterone levels increased in five out of the seven women whose hormone levels were measured, which may have explained why they were suddenly fertile.[21]

If you are a woman who has any kind of fertility issues, one of the first supplements you should take is vitamin B6. Birth-control pills almost completely eliminate this vitamin from the body. Deficiencies are linked to PMS, hormone imbalances, premenstrual acne and depression.

Vitamin B6 appears to be a key player in the oestrogen/progesterone balance. Usually, when oestrogen levels are found to be too high in a woman the knee-jerk reaction is to give her progesterone, rather than to question why her body is producing insufficient amounts. Without any side effects, B6 – a natural substance – can correct biochemical abnormalities caused by excess oestrogen and also balance out oestrogen-to-progesterone levels.[22]

B6 is also the hero of women who have been found to have high prolactin levels. This hormone is normally only released when a woman is breastfeeding, and inhibits ovulation. In some women this hormone is high without their ever being pregnant – thus rendering them infertile. Women who have been eating aspartame, in diet sodas, sugar-free gum or in other forms, may have high prolactin levels caused by the contraceptive effect of aspartame. The prescribed drug bromocriptine, which is meant to reduce prolactin levels, has a number of unpleasant side effects. Studies show B6 is as effective in reducing these prolactin levels but with no downside. Dr Jonathan Wright states: 'A review of the biochemistry of bromocriptine drugs shows that pyridoxine (B6) can do all the same jobs they do, and once again with fewer potential side effects.'[23] A Harvard study of women who had elevated prolactin levels, which caused their periods to stop, and who were actually lactating, demonstrated that, when given 200 to 600 mcg of B6 daily, returned to normal menstruation within three months. When the supplementation was stopped, however, all the symptoms and the infertility returned.

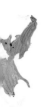

Like many other vitamins, B6 is depleted by a diet high in junk foods and sugar. Many foods contain vitamin B6, but the best fertility food sources are: alfalfa (again!), avocado, bananas, brewer's yeast (again), cabbage, cantaloupe, carrots, dulse, spinach, sunflower seeds and walnuts.

Vitamin B2

B2 – riboflavin – is helpful in preventing and improving hypothyroidism, which is linked with infertility and can be a symptom of excessive oestrogen.

Good fertility enhancing sources of B2 include: almonds, asparagus, avocados, broccoli, Brussels sprouts, dandelions, dulse, kelp, leafy greens, mushrooms, nuts and watercress.

PABA (Para Aminobenzoic Acid)

This nutrient plays a role in restoring fertility in some women, since insufficient oestrogen can be addressed by increasing intake of PABA, which is believed to stimulate the pituitary gland into producing more of this hormone. The best fertility food source is spinach.

Vitamin C

Vitamin C works like a miracle drug on sperm count, motility, viability and in preventing agglutination (the clumping up of the sperm together). Vitamin C works as well as a powerful antioxidant because it protects semen from damage caused by free radicals. Research on animals has shown that vitamin C deficiency severely harms the testes, resulting in defective sperm. Studies conducted on human beings by William A Harris of the University of Texas show that when men were given 1,000 mg of vitamin C per day for sixty days, their sperm counts soared by nearly 60 per cent, the sperm were 30 per cent more frisky and the percentage of abnormal and agglutinated sperm dropped. In fact, all of the men in this study had managed to impregnate their partner by the end of this two-month study, whereas none of the control group, who were not taking vitamin C, had managed to do so. In a further study, Dr Harris and his colleagues, Dr Earl Dawson and Leslie C. Powell, experimented with dosages and found that a higher dose of 1,000 mg worked the fastest, but a lower dose of 200 mg was just as effective, albeit over a longer period. Men who smoke or who are, or have been, exposed to toxic chemicals and pollutants should take at least 1,000 mg supplemental vitamin C every day.

A single orange, which contains 70 mg of vitamin C, could be sufficient to protect sperm from genetic damage.

One note of caution: while vitamin C is the number one sperm tonic and should be the first thing a man hoping to start or expand a family should take, women who are trying to conceive should avoid taking vitamin C in supplemental form. It is thought that high doses of vitamin C in a pill, as with an antihistamine, can dry up the precious cervical fluid needed for conception. Women should rely instead on a diet high in raw fruit and vegetables to profit from all the fantastic antioxidant and anti-ageing properties of vitamin C in its natural form, without any risk of impairing cervical fluid.

Vitamin C is found in high concentrations in berries – blueberries especially, but also strawberries and blackberries. It is important such fruit is organic, since berries can be a crop subject to very high levels of pesticides. Other good fertility food sources are: alfalfa, asparagus, avocados, beet greens, cantaloupe, dandelions, dulse, kale, kiwi fruit, onions, oranges, papayas and red peppers. Vitamin C cannot be stored in the body so it is necessary to get adequate amounts on a daily basis.

Vitamin E

Known as 'the sex vitamin', vitamin E is crucial for balanced hormone production. A powerful antioxidant that helps slow down the ageing process generally, it also helps increase sperm count. If vitamin C acts as the wonder tonic for men, then, for women, my pick would be vitamin E (and B6). Animal studies have shown that supplementation with antioxidants such as vitamins C and E and selenium in the diet reduces age-related ovulation decline to a marked degree. One study states: 'These findings may have direct implications for preventing or delaying maternal-age-associated infertility in humans.'[24] So, for older women, particularly if you are in your 40s and 50s, vitamin E and other antioxidants should be taken every day.

Men should not skip vitamin E – it has been shown to make sperm more fertile and able to penetrate the ova, and to correct sub-fertility caused by free radicals damaging sperm or interfering with sperm production in the testes.

Vitamin E is recommended for couples with unexplained infertility, since research has shown that giving vitamin E to both partners leads to a significant increase in fertility.[25]

The absolutely best way to get vitamin E into your diet is through raw sunflower seeds. Other fertility food sources of vitamin E include: alfalfa (as usual), brown rice, dulse, leafy dark-green vegetables, legumes, nuts, sesame seeds, sweet potatoes and vegetable oils (cold pressed and organic). More sources include eggs and oily fish such as tuna, sardines, mackerel and salmon.

Take sunflower seeds daily. Just one third of a cup gives you 100 per cent of the vitamin E you need and over 50 per cent of the selenium (and a whole bunch of other fabulous nutrients).

Essential Fatty Acids (EFAs)

Essential fatty acids are critical for normal glandular function and activity, especially in the reproductive system. The best sources of fertility-enhancing EFAs are as follows.

Borage Oil
Rich in omega 3 fatty acids

Choline
Improves the hormonal feedback system from brain to genitals and increases sex drive.

Evening Primrose Oil
Enhances the release of sex hormones. Since it promotes oestrogen in particular, women who know they have too much oestrogen relative to progesterone should not take evening primrose oil.

Flax Seed (Linseed)
A fertility power food. Flax seeds should be consumed daily to maximize your chances of having a baby.

Lecithin
Builds strong semen. Unless you have any inclination to eat raw egg yokes, then take lecithin granules derived from plant sources.

Fertility Action Plan

- Try to find a good herbalist in your area who can help you identify specific herbs to address any fertility issues.

- If you have not already had your vitamin and mineral levels tested, as suggested in Chapter 1's action plan, now would be a good time to find out if you have any deficiencies and to correct these through diet or supplementation.

- Make rosemary, parsley and sage your new best culinary friends (until you are pregnant – then dump the last two of them!).

- Visit the excellent website www.nutritiondata.com to find out what nutrients are in the usual foods you are eating. Supplement only those key vitamins and minerals you are deficient in.

Chapter 17
Amazing Amino Acids

At the cutting edge of nutritional research, as I write this chapter, is information not just on enzymes and glyconutrients but also on amino acids. The old schools of nutrition concerned themselves primarily with the division of food into the basic categories of carbohydrates, fat and protein; these will seem like the dietary Dark Ages when the full picture of the impact of amino acids on health, fertility and vitality is further known and can be fully appreciated.

What is clear already is that the chains of amino acids, which form proteins, are the second most-abundant substance in our bodies after water. They make up the biochemical structure of all body cells: genes, blood, tissue, muscle, enzymes, neurotransmitters and antibodies. Most importantly, for fertility purposes, they are a major constituent of hormones.

Twenty-four amino acids have been identified as necessary for the body to form more than 50,000 different proteins. The liver produces about 60 per cent of amino acids needed, and the remaining 40 per cent must be obtained from the diet from the consumption of protein-rich foods.

The amino acids that are most important for fertility are those that also enhance the secretion of growth hormone, which in turn raises the levels of all gonadal hormones and thus the sex hormones. You will remember from Chapter 3 that the pituitary does not stop producing growth hormones as we age, it just stops releasing it in such high amounts. Amino acids are the only nutrients able to increase the output of growth hormone back to its optimum, or previously youthful, levels. A brief summary of each of the most helpful amino acids follows.

Amino Acids to Increase Growth Hormone or otherwise Enhance Fertility

Arginine

The most important amino acid, together with lysine, for boosting growth hormone release. Indeed, one study found that arginine and lysine together were more effective in increasing growth-hormone release than the neurotransmitter dopamine.[1]

The head of the sperm contains a very high amount of this amino acid. If men are deprived of arginine for even just a few days, their sperm will not mature correctly.[2] Supplementing arginine increases sperm count, sperm quality and helps sperm motility.[3]

Arginine has been also used to treat impotency in men; it

has been found to increase the body's production of nitric oxide which helps penile erections.

Arginine is found in the fertility foods coconut, egg-plants/aubergine, oats, tomatoes and walnuts. It is also found in meat, dairy products and wheat.

Please note: if you suffer from the herpes virus, i.e. you have cold sores, be sure to take supplements of lysine, which balances arginine in the body, because arginine stimulates the virus.

Carnitine

While something of an impostor as an amino acid (since it is more like a vitamin B in fact), carnitine is one of my favourites: it boosts growth-hormone release and it pro-motes weight loss as well as enhancing fertility.

Carnitine is another important amino acid for men. While known more commonly for its role in assisting fat utilisation by transporting fats to the mitochondria (the power stations in each of the body's cells) for burning, it seems carnitine is also critical for the normal functioning of sperm cells. The higher the level of carnitine found in sperm cells, the better the sperm both in terms of sperm count and motility.[4] Carnitine supplements will prevent abnormal sperm being produced and will increase sperm count.[5] Carnitine has also been found to play a role in general anti-ageing. Your metabolism will improve, you will feel full of vim and vigour and your sperm will be produced in high quality, abundant amounts. Perfect for bedroom antics – go for it!

Carnitine is primarily found in meat, which is not a fertil-ity food. Supplemental forms are recommended.

GABA (Gamma Aminobutyric Acid)

GABA stimulates the release of growth hormones, but, as a natural Valium, has another side benefit of promoting feelings of calm and relaxation. It helps to stimulate sex drive. It is formed in the brain from glutamate and vita-min B6. Enzymes are key to this conversion so eating plenty of raw fruit and vegetables will help maintain optimal GABA levels, but it is widely available in supplement form. It is best taken at bedtime because of its sedative qualities.

Glutamine

Glutamine triggers the release of growth hormone and, together with the related aminos glutamic acid and GABA (see above), is involved with optimal brain function and mental activity. It is another amino acid that treats impotency. It is also very helpful in overcoming cravings for alcohol, sugar, sweets and all those ageing, high-glycaemic foods you should not be eating. Raw spinach and parsley are excellent food sources, but many foods contain it.

Glycine

Glycine is usually used in combination with arginine and ornithine in raising growth-hormone levels, although it does activate secretion of the hormone on its own. It seems to stimulate libido too. Glycine is found in brewer's yeast, pumpkin seeds, rice bran, sunflower seeds and wholegrains. It is also commonly available as a supplement.

Leucine

Leucine, isoleucine and valine are members of the branched-chain family of amino acids. They are all essential amino acids and have particular involvement with protecting muscle during times of stress and in maintaining muscle and skeletal health. They have been found to increase levels of growth hormone and are found in avocados, nuts and wheatgerm.

Lysine

Together with arginine and ornithine, lysine is one of the most important amino acids for stimulating growth-hormone release. It is also a valuable immunity booster, stimulating the secretion of thymic hormones and being a potent antiviral. It has a synergistic effect when used with arginine. As a side benefit, lysine is also very good for anyone suffering from recurring bouts of the herpes virus, such as cold sores or genital herpes, because it balances out any excess of the amino acid arginine, which can trigger an outbreak of this virus. Lysine is found in grains and beans, but the best fertility food rich in lysine is quinoa. Other food sources are eggs, dairy products, meat and potatoes.

Ornithine

Ornithine, which is not an essential amino acid, is a precursor to arginine and has many of the same benefits. One study found that taking 5–10 g on an empty stomach before sleep causes growth-hormone secretion to double overnight.[6] Ornithine also helps the immune system, regenerates the liver and is involved in maintaining and repairing skin tissue. It is derived from the breakdown of the amino acid arginine and can be found as a supplement.

Tryptophan

This amino acid, most useful for its role as a precursor to the neurotransmitter serotonin, has dual benefits for enhancing growth hormones. It not only promotes the secretion of growth hormones from the pituitary but, in addition, by relieving anxiety and stress leading to restful sleep, ensures that the powerful surge of growth hormones takes place during deep sleep. Tryptophan is found in bananas and nuts (and also chicken and turkey, which, if you are still eating these having read Chapter 4 on infertility foods, must be organic and free range of course!).

Following a contamination scandal in the late seventies in a factory in Japan producing tryptophan, this amino acid is usually only available as a supplement on a doctor's prescription. This is a great shame, since I believe it to be a totally safe and very beneficial nutrient; its only fault is to compete too well with antidepressant drugs, doing the same, but inexpensively and with no side effects. In its precursor form called 5-HTP (5-hydroxytryptophan) it is easy to find in health-food shops.

Depending on how 'wired' a personality you are, trypto-phan/5-HTP can make you feel quite snoozy. So, unless you are very on edge and need calming down, take any supplemental tryptophan/5-HTP at night.

Tyrosine

Tyrosine is the most powerful stimulant of all the amino acids. It is an essential amino acid that elevates the neurotransmitter dopamine – one factor in triggering the release of growth hormones.

The herb yohimbe (see Chapter 16) is thought to assist in impotency in men by prolonging the effects of tyrosine. This amino acid has an aphrodisiac effect. Large doses – 4 g or more – stimulate sex drive in men and women; this works apparently by increasing levels of dopamine (the pleasure, gusto and 'mojo' neurotransmitter).

Tyrosine is also one of the best stress-busting amino acids, and is therefore very helpful for overcoming all the fertility obstacles presented by stress. It is also the best one for overcoming infertility associated with hypothyroid.

A note: tyrosine also elevates blood pressure and is not recommended for anyone with hypertension, or who still drinks caffeinated beverages. It would be best to start with a lower dosage in any event, such as 400 mg in the morning and build up to 4 g. Research has found it to be safe in amounts even up to 7 g. However, when someone I know took this amount they started to have (very pleasant) day-time hallucinations. If you start to feel wired, hyper or anxious or start to get really vivid/crazy dreams at night, you are taking too high a dose.

Valine

Another essential amino acid, valine is found in large quantities (together with isoleucine and leucine) in muscle tissues. It promotes muscle strength and mass in addition to stimulating the release of growth hormone. It is found in avocados, nuts and wheatgerm.

Fertility Action Plan

- Decide what amino acids would most benefit you and start taking them as soon as possible.

- Take supplements of ornithine, arginine, lycine and glycine at bedtime to increase growth-hormone release by 20 per cent naturally as you sleep (see Chapter 3).

Part IV:
The Detox Plan

Chapter 18
Why Detox?

Insufficient sperm or ova, or low hormonal levels are caused not only by nutritional deficiency but also by too much retention of toxic wastes throughout the system, especially in the sexual glands. In the polluted world we live in, however, there is no guarantee that living in a Himalayan cave drinking only spring water and eating only organic home-grown vegetables means you will be free of toxins.

The role of the liver is not only to clean up the blood, but also, for regulating hormones, it is a key player in the bio feedback loop to the hypothalamus in the brain, which instructs the release of optimal levels of oestrogen, testosterone, FSH and prolactin. If your liver is overburdened with artificial chemicals, junk foods, saturated fats, pesticides, alcohol, cigarette smoke and caffeine (all the usual contraceptive substances), it will not be able to maintain the proper fertile hormonal balance in your bloodstream as well.

Cleaning out the accumulated toxins from a less-than-perfect diet in the past, as well as from the bombardment of chemicals from modern life, is critical to ensure that your body will be in its most optimal state for conception.

Detoxing can be a slow and steady process: simply eliminating all the obvious pollutants and fertility-robbing foods from your life will enable the organs of elimination (liver, kidneys, etc.) to catch up gradually on waste disposal. Depending how old you are, however, time may not be on your side. If you are already in your forties or older, you may have little time to lose. By far the quickest way to cleanse and rejuvenate your body is to undertake a fast.

At the Tree of Life Rejuvenation Center in Arizona in 2005, for example, Dr Gabriel Cousens conducted a one-week, green juice fasting pilot study with sixty people – all prospective parents seeking to conceive non-toxic babies. He also used a supplement of a liquid zeolite – an amazing mineral able to pull toxins and heavy metals out of the body. At the end of the study 88 per cent of the participants showed a 100 per cent reduction in heavy metals, chemicals and depleted uranium levels. For those participants who chose to continue to fast on green juices with zeolite supplementation for a second week, 100 per cent had a 100 per cent reduction in all heavy metals and toxins – yes, a 100 per cent removal rate! Since heavy metals, in particular, are so disastrous for fertility (not to mention health in general) isn't it great to know that a two-week juice fast with supplemental zeolite is likely to be sufficient to remove 100 per cent of these accumulated toxins in your body? This also means that your future babies will be very special indeed in the modern world – non-toxic babies.

'Having a non-toxic baby sounds lovely – but a fast?' I

hear you say. I suspect some people would far rather skip this chapter than skip the next meal. 'I could never fast', ' If I miss just one meal, I feel terrible', are a couple of the protests I have heard on the subject.

Until you understand the process of fasting or undertake a fast under supervision at one of the many excellent fasting centres around the world, then your fear of fasting itself will make the entire experience far worse, or even prevent you from beginning a fast in the first place.

We are like Pavlov's conditioned dogs when it comes to food – no matter whether we are really hungry or not, by the time breakfast, lunch or dinner time rolls around, we eat. The first world is plagued by the diseases of overeating, not of malnutrition.

What is fasting?

Fasting is a very ancient practice, which involves a period of abstinence from all food or just from specific foods. Fasting is nothing new. Many spiritual teachers are known to have fasted: Moses, Elijah and Jesus undertook forty-day fasts in the desert or the wilderness; in ancient Greece Plato, Aristotle and Pythagoras also fasted on water for forty days. Indeed, a forty-day fast was a requirement for any student who wished to study with Pythagoras.[1] Such varied historical figures as Zarathustra, Confucius and Leonardo da Vinci practised regular water fasting as well. In more modern times, Mahatma Gandhi fasted on numerous occasions, sometimes for as long as sixty days, to access the spiritual power and mental clarity he needed to succeed in leading India to independence from the British Empire.

Types of Fast

Water Fasting

Water fasting is a 5,000-year-old tradition, during which only pure water is consumed. No food, juices, supplements or anything other than water is taken. It is the most radical form of fasting and the one that cleans out toxins the fastest. On the other hand, it is the most intense and difficult: during the first days, as toxins flood into the bloodstream, a number of unpleasant symptoms such as headache, nausea, weakness and fatigue may be experienced. If you have never fasted before, it is better not to fast on water for longer than one day – which is manageable for anyone in reasonable health. I very strongly recommend, if you have never fasted before, that you undertake a few fresh juice fasts or the lemonade cleanse fast (see below) first before attempting a water fast.

If you are a kamikaze-type person who wants to try a water fast straightaway, then it would be easier to do so at a fasting clinic/under medical supervision, with experts on hand to advise you as to whether any detoxification symptoms are abnormal, as well as to be removed from the eating temptations or the stresses of home. The main advantages of a water fast is that it achieves the quickest detoxification and weight loss (if this is also a goal). The downside is that the organs of elimination (liver, kidneys, lungs, skin, etc.) could become overwhelmed and trigger an unpleasant healing crisis if your diet has been nutritionally empty beforehand.

Never fast on tap water. It is important to fast using the purest spring or mineral water you can find. Distilled water can also assist in the detox process since it is able to pull toxins out of the cells by absorbing and suspending them for elimination.

'Sole' (Salt Water) Fasting

As a variation on the traditional water fast, you could try a 'sole' fast of water saturated with Himalayan Crystal Salt. This miracle salt contains all natural minerals and trace elements, as described in Chapter 13. It is possible to water fast by adding one or two teaspoons of the sole solution to your spring/mineral/distilled water once or twice per day. This gives the body a mineral infusion, replaces electrolytes and balances energy. The sole solution helps the body to get rid of heavy metals such as lead, mercury, arsenic and excess calcium, since the crystal salt is able to breakdown their molecular structures.

Juice Fasting

Juice fasting involves taking only fresh pressed fruit or vegetable juices, preferably organic, and/or an organic vegetable broth. Packaged and tinned juices are not suitable for juice fasts: they are often little more than sugar water and are invariably pasteurized, meaning that all the enzymes have been killed off and many nutrients are depleted.

Juice fasting is recommended if you have never fasted before and is the perfect stepping stone to water fasting. The detox process is slower and less intense than that experienced on a water fast. Since a certain amount of calories are provided through the juice, there is not the same sense of weakness, and it is possible to continue your usual daily activities and even go to work, if you must.

Many people are also nutritionally depleted, so to begin a water fast from a nutritionally bankrupt state is not a good idea. The fresh juices consumed during a juice fast supply all the nutrients the body needs (living enzymes, vitamins, minerals, antioxidants and phytochemicals) and, thus, provide energy for the detox process. Juice fasting for a long weekend – three or four days – would not present a problem for anyone in reasonable health. If you want to undertake a longer juice fast then it would be helpful to do so at a fasting centre/health farm/spa or under the supervision of a medical doctor who is familiar with the fasting process.

The Lemonade Cleanse or ' The Master Cleanse'

The Lemonade Cleanse fast is one of my favourites. It consists of drinking a mixture of freshly squeezed lemon juice and water, to which small amounts of maple syrup and cayenne pepper have been added. The exact recipe is: juice of 1 lemon, 1 tablespoon of organic maple syrup (the darker the better), a small pinch (⅛ teaspoon) of cayenne pepper to 500 ml/8 oz of pure water. You can prepare the lemonade with either hot water or chilled water depending on the climate you live in/your preferences. At least two litres of lemonade should be consumed each day. Stanley Burroughs, who developed this cleanse, also recommends clearing the colon with a salt-water flush (see Chapter 19 on colon cleansing).

What Happens During a Fast?

I want to reassure you if you have never fasted before: the moment you stop eating, your body knows *exactly* what to do. During the first day of a fast the body will still be powered by glucose from food from the previous meal, as well as the immediate backup supplies of glucose, stored by the liver in the form of glycogen. There is usually enough of this excess sugar to keep the body going for 8–12 hours, but, within 24 hours, it is usually depleted. If you try a one-day fast, you will feel hungry, particularly around your usual mealtimes, but will not experience any other untoward symptoms.

After the first day, with all the glucose stores gone, the body switches over to its alternate fuel source – fat. This process called ketosis occurs on fasting days two to three, when an enzyme called lipase, which is present in fat cells, is activated by the liver and starts to convert fat to a useable fuel source: ketones/ketone bodies. These days are usually by far the hardest for anyone fasting. In some ways it is a pity to fast for less than four days, because the first three days are always the worst, as the body changes to fat burning and throws out huge amounts of toxins.

By day four, when the body is using ketones/fat-burning for energy, amazingly you do not even feel hungry – although you may still have food cravings.

As a veteran faster I am very familiar with this pattern: day one – OK, very hungry. Days two and three – feel like hell, awful, dying to eat something. Day four – awake feeling refreshed and reborn, having lost about 10 lb in weight already. Days four to seven, or longer, are never as bad as the first two days; just increasing feelings of lightness, of gentleness. The worst aspect, in my opinion, is boredom. It is boring not to eat, not to shop for food, not to cook, etc. (Of course, it is never boring not to have to do the cleaning up after eating!)

The difference between Ketosis and Ketoacidosis
Ketosis – fat burning and the release of ketones – is not the same as ketoacidosis, a serious condition found in Type I

diabetics, alcoholics, and those on the meat- and dairy-laden Atkins Diet!

Ketoacidosis occurs when the concentrations of ketones rise to abnormally high levels and, unlike ketosis, is not part of normal body functioning. With ketoacidosis, the levels of circulating ketones are too high for the body to maintain its delicate pH balance, and for the kidneys to excrete sufficient ammonia in the urine to balance that acid levels in the blood.

With ketosis from fasting, on the other hand, the body functions optimally. Indeed, some studies suggest that ketones might be the body's preferred fuel. Research has shown that ketones stimulate the heart, adrenal glands, skeletal musculature and brain to better functioning than glucose. Indeed, periods of fasting appear to have long-term beneficial effects on the brain, central nervous system and, most importantly, the endocrine system[2] (see the section below on fasting and rejuvenescence). Also, interestingly, babies spend the first few months of their lives in a state of ketosis, since breast milk has a relatively low carbohydrate but high fat content, so ketones are the primary energy source – the body's first fuel.

To me, one of the most amazing aspects of fasting is that, not only does not eating trigger the body to consume into its own stored fat, but also by a process called 'autolysis' the body begins to break down all diseased, dying and dead cells, mucus, tumours (including uterine fibroids), arterial plaque and toxic residues. The astonishing healing and youthing effects of fasting derive from the fact that it causes the body to cleanse itself of everything it does not need, yet leaves all the organs, muscle and vital lean tissue unscathed. This is called 'protein sparing' – the miraculous process by which the body preserves all healthy tissue while consuming and eliminating all accumulated fertility and health impairing detritus.

Dr Buchinger, founder of a world-famous fasting clinic in Germany, describes fasting as 'the burning of rubbish'.[3]

The Difference between Fasting and Starvation

Starvation occurs when there are no more reserves of fat, or superfluous tissues and unwanted molecules (bacteria, viruses, fibroid tumours, toxins, etc.) and the body is, as a last resort, forced to burn protein (stored in muscle and organs) for fuel. This is why anorexics die of heart failure – they have reached a point of such complete emaciation that the body turns to heart muscle (or protein from other essential organs) for fuel.

Most people, even slim people, could safely fast on water for 40 days, or on juice for 100 days, before the body will turn to its protein reserves. One pound of fat is the equivalent of 3,500 calories. If you have even 10 lb of spare fat on your body it is equivalent to 35,000 calories – plenty to live on for quite a while. According to A.J. Carlson, a Professor of Physiology at the University of Chicago, a healthy, well-nourished man can live from fifty to seventy-five days without food, provided he is not exposed to severe stress or harsh weather.[4] Other fasting specialists, such as Paavo Airola, state that a healthy, normal weight person can safely fast on water for up to forty days. The research from those who have undergone ultra-long water fasts (from sixty to one hundred and twenty days) under strict medical supervision, of course, shows that hunger diminishes after three days, then sharply returns, to a degree that is unmistakable, just as the body has used up its excess fuel reserves and is about to have to use essential protein. But these are very extreme examples. Unless you are very significantly underweight (in which case this too will be impairing your fertility), you can undertake a one- or two-week water or juice fast with no concern that you will be starving, literally.

Fasting and Rejuvenescence

My own particular fascination with fasting, having experienced a number of fasts of seven to ten days and one long forty-day fast (twenty-three days on water and seventeen on juice), is in its ability to turn back the clock, turbocharge the body, boost fertility and leave the faster looking and feeling more youthful and vibrantly alive.

One theory of the rejuvenating effect of fasting and of very low-calorie diets is based on the free radical theory of ageing. With fewer calories and less digestion, fewer free radicals are produced as the inevitable by-products of normal cell oxidation. In turn, this diminishes the risk of cell damage caused by oxidation.

While I have no doubt that the greater metabolic efficiency of fasting and the reduction of free radicals plays a role in the youthing effect, I find the research in the area of human growth hormone and insulin even more compelling in providing some answers as to why fasting may be nature's own best fertility treatment. It has now been discovered that fasting is one of the most potent inducers of growth hormone, and, as you learned earlier, growth hormone is one of the master hormones for boosting sexual function.

Of course, when you fast you will lose weight quickly. The loss of fat is another factor in the stimulation of growth hormone release by the pituitary and a corresponding rise in reproductive hormones.

So, to remain young, slim and fertile well into your forties, or even fifties, fasting on water or juice for a week to two weeks at a time, a couple of times a year is vitally important.

The Healing Crisis and Detoxification Symptoms

The first few days of any fast are likely to produce some uncomfortable detoxification symptoms. Fasting allows the body a breathing space. A chance to catch up on its own internal housekeeping: the organs of elimination are stimulated and metabolic enzymes, which would otherwise be used in the digestion of food, are redeployed by the body in the clearing out of accumulated wastes, toxins and debris. A water fast triggers a more intense detoxification than a juice fast or lemonade cleanse fast, and so may cause more unpleasant symptoms.

It is quite normal to experience any of the following symptoms during a fast, in particular in the first few days when toxins, previously stored in fat cells (the body's poison storage depot), flood into the bloodstream.

1. Headaches: major league headaches are common if you have consumed a lot of caffeine before the fast. Do not take any aspirin or painkilling medication. Drink plenty of water. If the pain becomes insufferable, take a magnesium supplement.

2. Other aches and pains, such as backache: hot or cold packs, or soaking in a long hot bath can help.

3. Fatigue: particularly if you are water fasting, you may feel very tired. It is important to rest as much as possible to facilitate the detoxification and healing processes under way in the body.

4. Weakness: this symptom will be more intense in a water fast than a juice fast. Try to rest as much as possible, and do not attempt any exercise, beyond very gently walking or stretching (if you feel up to it).

5. Dizziness: sometimes this is caused by dehydration – make sure you are drinking enough – or this can just be a sign of the fast lowering blood pressure. It is important to stand up very slowly from a lying or sitting position while fasting.

6. Chills/cold extremities: especially when fasting during the winter – wrap up warm and keep a hot-water bottle with you.

7. Nausea and vomiting: I always seem to get this once during a seven or more-day fast, but feel much better afterwards. This shows the body is in toxic-clearing overload, and can be alleviated by an enema or preferably a colonic irrigation treatment.

8. Coated tongue and halitosis (bad breath): you can bank on this symptom. Use a tongue scraper to remove a lardlike substance every morning. Clean your teeth at least twice per day, and brush the tongue, if you do not have a tongue scraper.

9. Dark urine with a strong odour: your kidneys will be working overtime to eliminate toxins; it is important to flush them out with plenty of water.

10. Strong body odour: it is important to bathe or shower twice a day. Also, to skin brush in order to allow the skin, the body's largest organ of elimination, to do its work; use only warm not hot water.

11. Acne: as part of the detoxification process, you make break out in pimples, like being a teenager all over again.

12. Sleep disturbances: in fasts of longer than three days, you may start to find your sleep patterns upset. You may experience insomnia, but be tired during the day. If the lack of night-time sleep is starting to bother you a lot, then you could take a supplement of melatonin – about 3 mg should be sufficient – one hour before your usual bed-time.

13. Emotional detox: many of us suppress our emotions with food, or we overeat for reasons other than hunger. During a fast, whatever feelings you have been numbing with food will present themselves with unmitigated intensity. There is a theory that, whatever emotion you were blocking out with food, will surface as the fat which represented that food is broken down and released.

14. Food cravings and fantasies: although feelings of actual hunger disappear by day three of the fast, unfortunately, cravings for different foods do not. During every fast I have ever undertaken, I have been tormented by images of different foods – sometimes things I have not even eaten in years.

I have a number of tips to alleviate any healing crises while fasting: drink plenty of water, rest, keep warm, go for a stroll in the fresh air or sit outside and sunbathe if the weather permits, and use a dry skin-brushing technique every day to help both the lymph and the skin.

Keeping the bowels moving is also certain to bring relief from any symptoms. The next chapter is dedicated to colon cleansing, so please read the detailed advice set out there. While fasting I recommend in particular aloe vera, the 'salt water flush', enemas and colonics if you are water fasting. In addition, prune juice could be taken by those on juice fasts. It is important to keep emptying the bowels while fasting, since they are of course the sewer of the body and will be having to deal with a higher than normal toxic load. At a

Natural Hygienist water-fasting clinic, which was opposed to colon cleansing (wrongly, in my opinion), I have witnessed at first hand the worrying results of auto-intoxication – when the filthy wastes accumulating in the colon start to be reabsorbed back into the body while fasting. It is my own personal experience that colon cleansing makes fasting easy, comfortable and pleasant.

Breaking a Fast

There is a saying that any fool can fast, but it takes a wise man to know how to eat again. After a fast, appetite returns strongly, and you may be tempted to rush out to eat any foods you have been craving: do not do so! Not only will you undo all the good work of fasting, it could actually be dangerous. In the hundreds of thousands of accounts of safe fasting in the literature, there are two instances of deaths by men gorging themselves on excessive food after prolonged water fasts (more than twenty days) and dying from this. The conventional wisdom suggests taking one day for every day you have fasted to come out of a fast. If you have fasted on water for four days, it would be wise to then fast on juice for two, then raw fruit and vegetables for two. If you have fasted on juice for six days, come out of your fast on raw fruit and salad for six days, and so on.

After fasting, the palate is incredibly clean, and, if your fast has lasted longer than seven days, your body will have removed a number of toxins too. This is a great opportunity to find out what food intolerances you might have, since the body will now react more strongly to anything it does not like. So, after you have had a few days on juice/raw fruit and vegetables, try eating bread or dairy and see what happens. Fasting, when practised wisely, offers you the opportunity to use it as a springboard to a whole new, better way of eating afterwards, one that will improve your chances of conceiving. Do not miss this chance, or throw away all the effort you have made to fast by reverting instantly back to your pre-fast diet.

Fertility Action Plan

- Reduce the liver's toxic load by discarding all household clean-ing and beauty products made from artificial chemicals – choose natural ones instead.

  If you have not done so already, eliminate toxic food and drink from your diet: non-organic foods, caffeine, alcohol, junk foods.

- Go on! Try a weekend/three-day fresh organic juice fast at home.

- Book a mini-break or week at a health farm/fasting clinic or spa and try a juice fast there, with pampering and support.

Chapter 19

Colon Cleansing and Colonic Irrigation

In our society, everything to do with the excretion process is off-limits for discussion. Yes, poo is taboo. Now, while I am happy about this when it comes to dinner-table conversations, it is a pity that more information about what constitutes a healthy colon and 'normal bowel movements' is not more openly communicated. The intestines provide four essential foundations to health and thus fertility:

- They are the first line of defence for the immune system when properly populated by 'friendly flora' bacteria
- They are where nutrients from food are absorbed into the bloodstream
- They produce hormones which feed back to the brain on the nutritional and emotional status of the body – you literally have 'gut feelings'
- They are, of course, the key organ of excretion, the sewer of the body, from where wastes and fertility-impairing toxins are eliminated

Colon Health and Fertility

As you know, the central hypothesis of this book is that fertility is a manifestation of radiant good health. If you have a sluggish or constipated colon, by permitting highly toxic faecal matter to be retained and reabsorbed into the bloodstream and, thus, into the neighbouring reproductive organs, you are creating an internal polluted environment that your body will register is an unsuitable one either for the gestation of a baby, or for the manufacture of healthy sperm respectively. Daniel Reid in his book *The Tao of Health, Sex and Longevity* records his experience treating couples with a background of ten to fifteen years' infertility, who were able to conceive after three to five seven-day fasts (see Chapter 19 on fasting) with daily colonic irrigations (which I shall describe later), followed by proper nutritional therapy.

Infertility can actually be caused by a collapsed colon, which puts excess pressure on the prostate gland in men, preventing the free flow of sperm, and on the Fallopian tubes in women, preventing the release of ova.

The Healthy Colon

So what is normal when it comes to colon functioning? To start with, having three bowel movements per day. Yes, each day. Look at babies, small children, and even your family pets: when healthy, they pass faeces easily and quickly, within half an hour of each meal. There are anecdotes of patients telling doctors they have 'regular bowel movements' and then it transpiring that they mean regularly once a week! To put it simply, unless you are pooing at least once per day, you are constipated. In a very healthy colon, you will be having a bowel movement after every single meal. If you are going entire days without a bathroom visit, you are seriously constipated and toxic wastes will be festering in your system, damaging both your fertility and your health in general.

The Scoop on Poop

The quality of your excrement is also informative: the ideal stool is a 'floater', which shows there is adequate fibre in the diet. If you look in the toilet bowl and see only 'sinkers', your faeces are too compact and without enough fibre. Another factoid while I am on this unsavoury subject. Faeces that leave 'skid marks' are a sign that there is too much sugar in the diet. If your poo is 'skinny' it also suggests the colon is lined with mucus or faecal matter. The ideal stool will be 'fat', i.e. at least 3-4 cm/2 in wide and long – yes, at least as long as 30 cm/12 in or longer – really! It will also be soft, breaking up easily in the toilet bowl and, as I said before, floating. If you are not used to inspecting the quality of your doo-doo, I seriously suggest you start looking, and notice what changes any alteration in diet brings. One other thing. If, after you have been to the bathroom, it is un-usable by anyone else (at least not without gas masks and oxygen tanks) then you certainly have internal toxicity, with far too much putrefying material in your colon.

Transit Time

The time between the consumption of a food and its elimination from the body is known as the transit time. Opinion varies on what constitutes a healthy transit time; I have read accounts from which between eight and twenty-four hours is normal.

Different foods are digested at different rates: fruit being the fastest through the system and shellfish the slowest. Your overall 'transit time' can impact on your fertility.

It is good to have an idea of your transit time, since it is possible to be going to the bathroom regularly, i.e. a couple of times a day, and yet still be constipated. There is a very easy test you can perform at home to find out. At one meal, eat a *lot* of sweetcorn and try to swallow the kernels whole, hardly chewing. Do not eat any sweetcorn again for at least two weeks. Now, start to pay attention to when the sweetcorn begins to come out the other end. Even more important, is to note when sweetcorn *stops* appearing in your faeces. This is the true measure of your transit time. The first sweetcorn could appear in the toilet after only a few hours, but, if it is still appearing a week or more later (and you have followed the test correctly and eaten no more sweetcorn), then you know you have a certain amount of congestion.

Colonic Crisis

If you would like to lose around 10 lb in weight effortlessly with no dieting and have the flattest stomach you have had in years – my top tip is to have a series of colonic irrigation treatments.

A poor diet of refined, processed, low-fibre foods and animal fats, and a lack of exercise, are the main reasons why many people's colons are not in great shape. Apart from constipation or diarrhoea, if you suffer from bad breath, body odour, bloating, gas, skin problems, headaches and backache – then it is likely your colon is clogged up. I can also tell who suffers from constipation by the presence of reading material in the bathroom. If there is a well-stocked library and the equivalent of Tolstoy's *War and Peace* has to be read before the bowels can evacuate, then the colon is definitely sluggish.

Hormones and the Intestines

Hormones also affect bowel movements. In the second half of the menstrual cycle, after ovulation and when progesterone is dominant, all women will find their bowel movements slow down/become less frequent. This is the body's way of trying to ensure that every nutrient possible is absorbed from food by slowing down its passage through the gut in preparation for a possible pregnancy. During this time of the month, I recommend an increase in the naturally laxative foods (see below) to keep the bowels moving. Both men and women who are hypothyroid will have a tendency to become constipated. Please see Chapter 32 on thyroid, and also follow the dietary recommendations set out there if you suspect that this could apply to you.

The intestines actually release hormones and feedback to the brain on the nutritional status of the body as well as on the emotions. Congested colons will be putting distress calls into the endocrine system, which will not help your chances of conceiving.

Natural Laxatives

The following foods and supplements can help encourage a natural bowel movement and support good intestinal health.

Water

One of the main causes of constipation is dehydration. Without sufficient water, the faeces become compacted and their passage through the gut is slowed. Drinking warm water (with a little fresh lemon juice) first thing in the morning is a good way to stimulate the bowels. If you are prone to constipation, the first thing you should do is massively increase your water intake. The body needs 1 oz of water for every 2 lb/1 kg of body weight. So if you weigh 160 lb (11 stone 6 lb) you should be drinking 80 oz of water – that's ten half-pint glasses. Do not drink any tap water, however. Most municipal tap waters have chlorine in them, which kills the helpful intestinal bacteria that are necessary for proper digestion of food and for good immunity, so either use some method of water filtration of the water you drink and use for cooking, or drink bottled mineral or spring water.

Almond Oil

Almond oil is high in essential fatty acids and magnesium and is another safe mild laxative. You can make up a salad dressing using almond oil, which is available in health stores and in speciality delicatessens, or, if you don't mind the taste of pure oil, simply take a spoonful straight.

Aloe Vera

Aloe vera is my number one recommendation as a laxative. The best way to take it is to find it fresh if you can – this is more of a problem if you live in a cooler climate – then cut open an aloe vera leaf and take out the jelly. Eat it directly or blend it into a smoothie with fresh fruit. Aloe vera juice is also widely available in health stores. I will be honest, it tastes very bitter taken fresh – I do not care for the taste at all – but it is fantastic for your bowels and health in general. Aloe vera can also be purchased in capsules, but please check that it has not had the aloin removed, since this is the laxative agent! As an added benefit, aloe vera contains eighteen amino acids, vitamins, minerals and other beneficial phytochemicals. It is known to be anti-inflammatory, antibacterial, immune stimulating and helpful to repair tissues generally.

Vitamin C

In nutritional literature there is often mention that vitamin C should be taken to 'bowel tolerance levels', i.e. the point at which it causes diarrhoea. For most people, this point will be reached with about two to four grams – that's between four and eight 500 mg capsules. Since vitamin C is such a wonder tonic for sperm, taking high amounts is ideal for any man who also wishes to improve his bowel regularity. For women trying to conceive, however, I do not recommend vitamin C in supplement form, since this can cause cervical mucus to dry out; instead it is better to get your vitamin C from high amounts of fresh fruit and berries, which are generally great for fertility as well.

Cacao/Dark Chocolate

In case you have ever wondered where the expression 'Montezuma's revenge' comes from, it is to do with the laxative side effect of consuming high amounts of that most popular of Aztec foods – cacao or chocolate. The Emperor Montezuma was observed by the conquistadors to consume some 50 cups of a cacao drink before visiting his harem of over 300 women. When the conquistadors themselves tried this 'Aztec Viagra' in high amounts they found themselves running to the nearest medieval 'bathroom'. Cacao contains very high levels of magnesium, which is a powerful muscle relaxant and alleviates abdominal cramping. But do not be rushing out to eat regular chocolate bars – only dark chocolate with a cacao content of over 70 per cent will be beneficial. Even better is to take raw cacao powder and make some superfood smoothies (see Recipes and Resources). Of course, cacao is a also powerful aphrodisiac; on the other hand, it does contain some caffeine, so moderation is the answer.

Digestive Enzymes

For anyone who suffers with intestinal upset – gas, bloating, constipation, diarrhoea or abdominal cramping – I recommend taking digestive enzymes with every meal. I suggest this anyway whenever cooked food is being consumed, since the natural enzymes in the food will have been destroyed by the cooking process. Digestive enzymes break down food completely making it very easily absorbed, digested and subsequently eliminated. Everyone I know who has bowel trouble, including someone I helped who had colon cancer, found tremendous relief and an improvement in their symptoms by taking digestive enzymes with every meal, whether cooked or not.

Flax Seeds (Linseed)

Flax seeds are wonderful for your intestines. The natural oils are very soothing to the lining of the intestines. It is also loaded with fibre. An amount of 50 g/3 tbsp of flax has approximately 20 g of fibre – that is three times that of beans, and four times that of wholegrain rice. You will be amazed at what it will do for your faecal bulk! Flax is also one of the richest sources of omega 3 essential fatty acids, which are needed by the body for energy production to maintain cell membranes and for optimal hormonal balance.

If there is one food to add to your diet for your fertility and health in general, then flax would be at the top of the list. I take it every day. I put about two to three tablespoons in little glass jars and top them up with mineral water. I store them in the fridge; overnight, the flax seeds soak up the water and developed a soft gel covering. I then spoon this superfood into fruit smoothies or stir into oatmeal. You can also grind up dry seeds and sprinkle them on top of cereal or salads or put them in smoothies.

Please note: if you are taking flax seeds, it is important to drink plenty of water to assist the fibre in its passage through the gut.

High-fibre Foods

When large amounts of fibre are eaten, the stools become bulkier, which, in turn, causes pressure on the colon wall, triggering the muscle contractions that herald 'the urge'. Good sources of fibre include flax seeds, psyllium seeds or husks (but take plenty of water at the same time), wholegrains, especially oat and wheat bran, and all fruits and vegetables. Raw fruit and vegetables have more fibre than when they are cooked.

Magnesium

As mentioned in the section about cacao, magnesium is a powerful muscle relaxant; it is, therefore, helpful as a mild laxative. In fact, magnesium is the key ingredient in the medicine 'milk of magnesia', which you might have been given as a laxative as a child. I would recommend the food and supplement choices mentioned in this chapter before any medication for constipation, but milk of magnesia is probably one of the better, gentler, over-the-counter remedies.

Probiotics

The typical European and North American diet is so loaded with sugar and yeast (from bread products and alcohol) that the balance of the healthy bacteria, a.k.a. 'friendly flora', in the intestines is often upset. A good probiotic (bacteria) environment is needed for the proper digestion of food and for good elimination. The bacteria in our intestines release chemicals that are essential for our health – such as vitamin B12. You may not know that the appendix is the body's B12-manufacturing zone; it is not just a useless appendage that can be amputated with impunity. If all the bacteria in our gut were killed off, we would not survive.

Everyone can benefit from a course in probiotics. Look for acidophilus and bifidus in your health-food shop. Food sources of good bacteria include organic natural yogurt (look for the words 'live culture' on the pot), fermented foods like sauerkraut and the drinks kambucha (fermented tea) and rejuvelac (made from fermented grains, usually wheat berries).

Prune Juice

Prune juice is a well-known, safe and mild laxative. It is also one of the least expensive. Prune juice contains a compound called dihydrophenylisatin, which is a natural colon stimulant. Prunes also contain high amounts of iron and are helpful if you are anaemic or low on iron (quite common among menstruating women who do not eat red meat). Prune juice can also be frozen into an ice lolly and eaten this way.

Salted Water

Before I describe how to undertake the salt water flush, I must warn you it is one of the most powerful and dramatic colon-cleansing techniques I know, so it is not recommended unless you have one to three hours to stay at home to be close to a toilet, since you may need to visit it several times.

Add two level teaspoons of uniodized sea salt (this technique does not work as well with iodized salt) to a litre of lukewarm water, and drink the whole litre first thing in the morning on an empty stomach. No, it does not taste good; it is like drinking sea water. According to Stanley Burroughs, author of *The Master Cleanser*,[1] the salt and water at this level of dilution will not separate, and will quickly and thoroughly wash the entire digestive tract in an hour or so. This is apparently because the salt water has the same consistency as blood and, thus, the kidneys cannot absorb the water and the blood cannot pick up the salt. Whatever the reason, having tried it a couple of times myself, I can say it works very effectively indeed!

Triphala

You may not have heard of this herbal remedy, which comes from the Ayurvedic tradition from India. A combination of three fruits (harada, amla and bihara), triphala is not only an effective laxative, but also functions as a blood and liver cleanser. It helps regulate bowel movements generally while at the same time it improves digestion, lowers cholesterol, improves circulation and liver function, reduces high blood pressure and has been found to be anti-inflammatory and antiviral. According to very recent research, it has cancer-treating properties too.[2]

Triphala powder is often available in Indian import shops in larger cities, and sometimes in health-food stores. There are a number of online sources by simply searching under 'triphala'.

Xylitol Water

Another very effective colon cleanser is xylitol sugar taken in moderately high quantities – such as 2 tablespoons dissolved in an 8 oz cup of hot water. I recommend xylitol as a sugar at various places in this book. It is a very low-glycaemic sugar (it only figures at 7 on the glycaemic index, compared with normal sucrose/table sugar which is 100), and is high in minerals, derived from birch trees and other fruits. Xylitol is also antibiotic and, in particular, inhibits the growth of bacterial plaque in the mouth. If you follow my general suggestion for your health – of replacing table sugar with xylitol – you may notice some improvement in the ease of your eliminations. To use as a laxative, however, xylitol needs to be taken in more concentrated amounts. When hot xylitol water is consumed on an empty stomach it will produce a number of eliminations in about a two-hour period. This is another beverage to consume in close proximity to a toilet.

Other Foods that Support Colon Health

Other foods, while not being strictly laxative, soften stools and help them to pass through the intestines. These are: almonds, apples (a combination apple and pear juice is very good), chicory, dates, endive, figs, grapes, mangos, papaya, pineapple and rutabagas.

Herbal Laxatives

Other plant-derived laxatives include cascara sagrada bark and senna pods. These are purgatives that contain a compound called anthroquinones which stimulates the peristaltic action of the colon. They are affective and safe for short-term use, but, if taken regularly, could irritate the colon, so are best kept for 'emergency use only' if all the other suggestions in this chapter have failed.

Another Reason to Abandon Tea and Coffee

Both coffee and tea are diuretics, i.e. they trigger water loss from the body. This in turn leads to dehydration and constipation. But tea has another strike against it: the tannins in tea help to bind stools and hold back bowel movements – it is even a treatment for diarrhoea. If you remember Chapter 5 on barren beverages, you will recall that caffeinated beverages are also an effective contraceptive. If you have had problems with constipation in the past, you have another motivation to give up tea.

Enemas and Colonic Irrigation

Colon hydrotherapy in various forms is nothing new. Even the Egyptians were great fans of the enema. Despite its ancient pedigree, however, most people are repelled by the idea of both enemas and, in particular, colonic irrigation. 'I'm not having a hosepipe stuck up my bum and five gallons of water poured into it,' said my cousin, when, somehow, this malodorous topic of conversation came up one day.

For those who have never had a colonic, the idea does sound distasteful – both sordid and embarrassing, if not painful – when, in fact, if administered by a skilled practitioner it is none of these things. The International Association for Colon Therapists (headquartered in San Antonio, Texas) describes colon hydrotherapy as: 'a safe effective method of removing waste from the large intestine, without the use of drugs. By introducing pure, filtered and temperature-regulated water into the colon, human waste is softened and loosened, resulting in evacuation through natural peristalsis.'[3]

You wear a hospital-type gown, vented at the back. The only embarrassing bit is exposing your bare backside to the gloved therapist (who will have seen hundreds of bums), who will gently insert a sterile speculum (with lubrication) into your anus. You then move gently on to your back and try to relax. There is normally a towel or sheet covering you as well. Most colon therapists will massage your abdomen over the fabric. They control water pressure, as purified water (up to five gallons) at an ambient body temperature is allowed to gently trickle into your colon. Dials on the machine register pressure and, when pressure builds up, the therapist will switch to the release valve. Although you might be convinced you are about to push out the speculum and deposit a big turd on the table, to your relief all the waste somehow pours safely through the tube and into a clear viewing tube of the colonic machine, before going down the pipes to the sewer.

Afterwards you feel fantastic, light and glowing. Your friends will demand to know why you are so radiant and your skin is looking so fantastic. Vanity aside, if you have been having trouble conceiving, a series of colonics, together with a radical detoxification programme, should be one of your first priorities. Colonic irrigation massively accelerates detoxification, allowing a huge amount of toxins and congested faecal matter to be flushed out rapidly. Colon hydrotherapy removes encrusted mucus from the wall of the intestines. A build-up of mucus feeds parasites, poisons the system and, in particular, prevents nutrients from being properly absorbed into the bloodstream. If you think of the intestines as the sewer of the body, it is obvious that, if the sewer is blocked up, then the 'drains', i.e. the lymph, kidneys and the liver, will be unable to get rid of accumulating waste. A clear colon allows the liver, lymph and kidneys to dump their toxins for excretion.

Colonic irrigation is a very effective cure for long-term chronic constipation, since it actually tones the bowel, and helps it to resume normal functioning.

Those who are opposed to colonic irrigation as an 'unnatural practice', such as those who vehemently adhere to the Natural Hygiene system of health, say that colonic hydrotherapy robs the colon of its friendly flora bacteria. To this criticism I would reply that the good bacteria in the gut need a clean environment; if they are overwhelmed by toxicity and parasites, which are typical in a congested colon, they will not be flourishing. In any event, as mentioned in the probiotics paragraph above, if this remains a concern, a good probiotic supplement will soon repopulate the intestines with all the healthy bacteria they need for optimal health and fertility.

Fertility Action Plan

- Start to monitor your bowel movements – both quantity and quality.

- Unless you are having daily eliminations, start to introduce laxative foods into your diet every day.

- Be adventurous – try colonic irrigation!

Chapter 20

Dental Health and Fertility

So what do teeth have to do with fertility, apart from the obvious fact that no one would want to kiss or go to bed with someone with horrible halitosis? You would be astonished to learn of the major impact of gum disease (also called periodontal disease or gingivitis) on your immune system and health in general. By now, you know the whole premise of this book: fertility and libido are a by-product of abundant good health. If your immune system is under par and fighting bacterial invasion in your mouth, your body will be saying, 'No, now is not a good time to have a baby; we are barely keeping things going around here.'

The older you are, the more this could be an issue: research suggests that 75 per cent of adults aged over 35 worldwide have gum disease. More relevantly, research now shows that gum disease can affect the health of pregnant women and their unborn babies. According to scientists at the University of Chile, women with gingivitis had an increased risk of delivering premature or low birthweight babies. It seems that the bacteria that cause gum disease also contribute to an inflammatory response of the placental membrane, which can lead to pre-term labour.[1] While there is no research presently available to prove a link between periodontal disease and impaired fertility specifically, it seems logical to me that any condition in the body that is known to harm your health generally and which has, in particular, been found to be harmful to pregnant women and foetuses, is certain to adversely affect your chances of conceiving. In the genetic race for survival of the fittest, a bacteria-infested environment, suppressed immunity and the likelihood of inflammation in the placenta, self-evidently would not add up to a safe bet for reproduction.

The following sections describe both lifestyle and nutritional solutions for preventing and treating gum disease.

Lifestyle Solutions

Fortunately, gum disease is entirely preventable and reversible through good dental hygiene, a healthy diet and periodontal treatment if necessary.

The first obvious step is to avoid or reduce gum disease by avoiding the build-up of plaque, an invisible sticky film that covers the teeth when the bacteria normally present in the mouth interact with sugars and starches from food. Brushing teeth properly twice a day and flossing has been found to be optimal for removing plaque, according to a review of fifty years' worth of clinical trial data.[2] If plaque is left on your teeth for more than a couple of days, it hardens under the gum line and is called tartar, which can only effectively be removed by a professional cleaning. Tartar can become a reservoir for bacteria; together with plaque, it irritates and inflames the part of the gum around the teeth, the gingiva. The mildest form of gum disease, known as gingivitis, is characterized by bad breath and swollen, red, bleeding or receding gums. Untreated, gingivitis progresses to a more severe form of gum disease called periodontitis, which can ultimately lead to tooth loss. Visiting the dentist and dental hygienist once every six months will ensure that any build-up of plaque and tartar can be kept in check before too much damage is done, and that if you do have gum disease it can be quickly treated.

My own top tip for dental hygiene is to find food-grade hydrogen peroxide in a spray, and squirt this round your mouth after brushing as a mouth wash – do not swallow! Hydrogen peroxide (available in all supermarkets, pharmacies and health stores) foams whenever bacteria are present. Swishing this in your mouth for a minute then rinsing will really help kill off bacteria lurking in those difficult to reach nooks and crannies of your mouth. It is amazing to see how you can have brushed your teeth vigorously and carefully, yet, after a little hydrogen peroxide mouthwash, then resemble a rabid animal – literally foaming at the mouth! Hydrogen peroxide is now proven to reduce gingivitis.[3]

Regular exercise also plays a role in your dental health: five sessions of moderate activity or three sessions of vigorous activity can reduce the chances of developing periodontal disease by as much as 40 per cent.[4]

If I have not yet managed to convince you to give up smoking, here's one more reason: it is estimated that smoking causes more than 50 per cent of adult gum disease – no wonder smokers have smelly breath.[5]

Nutritional Solutions to Gum Disease

Vitamin C
Foods high in vitamin C, most notably citrus fruit and berries, should be at the top of every dentist's recommended shopping list. Eating less than the recommended paltry 60 mg a day of vitamin C – that's about one orange – increases your chances of developing severe gingivitis by more than 30 per cent, compared with those consuming three times the

recommended amount – about 180 mg per day.[6] Like the collagen in your skin, the collagen in your gums needs vitamin C for its manufacture. Since some 20 per cent of the gum collagen is turned over daily, if you do not give your fibroblasts (collagen-producing cells) the raw material vitamin C they need to produce this collagen, you will not be building strong and healthy gums (and you will be getting prematurely wrinkly as well!).

For those who already have gum disease, a recent German study found that the consumption of two grapefruits a day for two weeks (that's about 185 mg of vitamin C from the fruit) had significantly less bleeding in the gums,[7] thanks to the increased levels of vitamin C in the bloodstream of the participants.

Professor Emmanuel Cheraskin, MD, DMD, has dubbed vitamin C 'The Invisible Toothbrush'.[8] In one study he found that 72 per cent of all dental patients could be deficient in vitamin C.

Calcium-rich Foods

Not surprisingly, calcium, the mineral that plays a key role in general building and repair of bones, is also essential for the health of the alveolar bone that supports the teeth. Those who are eating little dietary calcium have twice the risk of periodontal disease.[9] One of the best sources of absorbable calcium is sesame seeds: sprinkle them on all your food as a condiment, enjoy tahini (sesame seed butter) on bread or crackers, and even try delicious sesame seed milk. Other excellent sources of absorbable calcium are leafy greens, other seeds and nuts, broccoli and cabbage. The calcium in dairy products is not as easily used as calcium from plant sources so, contrary to what the milk marketing people would like you to believe, these are not the best source of calcium.

Co-Enzyme Q10

This supplement is my other top tip for healthy gums, one that I first learnt from a dental hygienist. Quite well known for its antioxidant heart health benefits, it is now shown that co-enzyme Q10 supplements may be effective in slowing gum disease by reducing bleeding and swelling.[10] Conversely, other research has found that those suffering from gum disease are often significantly deficient in co-enzyme Q10.[11] The main vegetarian sources are peanuts and spinach. It is also found in large amounts in mackerel, salmon and sardines. A supplement form is recommended in order to obtain a therapeutic dose.

Folic Acid

Of course, anyone trying to have a baby will know about the tremendous benefits of folic acid in preventing birth defects; I also strongly recommend it for its anti-ageing properties, which result from its vital role in protecting the DNA from damage during cell replication. But another reason to take folic acid supplements or to eat folate-rich foods, such as leafy greens, is that it reduces the risk of gingivitis, periodontitis and gum disease.[12]

Tea Tree Oil

Tea tree oil is well known for its antibacterial properties. Australian research has now confirmed that using a toothpaste containing tea tree oil twice a day, reduces the presence of gingivitis.[13]

Xylitol

This sugar substitute appears to prevent cavities by inhibiting the growth of the bacteria that cause cavities. One study comparing a toothpaste that contained xylitol with a standard fluoride toothpaste found that the children participants using the xylitol toothpaste had significantly fewer cavities over a three-year period.[14] A study with a gum containing xylitol also showed that it inhibited bacteria in saliva and dental plaque.[15]

Xylitol looks like normal granulated sugar and can be used in the same way for all baking purposes, etc. Xylitol is now widely available in the UK from health-food stores. It tastes great – and it will help your fertility too.

Mercury and Infertility

Far worse than gum disease is the serious damage to your health, that of your unborn child and your fertility in general caused by the mercury in amalgam fillings. As one writer puts it, 'Let's start with a straightforward fact: mercury is unimaginably toxic and dangerous. A single drop on a human hand can be irreversibly fatal. A single drop in a large lake can make all the fish in it unsafe to eat.'[16]

Until recently, nearly all dentists, and thus the public, accepted the general proposition of the dental authorities that the mercury in metal fillings stayed locked in, could not leak and presented no danger to human health. Mounting research has now shown this claim to be completely untrue. Amalgam fillings typically contain between 45 and 60 per cent mercury, together with other alloys. Research on extracted teeth containing amalgam fillings found that the mercury content of the fillings had been reduced by 10 per cent or more; the older the filling, the lower the percentage of mercury.[17] But where had the missing mercury disappeared to? Your body is the regrettable answer. It is now known that mercury vapour is released from amalgam fillings 24 hours a day, 365 days a year and continues to be released for as long as the filling remains in the tooth. Older fillings leak high levels of mercury vapour. A video released by the International Academy of Oral Medicine and Toxicology in March 2006 (go to www.iaomt.org/merc_release.swf) shows incredible footage of a dental mercury release demonstration made by Roger Eichman DDS at the IAOMT Symposium 2000 in Oxford, England, using a phosphorescent screen background. As shown by this video and a number of studies,[18] mercury comes off fillings every time you stimulate them; the stimulation causes the mercury to continue to leak out of the fillings for at least the following hour and a half. These are not small amounts of mercury either – since they are visible, they are, for example, more than 1,000 times higher than the Environmental Protection Agency (EPA) will allow in the air in the USA.[19]

It has also been found that between 80 and 100 per cent of this poisonous vapour inhaled into the lungs enters the blood and is subsequently deposited in the brain and all organs and tissues of the body.[20] Since over 75 per cent of the European and US populations are estimated to have amalgam fillings, this means millions of people of childbearing age are under constant, daily, exposure to a toxin known to be seriously damaging to both fertility and health in general. Research has shown that even tiny amounts of mercury can damage the brain, heart, lungs, liver, kidneys, thyroid, pituitary, adrenals, blood cells, enzymes and the endocrine system in general, as well as suppressing the immune system. Mercury crosses the placental membrane, is taken up by the foetus and is thought to cause, or contribute to, birth defects and miscarriage.

The conclusions of Sam Ziff and Dr Michael Ziff in their book *Infertility and Birth Defects – is mercury from silver dental fillings an unsuspected cause?* are that mercury toxicity causes hormonal disorders in women preventing conception and, in men, leads to defects in sperm.

Dental nurses have only a 50 per cent chance of conceiving thanks to their occupational exposure to mercury, compared to a 95 per cent chance for women without exposure to mercury.

There is such an increasing body of research on the link between heavy metal (including mercury) toxicity and infertility that, in Europe, the government of Sweden led the way in taking the issue of mercury poisoning very seriously: in 1987 it declared that mercury amalgam was toxic and unsuitable as a dental filling material. As a first urgent step, the use of amalgam dental work was banned in pregnant women to prevent damage to the foetus. A complete ban on mercury amalgam was implemented in Sweden to take effect by the end of 1997; Austria followed with a ban in 2000; Germany has a limited ban for children and women of childbearing age.

Mercury Removal and Detoxification

There are a number of nutritional supplements that help with the removal of mercury. The best is the mineral zeolite, which is available in liquid form, sometimes under the brand name Natural Cellular Defence. Secondly, the mineral selenium is very beneficial, together with the antioxidant vitamins alpha-lipoic acid and vitamin C. When you book your appointment to have your amalgam fillings removed, flood your system with vitamin C that day – take about 5 g. Some dental practices who are well versed in the dangers of mercury poisoning may even allow you to have a vitamin C intravenous drip during the amalgam filling removal procedure at an additional cost – this is definitely recommended if it is available.

Fertility Action Plan

- Visit your dentist and make sure you are not one of the 75 per cent of all adults over age 35 with gum disease, which could be undermining your fertility.

- Have your amalgam fillings replaced with safe 'white' (resin-ceramic) fillings as soon as possible.

- If you have had amalgam fillings for a long time or work as a dental professional, take liquid zeolite to remove fertility-impairing mercury from your system.

Part V:
Natural Living

Chapter 21
Sunlight

You have always known that holidays were good for you. Well, guess what? They are also good for your fertility. They combine the hormonal advantages of relaxation with the greater probability of being in sunshine or at least outdoors in natural daylight.

In recent times we have turned into sun-phobes, terrified of getting skin cancer or wrinkles from sun-damaged, prematurely aged skin. If you have been covering up every inch of your body for years and smothering impenetrable sunblock all over you, then I would highly recommend you read the book *The UV Advantage* by Michael Holick, PhD, MD and Mark Jenkins (ibooks, 2004). Dr Holick points out that the exaggerated warnings about the sun's harmful effects have led to a public perception that it is threatening to our overall health. This, in turn, is leading to a 'silent epidemic' of vitamin D deficiency.

Fertility, the Pineal Gland and Melatonin

Sufficient exposure to natural daylight is critical for optimum fertility. When the retina of the eye registers the presence of light, a signal is sent to hormone mission control in the brain – the hypothalamus. The hypothalamus then begins to produce hormones that stimulate the pituitary gland, which, in turn, releases the gonadotrophic hormones that activate the ovaries or testes to produce the male and female sex hormones. At least twenty minutes of natural daylight is required to set this vital hormonal sequence in motion. Living in a northern climate like the UK with limited sunlight, three hours or more of exposure to full spectrum light is needed daily to ensure the proper functioning of the whole endocrine system.

If you are stuck in an office all day working under only artificial light (about which, more below) or always wear sunglasses the moment there is a glimmer of sun, insufficient light will be getting to the retina and your fertility will be impaired by correspondingly low levels of hormones.

Of course the brighter the light the more the retina can absorb, and the stronger the impulse to the hypothalamus to get those hormones going. Researchers have also found that sunlight, through the retina–pineal connection, stimulates the release of growth hormones. I have direct proof of this. At the age of 33–34, the first year I lived in the Cayman Islands, I grew an inch and a half taller, from 5 ft 10 in. to

5 ft 11½ in., having not budged an inch since reaching my previous height at the age of 16, when I thought I had stopped growing. I have since met a woman who also grew nearly two inches in her mid-twenties when she moved from chilly Scotland to Florida, 'the Sunshine State'. You will remember from Chapter 3 that higher levels of growth hormone, as the master hormone of youth, ultimately lead to the higher levels of sex hormones needed for both sex drive and fertility itself. Tempted to rush to get some travel brochures? Off you go! Taking a trip to the sun is a much nicer way to make a baby than a trip to your local, artificially lit fertility clinic. But do forget those sunglasses!

There is another compelling reason to allow your eyes to get a good daily fix of light. Light to the pineal gland helps set your circadian rhythms. However, darkness stimulates the pineal gland to produce melatonin, the hormone that tells the brain it is time to fall asleep. In the dark winter months, our melatonin level naturally increases and, in women, fertility undergoes a corresponding dip. In one study of women undergoing IVF, fluid samples were taken from the largest pre-ovulatory follicles of 120 women and checked for melatonin levels. Both melatonin and progesterone levels were found to be significantly higher in the dark months during autumn and winter, and oestrogen levels were lower. In contrast, in spring and summer, the lighter months, melatonin levels were lower and oestrogen higher. Anecdotal evidence suggests that Eskimo/Inuit women cease menstrual cycles in winter. At the other end of the light spectrum, in Finland's summer months with almost twenty-four hours of daylight, there is the highest rate of conception. The conception rate then drops significantly in the long, very dark months of November to February.[1] It seems that women are not so different from animals in having seasonal breeding patterns. You are more likely to conceive in spring and summer, or, if you take yourself off to a part of the world enjoying such seasons.

Since there is a clear link between depression and infertility, or at least sub-fertility, women who become depressed in the winter may have impaired fertility unless they undergo light therapy (exposure to bright, full spectrum lights for extended periods – such as three hours daily).

Studies have also found that women's melatonin levels drop around ovulation and increase with menstrual flow, and very high levels actually cause infertility. Female athletes who exercise to the point that they are no longer getting their period have melatonin levels twice as high as normal. Melatonin is, for this reason, being tested as a form of birth control; women are taking 75 mg (a massive amount – a normal supplemental dose is 3 mg) a day as part of a long-term study of its effectiveness as a contraceptive.[2]

The Vitamin D Connection

Sunshine does not just hold fertility benefits for women, it also makes men more fertile. The body uses sunlight to make vitamin D. This is not a nutrient, but a hormone. Researchers from the Dartmouth–Hitchcock Medical Center, New Hampshire, studied links between fertility and vitamin D. The study looked at semen samples from eleven fertile and twenty infertile men for levels of the vitamin D receptor, and found that fertile men had higher levels of vitamin D. It seems the vitamin boosts sperm counts. This finding is also supported by animal studies which have found that vitamin D plays a role in male fertility: animals with vitamin D deficiency have less active sperm.

Vitamin D Deficiency

Both men and women should note than studies have shown that sun cream with SPF8 reduces vitamin D production by 97.5 per cent and SPF15 reduces it by 99.9 per cent. The darker your skin, the more exposure to sunlight you need to maintain optimal levels for health and fertility.

No supplement or edible form of vitamin D compares to that obtained from natural sunlight; it stays in the body for a longer time, and sunlight causes the body to make not only vitamin D itself but also related substances, photoisomers, which are very beneficial to health.

The Feel-good Factor

According to the research of Dr Michael Holick and his team at the Boston University Medical Center, it is not just the brain that causes 'feel-good' beta endorphins to be released. The skin also makes beta endorphins when exposed to ultraviolet radiation. Add to this the sun cure for Seasonal Affective Disorder and we can see that science has now explained why lying on a beach makes you feel so good! The success of bright light therapy as a remedy for Seasonal Affective Disorder has led scientists to investigate the use of sunlight and bright light therapy for non-seasonal depression. A number of studies have proved that bright light therapy alone is as effective as antidepressant medications in reducing symptoms of non-seasonal depression.[3]

Everything that elevates mood and lifts depression is very good for fertility – we know why so many babies are conceived on vacations.

Artificial Light

Artificial light does not radiate a complete spectrum of light, like natural sunlight. Incandescent light emits mostly yellow, orange and red light. Fluorescent light (cool white) is in fact mostly a yellow-green light. The light from sunlamps is also unbalanced, having either too much ultraviolet or too much infrared light A number of studies have shown that the use of artificial light adversely affects reproduction in both plants and in animals. In experiments on mice, those under pink fluorescent bulbs stopped breeding earlier than mice under natural daylight, and their offspring were much smaller than the babies of mice exposed to a natural, full spectrum of light. Research shows that light has a reaction on the entire hormonal system of animals via the nerve impulses from the retina to the pituitary. Artificial light can therefore play havoc on the endocrine system.

Most importantly, it has been found that fluorescent lights impair the function of the pituitary gland and only natural daylight allows the ovaries to produce appropriate levels of oestrogen and progesterone.[4] The ability of artificial light to interfere with circadian rhythms has also been termed 'light stress'.

You are also more likely to miscarry if you sleep with an illuminated alarm clock next to your bed according to one study, presumably because of the ill effects of artificial light entering through the eyelids to the retina during sleep. I strongly recommend replacing such a clock with a non-illuminated battery-operated clock.

Heliotherapy – Vitamin S

Heliotherapy – using the sun for healing – is not new. The ancient Babylonians, Egyptians, Syrians, Greeks and Romans were all aware of this, and their cities all had sun gardens. Indeed, the sun was worshipped as a god and a number of temples to the Sun god were erected. In European pagan cultures temples were round and the holy sites of standing stones were constructed in a circle shape, in homage to the sun.

Thousands of years later, fascinating research in the areas of quantum mechanics, physics, biochemistry and physiology has found that *we are human photocells whose ultimate biological nutrient is light*. When I saw that sentence in Gabriel Cousens' book *Conscious Eating*[5] I re-read it three times. Imagine the implications. We are beings of light, we need light for our health, for our very lives. But this is not just some kind of New Age hocus-pocus; scientists now know how the photon energy of sunlight is carried into our bodies and thereafter used as energy. Research carried out by Dr Hans Eppinger found that all the trillions of cells in the body are essentially batteries that appear to be charged up when someone is healthy, but depleted or discharged when we are literally 'run down' or sick. The cellular batteries are fed on their positive poles by oxygen and on their negative poles by photon energy collected from the sun or from raw plant foods we eat. The energy manufacturing mechanism of the cell acts like a step down transformer, turning the sun's energy into volts we can use, namely converting the electrons into adenosine triphosphate (ATP), which is the primary energy fuel of the cell.

Incredible research carried out by Dr Johanna Budwig in Germany has found that, not only do raw plant foods carry sun electrons into the body to supply the cellular batteries, but also, amazingly, '*electron rich foods act as solar resonance fields in the body to attract, store and conduct the sun's energy in our bodies*'.[6] It seems that, when we have these sunlike electrons from uncooked fruits and vegetables (they are called 'pi-electrons') in our cells, they call out to their friends, the photons in the sun, to 'come on down' into the body. According to Dr Budwig, the pi-electrons not only attract the sun photons, they actually activate them. She believes the energy we derive from these solar photons acts as anti-ageing energy.

To be at your maximum reproductive potential, no matter how many times you have been around the sun, you need to have all your cell batteries charged up and firing. You want the ever-youthful sun electrical energy coming into your body. For this, you should eat electron-rich, raw fruit, vegetables, nuts and seeds and get out into the sun to absorb those anti-ageing electrons whenever you can. Further, you need to be outside in natural daylight, without wearing sunglasses as much as possible; aim for three hours a day in a cooler climate. Finally, to be clear, I am not suggesting you fry yourself to a crisp at any given opportunity. I am simply suggesting allowing natural sunlight to penetrate your skin as much as possible without burning, and allow sunlight to reach the pineal gland via the retinas of the eyes, by removing sunglasses from time to time.

Fertility Action Plan

- Get outside in natural light as much as possible.

- If you work in an office/under artificial light, go for a walk outside during lunch and break times

- If finances permit, take holidays in sunny places during the grey winter months.

- Get rid of any illuminated alarm clocks.

Chapter 22

Lunaception and Night Light

Having considered the impact of the sun on fertility, I need to consider the moon, whose influence is almost entirely disregarded by people in the Western world. No, I am not talking about astrology, but rather the subtle but clear biological effect of any light on women's fertility – whether from the sole natural source, the moon, or from artificial lighting during the night.

The flip side to having adequate sunlight during the day, is to ensure that, at night, you are sleeping in a room that is as dark as possible. As mentioned in the sunlight chapter above, bright light suppresses melatonin secretion from the pineal gland.[1] The hypothalamus gland – hormonal mission control – is loaded with melatonin receptors. It is likely that the ovaries and testicles are as well.[2] Melatonin, therefore, directly affects the hormonal balance of the whole body and, in particular, the menstrual cycle.

Traditionally, women's menstrual cycles have followed the cycles of the moon. The native American Indian expression (my favourite one) for a woman's period is 'moon time'. Tribes such as the Mandingos, Susus and Congo call menstruation 'the moon' and, in some parts of East Africa, menstruation is actually thought to be caused by the new moon. In primitive or indigenous societies without electricity, the amount of light affecting the pineal gland and, thus, melatonin production comes from the phases of the moon. Even today, many women notice that they ovulate on the full moon and have their period on the new moon. Farmers know that the new moon is the best time to sow seeds for maximum root growth; by amazing coincidence, this is just about the time, if conception has occurred, that the embryo will be implanting itself into the uterus lining. Even some primates seem to show peaks of sexual activity in sync with the lunar cycle.

In the 1960s some extraordinary research was carried out on the effect of night light on the menstrual cycle. It was found that women's menstrual cycles would become regular by sleeping in complete darkness on days one to thirteen, then sleeping with a 100 watt light bulb (covered by a lampshade) on all night – to imitate the full moon – on days fourteen to seventeen, then returning to sleep in complete darkness for the remainder of the cycle.

Louise Lacey, a writer who coined the wonderful term 'lunaception', decided to try variations on this experiment on herself to try to regularize her menstrual cycle, which had become chaotic after being on the pill. She found that, by sleeping in complete darkness for all except three nights each cycle (when she would keep a light on in the room with a 45 watt bulb, or a brighter light on in the bathroom nearby with the door open), that this reliably triggered ovulation – as verified by charting her temperature. Ms Lacey and twenty-seven of her friends used this as a contraceptive approach. They all developed totally healthy, regular menstrual cycles and avoided having sex on the days they slept with the light, effectively preventing any pregnancy until they were through menopause.[3]

Other clinical research has produced impressive results for women sleeping in complete darkness or with the introduction of light for a few days mid-cycle. Women who were having anovulatory cycles began to ovulate regularly. Women with less obviously fertile cervical mucus began to have discernible, healthy mucus levels. Short cycles (twenty-six days or less) became optimally longer; and very long cycles (thirty-five days or more) settled into a pattern of twenty-seven to thirty-one day cycles. Levels of both progesterone and follicle stimulating hormone became normalized. Mid-cycle spotting was reduced and women who had had a history of miscarriage were able to sustain a pregnancy. Finally, pre-menopausal women were able to develop a fertile mucus pattern and relief from menopausal symptoms such as hot flushes, insomnia and mood swings.[4]

It is important to note that having an illuminated alarm clock, or other small lights in your bedroom such as from a stereo system or TV on all the time will all be affecting your pineal gland and, thus, your melatonin levels. There is a link between having an illuminated clock by the bed and a higher incidence of miscarriage.[5] Find an alarm clock that is not illuminated or on which you have to press a button to see the time. Cover up any small lights from electrical appliances with tape. Invest in blackout blinds (later on these will also be great for the baby's room), or heavy curtains. I strongly recommend using Fertility Awareness techniques (see Chapter 34) together with these modifications to your sleep environment to maximize your chances of having a baby the good old-fashioned way.

Fertility Action Plan

- Try lunaception by sleeping with your curtains or blind open around the three days of the full moon.

- Otherwise, sleep in complete darkness, removing all illumination in the bedroom, including clocks and electronic appliances.

Chapter 23
Exercise

Multiple studies in recent years have pointed to metabolism, not genetics, as the key to ageing – the so-called metabolic model of ageing.[1] In an nutshell, this theory states that high muscle mass and physical activity send longevity signals to the body which, in turn, prompts a sequence of rebuild, repair and restore instructions to the cells. As mentioned in Chapter 3, exercise sends a wake-up call to the pituitary to secrete growth hormone and in turn elevate all sex hormone levels. On the other hand, with low muscle mass and no physical activity, the body signals the brain that you are 'over-the-hill', so wear down, tear down, break down ageing messages are dispatched to the cells. And as for reproducing? Forget it!

For prolonged youthfulness and procreation (or regeneration if you feel yourself beginning to slow down) the answer, apart from an excellent diet, is to exercise!

Professor Ronald Feinberg of Yale University School of Medicine recommends three to seven hours of exercise a week to boost metabolism, self-esteem, overall health and, most importantly, reproductive function.[2] Dr Mark Perloe, author of *Miracle Babies and Other Happy Endings* suggests twenty to thirty minutes' walking a few times a week for those who have got out of the habit of exercising.[3]

Infertility and Excessive Exercise in women

There can, however, be too much of a good thing, particularly for women who are fitness fanatics or whose career is very physical – such as ballerinas, gymnasts, skaters and athletes – since this leads to very low body fat levels and causes the ovaries to shut down. As early as the first century AD, Soranus of Ephesus noted that women who took too much exercise did not menstruate.[4] Women who exercise too much have a similar reduction in fertility to underweight women: too little body fat (under 22 per cent) leads to a production of anti-oestrogens and reduced fertility (see Chapter 9 on weight).

More than one hour of strenuous aerobic activity per day can reduce your chances of conceiving. Research on female runners has found that more than 50 per cent of serious runners who still have periods have shorter cycles that are not ovulatory or are deficient in progesterone.[5] Dr Ralph Hale at the University of Hawaii found that twenty miles of running per week was the cut-off point at which menstrual changes will occur in most women.[6] Other studies show that there is a higher miscarriage and lower fertility rate among athletes due to luteal phase deficiency, characterized by very short cycles. Research undertaken by Dr B.A. Bullen of Boston University followed twenty-eight healthy women, who gradually increased their daily running mileage from four miles per day to ten miles per day. Thirty-three per cent of the women who managed to maintain their weight had a luteal phase deficiency and 63 per cent of those who lost weight had a luteal phase defect by the end of the study.[7]

Research from Boston University has found that even relatively mild exercise can disrupt normal menstrual cycles if it is started abruptly. For fertility, do not turn into a couch potato but start gently into a moderate exercise programme.

If you are engaged in a high level of physical activity, competitive sport or sporting professions and you have irregular, absent or very short periods, and/or have had a miscarriage, then it is likely that your exercise levels are impairing your fertility. Increasing your body fat to at least 22 per cent (a BMI of 20 or higher – see Chapter 9) may help, but the best solution for fertility is to ease off. Run absolutely no more than twenty miles per week (preferably no more than ten) and strenuously exercise for no more than one hour a day. Another option is to take days off during which you do not exercise at all. Keep tapering off your training schedule until you have a return to regular monthly menstrual cycles of twenty-six days or longer.

Over-exercising and Men's Fertility

The research suggests that men can exercise very strenuously with no adverse impact on their fertility (except that they might be too worn out to make love – exhaustion is a powerful contraceptive!). Nevertheless, since very low body fat levels can impair the quality of sperm it is also suggested that men do not overdo it when you are trying to conceive. Bodybuilders and weightlifters also need to bear in mind that steroids can seriously damage your sperm count. Natural alternative nutrients instead of steroids are included in Chapter 11 on medicines.

Fertility Action Plan

- If you are a couch potato, start walking from twenty to thiry minutes at least three or four times a week.

- If you are an exercise fanatic, cut down to about one hour per
  day.

Chapter 24
Sleep

Good-quality sleep is essential for hormonal health, fertility and general well-being. Sleep deprivation raises stress hormones and causes hormonal imbalances, which increase the chances of infertility.[1]

Our sleep consists of a number of different stages, quaintly referred to as 'sleep architecture' in the medical jargon. By monitoring brainwave patterns and eye movement, scientists have noted we have the following sleep states:

NREM sleep stage 1 (REM stands for 'rapid eye movement' and the N for 'non'). This is the first stage of light sleep shortly after falling asleep. The brainwave patterns are in a relaxed state, less than 50 per cent awake, alert, focused brainwaves. Heart and breathing rate slow down and the blood pressure falls.

NREM sleep stage 2. A deeper level of sleep, with only relaxed brainwaves – the typical pattern found when in deep meditation or trance. Breathing and heart rate are even slower and blood pressure is low.

NREM sleep stage 3. This is the first stage of deep sleep, characterized by the presence of the slowest brainwaves. Eye movement is very slow and the body is totally relaxed. This is when the anterior pituitary gland kicks in with a burst of growth-hormone release – to keep you young and fertile. The body can carry out repair and regeneration in this stage of sleep.

NREM sleep stage 4. The deepest sleep of all. This is the stage where maximum growth hormone is released by the pituitary and where most repair and renewal can take place on a cellular level.

REM sleep stage 5. Dreaming. This stage of sleep, typified by rapid eye movement, amazingly shows brainwaves similar to a waking state. Yet the body shows an almost paralysed muscle state – except that this is the phase when a man can have an erection and a woman can have a clitoral engorgement (I guess it depends on how raunchy your dreams are!).

We each go through each of the stages of sleep in cycles, with more NREM, i.e. stages 1–4, in the first half of the night and more REM in the second half of the night and towards morning, each cycle lasting on average about 90 minutes. Since the most crucial sleep for repair of wear and tear in the body (including the cells of the ovaries and testes) and general anti-ageing are stages 3 and 4 – deep sleep – the importance of getting to bed earlier becomes obvious. It is not just an old wives' tale that 'early to bed, early to rise, makes you healthy, wealthy and wise', or that there an old adage that 'an hour's sleep before midnight is worth two after'. If you are only getting to sleep in the wee hours of the morning, you will have more of the crazy dreams in REM and light sleep and less of the deep, healing and restorative sleep of stages 3 and 4.

Most people need between seven and eight hours' sleep to stay healthy, fertile and function at optimum levels during the day.

But, no matter what type of sleep you might be skimping on, according to Dr Eve Van Cauter of the University of Chicago Medical Center, 'Chronic sleep loss has a profound effect on metabolism and hormonal function . . . Ongoing research suggests that the effects of chronic sleep loss may be as profound as the lack of physical activity.'[2]

Sleep-deprived Men

Dr Van Cauter's team carried out an experiment to see what would happen if they restricted, then extended, the sleep of eleven healthy young men. For the first three nights, they slept eight hours. For the next six nights in a row, they got a meagre four hours and, for the last seven nights, they spent a lazy twelve hours per night in bed. At the peak of their sleep deprivation, the physical deterioration of the participants was marked: 'What we found suggests that these young men had metabolic and hormonal profiles that in some ways resembled those of men in their sixties,' said Dr Van Cauter.[3]

Their ability to regulate their blood sugar after a high carbohydrate meal was particularly affected; their bodies' ability to secrete insulin fell significantly. They also had elevated levels of cortisol – the stress hormone. While the University of Chicago researchers did not look specifically into what happens to the fertility of men who go without sleep, what we do know is that anything that adversely affects the balance of hormones, including the stress hormones and glucose-regulating hormones, is definitely going to have a detrimental impact on the sex hormones. We also know that lower levels of growth hormone, released during deep sleep, leads to lower levels of male (and female) sex hormones. What is worrying is that all these symptoms can be seen after just a few days of lost sleep, and the health consequences to men who have a career involving long working hours (like very many busy professionals I know), and/or are proud to 'get by on five hours a night', will be proportionally worse for as long as the sleep loss continues.

Sleep-deprived Women

In women, the hormone estradiol produced by the ovaries is one of the primary hormones regulating the brain's sleep centre. If estradiol levels fall or are out of balance with progesterone levels, this will disrupt normal sleep patterns. This is dealt with under the section concerning hormonal changes and insomnia below.

Disrupted sleep patterns and lack of sleep will mean impaired fertility in both men and women.

Sleep and Anti-ageing

Growth hormone is released in bursts or pulses from the anterior pituitary about one to two hours after we fall asleep and achieve a deep NREM sleep state. If sleep is disturbed, broken or fitful, then a vicious circle occurs: fatigue from the lack of sleep causes less growth hormone to be released; lower levels actually lead to insomnia. Studies show that the decline in sleep quality associated with ageing contributes to growth hormone deficiency and, conversely, measures to improve sleep quality can produce significant increases in growth hormone.[4] The research carried out by Dr Van Cauter at the University of Chicago shows that, if deep sleep can be restored, the ageing process can be slowed thanks to higher levels of growth hormone.[5]

Causes of Insomnia and Some Solutions

Insomnia takes a number of forms. It can mean difficulty falling asleep, waking up in the early hours unable to get back to sleep, waking up frequently during the night/having very restless sleep or having very poor quality sleep, such that you do not feel at all rested or refreshed on waking up. Having an occasional 'off' night, tossing and turning is perfectly normal. Having sleep difficulties or missing sleep for more than three weeks, however, is termed 'chronic insomnia' and has serious health consequences.

There are many causes of insomnia:

Hormonal Changes

Changes to the balance of the hormones released by the ovary, testes, thyroid, adrenal and pituitary gland can lead to sleep difficulties. Stress and illness are the two biggest causes of these hormonal changes.

Stress and Clinical Depression

It is difficult to get a good night's sleep in times of stress. Your hormones actually conspire to keep you awake since, so far as your body is concerned, this is a time of danger. For women, stress suppresses the ovaries, which produce less estradiol, in turn causing insomnia. In men, stress will also cause hormone levels to fall, disrupting sleep and growth-hormone release. As explained in Chapter 3, lower growth hormone also ultimately leads to lower sex hormones – and another vicious circle.

When both men and women endure long-term stress, the adrenals also release cortisol – a hormone that is also responsible for disrupting the sleep cycle – with the knock-on effect of further metabolic and hormonal disturbances. Finding ways to handle stress, in particular by allowing adequate time to wind down before bedtime, will lead to more restful sleep.

Insomnia is common in people with depression and anxiety disorders. In fact sleeping too little (or sometimes sleeping far too much) is a classic sign of depression.

Caffeine and Other Stimulants

Drinking caffeinated drinks (coffee, tea, hot chocolate, sodas) and taking any other kind of herbal stimulants such as guarana, kotu kola, ephedra/mahuang or other weight-loss products all interfere with quality sleep and, in the case of caffeine at least, significantly impair fertility.

Alcohol

Since alcohol makes you drowsy and helps you to fall asleep, most people do not associate it with disrupted sleep patterns. Yet, whenever you drink alcohol, this stimulates noradrenalin release in the night. So you may fall asleep easily but wake up in the middle of the night unable to get back to sleep, or you may have light restless sleep. Apart from giving up alcohol for your fertility, you will be amazed what going to bed sober will do for the quality of your sleep.

Medical Disorders

Certain disorders such as arthritis, kidney or thyroid disease, asthma, allergies, other types of breathing disorders, sleep apnoea, heart disease, narcolepsy (sleeping sickness – falling asleep at any moment), restless leg syndrome and many others all interfere with good sleep. It is outside the ambit of this book to explore how nutrition could help in these particular cases, but the nutrition and lifestyle tips set out below ought certainly at least to improve sleep patterns.

Medication

Certain medications can upset sleep, particularly if they contain caffeine. Decongestants in allergy and cold medicines, anti-depressants, and theophylline for asthma are particular culprits.

Jet Lag/Disruption to Your Body clock

International travel, as well as working shifts, can play havoc with your sleep patterns. I recommend supplemental melatonin (on an occasional basis) to help you fall asleep when you need to.

Sleep-promotion Nutrients

The top nutrients to promote restful sleep are the minerals calcium and magnesium and vitamins niacin (B3), B6 and, in particular, B12. Japanese researchers found that a supplement of 1.5–3 mg of B12 every day restored normal sleep patterns. Vitamin B12 appears to helps by working with the sleep hormone melatonin.

The amino acid tryptophan (available only on prescription) as well as its precursor 5-HTP (5-hydroxytryptophan) are fantastic for good sleep. They naturally lead to increases in serotonin levels – the 'don't worry, be happy' brain chemical. If you are a wired/hyper-type of personality, you can take them at any time of day (they never make me drowsy!); if, on the other hand, you are more mellow in temperament, they could make you immediately sleepy, so it might be better to take them in the hour before your usual bedtime.

Supplements of melatonin can be purchased everywhere in the USA and online, but, annoyingly, not from shops in the UK, despite the excellent safety record of this form of the pineal sleep–wake hormone. I take melatonin whenever I am travelling internationally or whenever, for any reason, I am unable to fall asleep. I love it. A dose of about 3 mg sends you naturally to sleep within an hour of taking it, you sleep a normal sleep cycle and wake up feeling wonderful. It is a powerful antioxidant. If you have persistent sleep problems I recommend buying melatonin online.

The herb valerian acts like mild sedative on the central nervous system, like a weak form of valium. A number of studies have shown that taking about 400–900 mg (about an hour before bed) has led to huge improvements in sleep for those suffering with insomnia. If you wake up groggy, you will need a lower dose.

Final Lifestyle Tips

Winding down

Avoid eating for at least two hours before going to bed. You may be kept awake by the digestion of your meal. If you drink, even water, close to your bedtime, you may have your sleep disturbed by having to go to the bathroom in the night. It is better to stay well hydrated in the day and chug down a litre of water when you wake up, but not to drink anything at all in the hour or so before you would normally try to fall asleep.

Exercising shortly before sleep can also contribute to keeping you awake, since this will stimulate metabolism.

Exercise

One study involving 700 participants found that those who took daily walks were one-third less likely to have trouble sleeping until their normal wake-up time. Walking at a brisk pace is even better – this reduces the chances of any sleep disorder by 30 per cent.[6] Exercise is, of course, a perfect antidote to stress and helps promote relaxation, both of which make for good sleep.

Timing exercise appropriately can help with sleep problems. For those who have difficulty falling asleep before 2 a.m., an early morning walk at first light will help strengthen the circadian rhythms. For someone who falls asleep easily but finds him or herself wide awake in the middle of the night, walking in the late afternoon is recommended by Dr Joyce Walsleben, director of the Sleep Disorders Center at New York University.[7]

Oxygen

Keep fresh air circulating in the bedroom. If possible, sleep with a window open.

The Light Factor

Sleeping in complete darkness triggers the natural release of melatonin, the hormone that governs circadian rhythm. Light in the bedroom can interfere with melatonin release and impair fertility (see Chapters 21 and 22). Finding blackout blinds or heavy curtains, or even sleeping with eye shades, is strongly recommended.

Meditation

This is one of my favourite techniques to help me sleep on nights when unwritten paragraphs in this book are churning around in my head and keeping me awake. I just repeat the phrase 'breathing in, I am breathing in [take a deep breath], breathing out, I release and relax completely [exhale completely]'. Within about ten minutes I am sleeping soundly. Deep breathing is known to oxygenate and calm the body. All kinds of meditation will quiet the mind.

Final tips

Hop-filled pillows and lavender oil are also wonderful relaxants. I like to sprinkle lavender oil on my sheets and pillows anyway, just because I adore the smell. A warm bath with lavender oil will also be conducive to a good night's sleep.

Sweet dreams!

Fertility Action Plan

- If you have been skimping on your sleep or going to bed late, make quality sleep a priority. Switch off the TV and aim to be asleep by 11 p.m.

- If you have sleep problems, avoid all stimulants and take melatonin, niacin, B6 and B12. Also try valerian.

- Wind down for sleep, starting at least two hours before bedtime.

Chapter 25

Your Fertile Imagination – the Power of Feeling Good

One of the most astounding discoveries in medicine in very recent years, and a fact known by a minimal percentage of practising doctors, is that *the heart is an endocrine gland*. Yes! I will repeat that for those of you who can't believe your eyes. The heart is an endocrine gland, which produces at least five hormones that affect all the other hormones in your body including all the sex hormones. It has recently been discovered that the heart produces at least five hormones.[1] These hormones affect the functioning not only of the heart, but the brain and body in general as well.

Here's the next bombshell: the heart has neural cells, the same as the brain, and, therefore, is a seat of consciousness. Chinese medicine and Buddhists, who believe that consciousness lies in the heart not the head, may have been right all a long. The food for your heart? Your feelings. Your emotions affect your heart, the hormones it releases and, in fact, every single cell in your body. Excellent plant-based nutrition will prepare the foundation for super-fertility but the answer to having a baby may lie in a place you always half suspected: your heart, your feelings.

The field of psycho-neuroimmunology is exploding as the connection between mind and body is explored by medical researchers. How you feel has a direct impact on your health and your fertility. Happier feelings lead to a happier biochemistry and a better hormonal balance. Negative feelings and depression will measurably damage your fertility – even if, ironically, those negative feelings have been triggered by your fertility challenges. Researchers have noted that couples struggling to have a baby can be as depressed by their infertility as patients suffering from terminal illnesses. A vicious emotional cycle is then set up, since the depression and negative feelings then reduce the chances of conceiving even more.

Depression and Women's Infertility

Women who are depressed are twice as likely to experience infertility as women with a positive outlook.[2] Their chances of IVF succeeding are reduced to a mere 13 per cent compared with women who are not depressed, whose chances of pregnancy are 29 per cent.[3] Hormonal imbalances triggered by depression in turn cause irregular or missing periods, a reduction in egg quality, delay in the release of the egg and prevent the egg from implanting. Depression and stress can cause the Fallopian tubes and the uterus to contract and, thus, to inhibit movement of the egg.

Depression and Men's Infertility

Men who are depressed are likely to have low sperm counts and abnormally shaped sperm caused by hormone imbalances.

Eating for Mental Health

Far too few people really appreciate the extent of the connection between the food they eat and their physical health. Even fewer are aware of the connection between nutrition and mental health. It is not just that you are what you eat, as the old saying goes, but you literally think and *feel* what you eat!

Food is itself a powerful drug, literally a mind-altering substance that can have a dramatic impact on your mood and mental health in general. Did you realize that, if you had a carbohydrate breakfast such as fruit, you are likely to be feeling calmer and more relaxed reading this than those who ate a high-protein breakfast like eggs or a nut milk? The latter, however, may be more alert and focused (and absorbing what I write!).

It's all a matter of biochemistry. Independent of the stresses and upsets of day-to-day living, our happiness is determined by certain brain chemicals – given the fancy name 'neurotransmitters'. These brain chemicals broadly fall into two groups:

1. The first group includes the neurotransmitters serotonin and GABA (gamma aminobutyric acid). These are the chill-out, be happy, relax, don't worry brain chemicals. Basically, they have calming and anti-anxiety effects. They help maintain emotional stability, healthy sleep patterns and an overall sense of well-being. If you are running low on serotonin and GABA, you may have bitten fingernails, be prone to worry and anxiety, panic attacks and general fearfulness, you may not be sleeping well and have a tendency for both obsessions and cravings – typically sugar and alcohol. Depression resulting from too little serotonin

and GABA is what is popularly viewed as being 'neurotic', 'highly strung' or 'wired'.

2. The second group of neurotransmitters includes dopamine and norepinephrine. These brain chemicals are what give us our gusto, joie de vivre, energy, motivation, power, alertness, focus, and feelings of well-being and pleasure. If your dopamine and norepinephrine levels are not at their optimum, you will be feeling apathetic, unable to drag yourself out of bed in the morning. Depression resulting from a lack of these brain chemicals is characterized by a lack of energy and melancholy, in many ways the symptoms of what we might think of as the typically depressed, low-spirited person.

You may recognize in yourself a tendency towards a serotonin deficiency or you may be more likely to get stuck in a lack of dopamine blues. You may have symptoms of both types of depression. But it is possible to eat yourself happier. What most people notice when they go to health farms or spas or healing centres is not just that they feel healthier after a week of a pure diet, relaxation, fresh air and exercise, but that they actually feel much more positive mentally too. Being happy and feeling good, is one of the easiest ways to improve your fertility – and there are foods that can help.

> You can eat yourself to a happier state of mind and improved fertility.

Anti-anxiety Nutrition

The natural amino acid l-tryptophan and its precursor 5-hydroxytryptophan (called 5-HTP) are the raw material of serotonin manufacture in the brain. So, if you need to chill out and relax, you should focus on foods naturally rich in tryptophan such as almonds, avocados, bananas and wheatgerm, and emphasize food that encourages the release of tryptophan. This is unrefined carbohydrates, such as fruit and starchy vegetables (potatoes, parsnips, turnips, swedes, carrots, sweetcorn) and wholegrains – you always knew pasta made you feel happy! Cravings for sugar and alcohol are a classic attempt by the body to raise tryptophan levels by getting you to eat carbohydrate-rich foods, but will directly impair your fertility.

Of course, excessive consumption of refined sugars, sweets and alcohol leads to high levels of insulin and a blood-sugar crash, that ultimately will lead to even lower tryptophan/serotonin levels – another reason to stick to the healthy carbohydrates that enhance fertility.

The amino acid tryptophan is only available on prescription. 5-HTP is, however, generally available in health-food stores, and is a totally safe supplement I strongly recommend if you want to be serene and relaxed. It is also a natural appetite suppressant. The only side effect of taking too much is that you will become sleepy.

Pep-you-up Foods

For pleasure and gusto, you need to eat foods rich in the amino acid phenylalanine. Phenylalanine is found in the fertility foods brown rice, lima beans, nuts, peanuts and sesame seeds as well as eggs. Chocolate with high cocoa content is a great source of phenylalanine. The main ingredient of aspartame (diet sugar) is phenylalanine, but, for the reasons already set out in Chapters 4 and 5, it is not recommended.

There is also a clear link between low levels of the omega 3 essential fatty acids and depression. Taking the fertility power food flax seeds daily will help with this, as will pure fish oil capsules, which, unlike fresh fish, will not be contaminated with fertility-harming pollutants like mercury and PCBs.

The Secret to Fertility: the Law of Attraction

As quantum physics now proves, we know that the whole world is vibrating. We know that thoughts vibrate, and that our consciousness affects our environment. The concept of the law of attraction states that what you think about most you will manifest in your life. So most of us manifest by default, by thinking about what we don't want: infertility, debt, ill-health, no partner, work challenges, etc. And guess what we find ourselves dealing with? So, if you are mostly thinking about the *lack* of a baby in your life, if all you are noticing is that you are *not* pregnant and feeling bad about this, then what you will be attracting to you is more of the same, possibly amplified: the lack of a baby, the not-pregnancy. Never underestimate the power of positive thinking.

About a year ago, I watched an amazing film called *The Secret* on DVD, and later I read the book of the same title, written by Rhonda Byrne. One of the most amazing stories in this is the account of a man called Morris Goodman, who was completely paralysed in a plane crash. He could only blink his eyes; he could not swallow, or even breathe unassisted. Within nine months, by the power of his mind, by focusing only on walking out of the hospital, visualizing placing one foot in front of the other, and ignoring all the medical professionals who were telling him that a cure was impossible, he healed his ruptured spine – and walked out of that hospital on his own two feet, unassisted! This miracle story made me think just what the human mind can do when focused with positive intent.

Start to feel really excited about the baby you are going to have. Have you bought them a little toy, or a little outfit? Are you really anticipating their arrival? Monitor your thoughts, and any time you find them drifting in the direction of why you might *not* have a baby, stop! Replace that image with one of you/your partner patting a fat pregnant belly, of preparing for the birth, of holding your healthy newborn in your arms. The body cannot distinguish between what is only imagination and what is real, so visualising the new baby will trigger hormonal changes that will make this a reality.

I wish with all my heart for everyone reading this who wants to have a baby (including myself) that we maintain the clear, focused intent and positive feelings that turbocharge both hormones and fertility, and now joyfully anticipate the birth of a wonderful healthy baby/babies.

Fertility Action Plan

- Buy 5-HTP, GABA or phenylalanine supplements if you have been feeling depressed.

- Go to the website www.thesecret.tv to find out more about this amazing film and book that can inspire you to think positively and to make your baby dreams come true.

Part VI:
Nutritional Treatment of Particular Conditions

Chapter 26
Miscarriage and Luteal Phase Defects

There can be few experiences as heart-wrenching as miscarriage or the trauma of a stillborn delivery. The tender hope for a baby is vanquished, your body has betrayed both you and the baby's father and, for nearly all women who lose a baby, the overwhelming grief is mixed with guilt: 'What did I do wrong?'

It is of little consolation to those who have suffered the loss of a miscarriage to know just how common an occurrence it is. Some studies using highly sensitive pregnancy tests suggest that as many as 50 per cent of all fertilized eggs die and are spontaneously lost before implantation in the womb occurs and the woman knows she is pregnant.[1] The rate of miscarriage prior to days 35–50 (the point at which a pregnancy may be clinically recognized) is estimated to be 30 per cent.

It is my impression that the medical community offers little to comfort the grieving woman. Women over thirty-five are likely to be informed that the miscarriage was almost certainly caused by 'chromosomal damage' to the foetus – after all, what can you expect at your (advanced) age? – and that one ought to be grateful for its loss compared with the difficulties of having a child with birth defects. Women are often told just to 'try again'. There are few traditional medical treatments to prevent any future miscarriage.[2] However, there is a lot you can do nutritionally to help.

It is now pretty much accepted that the overall rate of miscarriage for clinically recognized pregnancies is one in four.

The Causes of Miscarriage and Nutritional Solutions

Chromosomal Abnormalities/Damage

The first thing I would like to remind all women reading this is that half of every baby's DNA comes from the father. Chromosomes are the tiny threadlike structures in each cell which carry the genes – the blueprint of life. We all have 23 pairs of chromosomes – one of each pair donated by our mother, the other by our father – a total of 46 in all. It has been found that, up to 70 per cent of all first-trimester miscarriages are caused by chromosomal abnormalities in the foetus.[3] Other recent research indicates that chromosomal damage could also cause 50 per cent of repeated miscarriages too.[4] But, remember, when the usual 'chromosomal damage' pronouncement is made by a doctor as the cause of the miscarriage, there is a male person who can take 50 per cent of the responsibility for this.

White-coated persons will also tell you that 'maternal age'

is the problem here. No, I am not in denial, the statistics are gloomy: the clinical miscarriage rate for women under thirty-five is almost three to four times lower than for women over thirty-five. However, as I hope is very clear to anyone reading this (remember Chapters 2 and 3) your chronological age and your biological age do not necessarily equate to the same number. When my sister Jude was expecting her third baby at age 37, her doctor hummed and hawed about her 'triple test' – the blood test for Down's syndrome (a birth defect caused by a chromosomal abnormality) – warning her that at her geriatric age the chances were now 1 in 250. Her results? In fact, a chance of one in 4,000 that my then unborn nephew would have any birth defect. This is the same as a woman in her late teens or twenties could expect – so much for maternal age and chromosomal damage. In fact, baby George was born on 3 July 2006 – the day after my sister's 38th birthday – weighing 8 lb 11 oz; a perfect bouncing baby boy.

Let me spell out my philosophy on genetic damage to your cells (including those forming eggs and sperm) and ageing in general once again: if you drink alcohol and caffeine, smoke, eat pesticides, GM or junk foods, and a diet high in sugar and refined carbohydrates, you will *definitely* accelerate your ageing, such that your biological age could even exceed your chronological, i.e actual, age. Poor dietary choices will directly contribute to DNA damage to your cells and massively increase your (or, if you are a man reading this, your co-parent's) risk of miscarrying. The older you are, the more it behoves you and your partner to clean up your acts when it comes to lifestyle and diet. The very good news is that if you follow a pure whole-food plant-based diet, such as the Fertility Diet, eliminate the obvious toxins and make a concerted effort to detoxify your body before conceiving, then the genetic material in both the sperm and the egg at the critical moment of conception when the genes cross over will be of a relatively better quality and the prospects of a successful pregnancy and a healthy baby are enormously increased.

I believe that a study on pre-conceptual care and pregnancy outcome, carried out between 1990 and 1992 by the UK charity Foresight, demonstrates the assertion I make in the above paragraph very clearly. A total of 367 couples participated in the programme; they had age ranges of 22–45 for the women (average age 34) and 25–59 (average age 36) for the men. Ninety per cent of the males and 60 per cent of the females regularly drank alcohol. Forty-five per cent of the men and 57 per cent of the women smoked. There were numerous fertility issues plaguing these couples: 59 per cent had a previous history of reproductive problems; 37 per cent had suffered infertility for between one and ten years; and 139 of the couples (38 per cent) had experienced between one and five previous miscarriages. Eleven couples had had a stillborn child, seven had had babies with birth defects and three had suffered the terrible trauma of infants who had died of sudden infant death syndrome.

During the two years of the study, all the couples gave up alcohol and smoking completely, followed a wholefood diet and were given mineral supplements to correct any deficiencies discovered through blood, hair, sweat and/or semen analysis. Their results were stupendous! A massive 327 women (89 per cent) had become pregnant and given birth to 327 normal weight, healthy babies.[5] There were no miscarriages among this previously high-risk group. Not a single one! On general statistics alone, there should have been eighty-one miscarriages (one in four), not zero. In fact, the scientists who conducted the study predicted that an identical cross-section of British couples not following the Foresight guidelines would experience ninety-two miscarriages, eleven malformations and five stillbirths. None of the babies in this study was stillborn, had birth defects or had died through sudden infant death syndrome – well worth the sacrifice of wine, beer, cigarettes and a poor diet on the part of the parents, I would suggest.

For any of you who think the zero miscarriage rate of the 327 couples – sorry, I mean, 654 parents – on the Foresight programme was a freak event and just 'luck', contemplate the following.

Smoking

Research shows that, when either parent smokes, there is an increased risk of miscarriage.[6] For women who smoke, the risk of miscarriage is 27 per cent (more than the average 25

Ideally, both men and women should stop smoking four months prior to trying to conceive, if they want to have a healthy, full-term baby.

per cent risk) compared with non-smokers.[7] According to a report issued by the British Medical Association in February 2004, smoking is responsible for up to 5,000 miscarriages a year in the UK. Remember, too, that, if your biological clock is ticking, research carried out by Dr David Torgerson at the University of York in the UK in 1997 showed that women who smoke have a six times higher risk of an early menopause, i.e. before the age of 45.[8] Three other studies demonstrate a clear link among women who smoke between the early onset of menopause and infertility.[9]

Smoking reduces fertility in both women and men, and gives a higher risk of miscarriage. Do you really want that nicotine fix more than you want your baby?

As a woman who smokes, you cannot even be complacent about miscarriage once you have got through the first trimester: smoking increases the risk that your body will reject the baby at *all* stages of pregnancy and increases the risk of bleeding – a sign of a threatened rejection.[10] You are also more likely to suffer from a condition called placenta praevia, in which the placenta is abnormally close to the opening of the cervix, which has been related to miscarriage.[11]

Men, if you smoke, apart from the likelihood of having erectile dysfunction, you will have decreased sperm count and density, a lower proportion of motile sperm and an increase in abnormal sperm – a direct cause of foetal malformations.[12] In other words, since nature's way of eliminating a malformed foetus is to cause it to abort spontaneously, dodgy sperm produced by a smoking father will increase the chances of a miscarriage in his partner, even if she is a non-smoker. If you have been deluding yourself that a miscarriage is just a body malfunction of a woman, you really need to grasp that your smoking could well cause or already be to blame for the loss of a baby.

Alcohol Consumption

Imagine you witness the following scene: a mother in her kitchen uncorks a bottle of wine or pops the top off a beer and pours the alcoholic beverage into a baby's bottle and gives it to her infant. You would be horrified, right? Straight on the phone to social services to report child abuse. Yet this is exactly what happens when a pregnant woman drinks, and that includes a woman who does not yet know she is pregnant. All alcohol is a low molecule liquid, meaning it is able to shimmy on through the placental barrier and to enter the foetus at almost the same level that it is in the mother. If you are planning on giving up drinking once you know you are pregnant and, in the meantime, are partying as usual, then you need to know that the consumption of a substantial amount of alcohol before the embryo has embedded in the uterus can cause a miscarriage.[13]

Generally speaking, alcohol is a 'teratogen'. This is a fancy scientific word meaning something that can cause developmental malformations. In the first few weeks of life an embryo goes through massive growth and cell development. By the thirty-sixth day, the neural tube is clearly present and open, and most of the organs have begun to be formed: brain, heart, limbs, eyes, digestive tract, etc. Drinking at this point can irreparably damage the foetus and, if it survives, it could have a number of malformations such as a defective heart, musculoskeletal abnormalities and mental retardation. It could have a birth defect called 'foetal alcohol syndrome' characterized by growth, facial, cardiac and mental abnormalities. More often that not, a poorly formed or defective foetus will not survive, and will miscarry.

Paternal drinking also plays a role in miscarriage. Alcohol is a testicular poison and, like smoking, leads to an increase in abnormal sperm.[14] It's ironic that, in our culture, heavy drinking is at the core of male socializing, yet leads to serious reproductive harm: sperm samples taken from men consuming excessive amounts of alcohol show clear abnormalities.[15] With defective sperm there are three possibilities: no conception; conception of a foetus with chromosomal damage which will miscarry; conception of a child with birth defects. Not really worth a boys' night out? Preparation for pregnancy is a joint responsibility in every way. Sperm take three months to mature, so a minimum of three months' pre-conception abstinence is strongly recommended. If your male partner has continued to drink and you have a history of miscarriage, then one cause could be his alcohol-damaged sperm. But men, you are lucky, unlike women you only need to join the temperance movement at the pre-conception stage. As soon as junior, with perfect chromosomes, is on the way you can hit the bottle (moderately!) to celebrate if you want to.

Caffeine

One study from McGill University, Montreal, found that drinking the equivalent in caffeine to more than three cups of coffee per day during pregnancy more than tripled the rate of miscarriage.[16] Since caffeine consumption can also lead to chromosomal damage (see Chapter 5) switching to herbal teas, or, second best, naturally decaffeinated (i.e. through a water process, not chemicals) beverages should be a priority. Note: even decaffeinated coffee has 3 per cent caffeine; it is a massive improvement, but, personally, if I were at last pregnant with the baby I have longed for, I would not be willing to risk it.

Hormonal Imbalances and Luteal Phase Defect

If you have a short cycle, such as twenty-four days or less, you may have a short luteal phase. This refers to the time after ovulation until menstruation takes place, if there has been no conception. This is the time during which progesterone is released from the remains of the follicle left behind after the egg has been released from the ovary – the so-called corpus luteum or 'yellow body'. This corpeus luteum usually lasts between twelve and fourteen days. In some women, however, it lasts less than twelve days, and this can be problematic, since, unless there is sufficient progesterone released until such time as the egg can implant and mature, a miscarriage can result. Research from Germany found that low progesterone was the cause of infertility in 63 per cent of the 753 infertile women studied.[17]

Luckily, there is *a lot* you can do naturally to raise progesterone levels. The key supplements are B6 and magnesium and the key herb to raise progesterone is vitex (wild chasteberry). The herbs false unicorn root (*Chamelirium luteum*) and cramp bark (*Viburnum opulus*) are also recommended to prevent miscarriage.

Flax seeds (linseed) can also help. The lignans enterodiol

and enterolactone – plant compounds found in flax seeds – have been shown to increase ovulation rates and lengthen the luteal phase in women with normal menstrual cycles; it further increases the luteal phase level of progesterone relative to estradiol.[18] I eat flax seeds every day for all their amazing health benefits and I strongly recommend them to all women wishing to conceive.

If you are a fitness fanatic who has had a miscarriage, your chances of a successful pregnancy will be greatly increased by easing off your training schedule to no more than ten miles per week or one hour per day, or whatever level is sufficient to allow your periods to stabilize at regular cycles lasting twenty-six days or longer. (See Chapter 23 for details of appropriate levels of exercise for fertility.)

My absolutely top tip for anyone who has had a miscarriage and is pregnant again, or who seeks never to have a miscarriage, is sweet potato! This is the richest natural plant source of progesterone. It is also one of the best sources of beta-carotene, a great antioxidant. I have given nutritional counselling to a number of women who have had between one and three miscarriages. Apart from the rest of the advice in this chapter, when they were pregnant again, I insisted that they eat as much sweet potato as possible – yes, lunch and dinner every day. By the time they were about four months' pregnant and patting fat bellies, they each begged me to let them stop eating the sweet potato, which by then they loathed, and I let them. All the women who have followed my magnesium and sweet potato anti-miscarriage cure are happy mothers today.

Eat as much sweet potato as you can to avoid miscarriage.

Exposure to Mercury and other Heavy Metals

In a nutshell, exposure to mercury vapour, whether by occupational exposure (such as dentists, dental assistants) or from having mercury amalgam fillings, leads to an increased risk of miscarriage. This topic is dealt with in more detail in Chapter 20.

I particularly recommend the mineral supplement zeolite, which is very effective at chelating heavy metals such as mercury and toxins and drawing them out of the body.

Time Spent at Visual Display Unit (VDU) Screens

One worrying study from 1988 reported that women who spent more than twenty hours a week in front of a VDU screen, such as a computer monitor or TV screen, had twice as many miscarriages as women who did not work with computers.[19] If you are pregnant, try to limit the time spent in front of the computer or the TV. Try to take any breaks at work away from the computer, and take breaks at least every half an hour – for just 5 minutes. It will also help to switch the VDU off rather than using the screen saver, and sit as far away from the computer as you can while working. The electromagnetic radiation from the screen is to blame for the miscarriages. I once read that walking along sand on a beach in bare feet was the perfect antidote to electromagnetism from computers and the electromagnetic fields of modern technology surrounding us (the reason was to do with silica in the sand). If you are lucky enough to live near a beach this is worth bearing in mind, but I am sure any walk in nature would help!

Exposure to Solvents and Toxic Chemicals

In preparing to become pregnant, it is vital to avoid exposure to solvents and toxic chemicals which have been linked to miscarriages, stillbirths, birth abnormalities and congenital defects. A number of studies from both Finland and the USA found that women who had miscarriages were two to four times more likely to be exposed to organic solvents at work compared to women with healthy pregnancies.[20] If you live in a rural area surrounded by non-organic farms where pesticides are sprayed, or near waste sites and landfills where toxins are buried, the chances of your miscarrying, or of harm to your unborn child, are significantly increased. This means you need to take every effort to avoid freshly painted buildings (unless non-toxic paint has been used), non-ecologically safe cleaning products – especially ones such as oven cleaners – and go nowhere near insecticides and pesticides. Stop putting any toxic chemical weed suppressant on your garden. Replace all beauty and cosmetic products with the most natural, organic ones you can find. If you dye your hair, you will need to switch to a safe vegetable dye alternative or revert back to your natural colour.

Avoid Dry-cleaners/Wearing Clothes that Have Been Dry-cleaned

The main chemical used in the dry-cleaning process called perchloroethylene is a spermatotoxicant and ovotoxicant. A number of studies have shown that, not only do men and women working in the dry-cleaning business take significantly longer to conceive than those who do not, there is a very high reported rate of miscarriages among women working in or even living near dry-cleaning shops.[21] While pregnant or hoping to conceive, it is important to avoid going near dry-cleaners and to avoid wearing clothes that have been recently dry-cleaned since these may still emit some of the chemical used in the cleaning process.

Herbs to Avoid when Pregnant

There are certain herbs that can be very beneficial to reproductive health prior to conception, for example in balancing hormones and helping to make periods regular, which must then be avoided during pregnancy since there is a risk they could stimulate a spontaneous abortion. These are rue (*Ruta graveolens*), mugwort (*Artemisia vulgaris*), parsley (*petroselenium crispum*) and sage (*Salvia officinalis*). All of these herbs are uterine stimulants and might have been prescribed by a herbalist to restart stopped periods, for example. They are, however, known abortifacients – which is why they must only be taken under the supervision of a qualified herbalist if you are pregnant. Taking an incorrect dose can damage the foetus without aborting it. Other herbs to be cautious of once pregnant are black cohosh, blue cohosh, fenugreek, liquorice and red raspberry leaf. They may also be too stimulating to the uterus to be safe, when pregnant.

Uterine Abnormalities and Fibroids

One potential cause of miscarriage is uterine fibroids – tumours that grow from muscle tissue in the uterus, which can vary in size from that of a pea to that of a basketball. Please see Chapter 27 on Uterine Fibroids for a full account.

In respect of other instances of uterine abnormalities – such as a so-called incompetent cervix (only a man could

have come up with such a disparaging term), namely a
cervix that dilates too quickly, so the uterus cannot hold a
baby – I am afraid I have no nutritional solution to offer.
However, I would recommend strengthening and toning the
pubococcygeus muscle, a.k.a. the PC muscle, that is located
in the genital area between the vagina and the anal opening.
You can do this with an exercise called Kegeling. Kegeling
basically involves rhythmically contracting and relaxing the
PC muscle as if you were trying to stop the flow of urine.
Kegel exercises, which can be carried out anywhere, will definitely benefit the overall health and condition of the uterus.

PCOS and Diabetes

Unfortunately, approximately one third of pregnancies in
women with PCOS end in miscarriage. They also suffer the
additional risk of other pregnancy disorders such as pre-
eclampsia, gestational diabetes and stillbirth. Diabetic
women also need to maintain strict control of their blood
sugar levels during pregnancy. If levels of glucose fall too
high or too low, this can lead to birth defects in the developing foetus, especially in weeks five to eight of pregnancy. My
advice to women with PCOS and with diabetes is to follow
the nutritional guidelines set out in the PCOS chapter that
follows in order to minimize your chances of a miscarriage.
Supplemental magnesium, zinc and chromium are strongly
recommended.

Thyroid Problems

Untreated and unrecognized hypothyroidism (underactive
thyroid) doubles the risk of miscarriage, stillbirths and premature births, as well as tripling the risk of birth defects.[22]
Thyroid hormones not only play a key role in our own brain
functioning and mental health, they are also crucial for
foetal brain development during pregnancy. If adequate and
balanced amounts of thyroid hormones and the mineral
iodine are not present in the mother, permanent brain
damage can be caused to the baby – this ranges from severe
retardation to less obvious learning and neurological challenges. A 'damaged' foetus is more likely to spontaneously

abort. Fortunately, when thyroid conditions are treated, whether by diet or drugs, so that thyroid levels are balanced, women with thyroid diseases enjoy the same likelihood of a successful pregnancy as women who are not facing any thyroid challenges.

Women with levels of thyroid hormones that are either too high or too low are at far greater risk of losing their babies.

Obesity and Miscarriage

Australian researchers have found a link between being overweight and miscarrying. They studied 67 women who had had a 75 per cent miscarriage rate in previous pregnancies; they were put on a weight loss intervention six months prior to conceiving with intense diet and exercise. Following their weight loss, the miscarriage rate was down to around 18 per cent – below average.[23]

Infections/Fever over 100°F

When a woman becomes sick and gets a fever over 100°F this can stimulate miscarriage. Certain infections are documented to cause miscarriage – these include toxoplasmosis (why pregnant women should not eat soft cheeses, or empty cat litter trays), listeria and malaria. The most notorious viruses endangering a pregnancy are German measles (rubella), mumps, measles, hepatitis A and B and parvo virus. If the first-ever herpes viral attack takes place in the first twenty weeks of pregnancy, this also could harm the unborn child.

Fortunately, the more common ailments of coughs, colds and the flu, even accompanied by fever, do not normally harm the baby, but, of course, you must be certain to take only medications that are safe for pregnancy. If you can, preferably take only food remedies, like ginger tea, hot lemon and honey and drink plenty of water until you feel better.

Excessive Heat

Raising body temperature to high levels, for example with very hot baths, an electric blanket or the heating mechanism of waterbeds could also be a risk for sustaining a pregnancy.

Some researchers have considered whether electromagnetism from electric blankets could also be responsible for decreased fertility. I recommend not using any devices that heat up the bed and, in general, do not allow yourself to overheat, in order to avoid miscarriage.

Genito-urinary Infections

The sexually transmitted disease chlamydia (see Chapter 16) has been found to be directly responsible for spontaneous abortions.[24] This is easily detectable with a blood test and often treatable with antibiotics.

Fungal infections (called genital mycoplasmas) in the cervix are associated with a considerable higher incidence of miscarriage compared to women without such infections.[25] An imbalance in the friendly protective bacteria in the vagina triggered by an overly acidic diet (meat, sugar and dairy products being the most acidic foods) can lead to inflammation and an overgrowth of a bacteria called gardnerella vaginalis – leading in turn to an infection called bacterial vaginosis. Bacterial vaginosis is linked to miscarriage (as well as premature births).[26]

I strongly recommend testing to ensure you do not have chlamydia or any other fungal or bacterial genital infection before trying to conceive. If you have had a miscarriage, please insist upon a blood test to rule out the presence of any genito-urinary infections as a cause.

The S factor – Stress, Anxiety and Miscarriage

As I am sure you are aware by now if you have read Chapter 18, acute stress throws all sex hormones off balance. This then gives abnormal feedback to your pituitary, and could unfortunately signal that now is not a good, or a safe, time to be having a baby. Your body will respond to this message by terminating the pregnancy.

According to the Harvard doctors, Robert Barbieri, Alice Domar and Kevin Loughlin, who wrote the book *Six Steps to Increased Fertility*, anxiety is associated with spontaneous abortions.[27]

If you have been lucky enough to get pregnant, now is the

time to look after yourself and your unborn child. This is *your* time. Ask for support and help from family, friends and co-workers. Shed as many burdens and stresses in your home and workplace as you possibly can; the life of your baby could depend on it.

Night Lighting

I was amazed to discover that something as innocuous as an illuminated alarm clock near to the bed as you sleep could be a cause of miscarriage.[28] Any light at night will penetrate the eyelids and, through the retina, have an impact on the pineal gland and affect the levels of the hormone melatonin, which governs circadian rhythms. This, in turn, will have an influence on all hormonal levels. Please see Chapter 22 for a fuller discussion of this issue. For a healthy pregnancy it is better to sleep in complete darkness. Replace any bedside clock with one that does not have an illuminated face.

Deficiencies in Key Nutrients

Folic Acid

Since folic acid prevents DNA damage and the occurrence of neural tube defects in foetuses during the first few weeks of pregnancy, a deficiency in folic acid also increases the chances of miscarrying. This is the number one vitamin to be taking while trying to conceive and throughout pregnancy. A supplemental dose of 800 mcg is recommended, as well as eating folate-rich foods: beans, black-eyed peas, citrus fruit, leafy greens, lentils, mustard greens, spinach and turnips.

Vitamin B6 (Pyridoxine)

Women with a history of miscarriages could be deficient in B6 – a vitamin that is depleted with the consumption of alcohol and caffeine, as well as if contraceptive pills have previously been taken. Alcohol deactivates B6 and caffeine causes more of the mineral to be excreted in the urine. B6 is the key nutrient to raise progesterone levels. Low progesterone is, of course, the main hormonal imbalance behind luteal phase defects which prevent a pregnancy from being sustained. It is preferable to take B6 in a combination vitamin B supplement rather than on its own. The best food sources are: brewer's yeast, carrots, peas, spinach, sunflower seeds, walnuts and wheatgerm. Non-plant sources include fish and eggs. Other foods containing some B6 are: avocado, bananas, beans, broccoli, cantaloupe and brown rice. Note: the mineral zinc is needed to convert B6 into its active form in the body (see below).

Vitamin C

There has been significant research showing that adequate levels of vitamin C with bioflavonoids can prevent miscarriage. In one study 45 per cent of a group of 1,334 women who had had a miscarriage had low levels of vitamin C and bioflavonoids. When 100 pregnant women in this group were given 350 mg of vitamin C each day, 91 of them gave birth to healthy babies.[29] In a second study, eleven out of thirteen women who had miscarried went on to have babies when they were given supplemental vitamin C with bioflavonoids.[30] You can obtain plenty of vitamin C from food by eating plenty of brightly coloured fruits and vegetables.

Copper

Turkish researchers at the University of Ankara have also found a connection between a deficiency in the mineral copper and risk of miscarriage. Women who have had a miscarriage were found to have low copper levels.[31] Copper and zinc work synergistically together. Note that copper can be toxic in high doses so *never* exceed the amount suggested on the bottle/packet. Foods that include trace copper are: almonds, avocado, barley, beans, beets, broccoli, garlic, lentils, mushrooms, nuts and oranges; it can also be found in seafood.

Vitamin E

Some fascinating studies were carried out in Germany in the late 1980s on the link between a vitamin E deficiency and miscarriage. A group of 100 fertile couples who had previously had, collectively, 144 conceptions without a single live birth, were given supplemental vitamin E each day (100 iu for men, 200 iu for the women). On this protocol they went on to have seventy-nine babies – and only two further miscarriages.[32] When the experiment was repeated with a second group of one hundred couples (who had collectively had sixty-three previous miscarriages), forty-one babies were successfully carried to term, with no miscarriages occurring.[33] Other Canadian research showed an 86 per cent success rate in treating women with a history of miscarriage using vitamin E therapy. It is, therefore, highly recommended – a supplement of 200 iu is good. Good food sources of vitamin E are leafy dark-green vegetables, nuts, seeds and wholegrains.

Magnesium

A magnesium deficiency is suspected to be a common cause behind miscarriage since low magnesium levels are associated with low progesterone. Together with B6, magnesium is my top recommendation for women who have suffered a miscarriage. The best food sources are almonds, leafy green vegetables and raw cacao (raw chocolate), but note that cacao also contains caffeine so should be consumed in strict moderation.

Zinc

A number of animal studies have shown that a zinc deficiency causes miscarriage, and there is no reason to suppose this is not true in humans too. Dr Carl Pfeiffer stated that, since male babies need higher zinc levels than female, if a woman has been able to have a daughter but miscarried a son, low levels of zinc could be the reason why.[34] Zinc and B6 work together – zinc converts B6 into its usable form and B6 helps with zinc absorption. They make an excellent anti-miscarriage duo. Zinc can be found in brewer's yeast, carrots, pumpkin, seaweed and sunflower seeds. Oysters are the richest non-vegetarian source.

Fertility Action Plan

- Follow the Fertility Diet guidelines – be sure to eliminate alcohol and caffeine from your diet.

- If you smoke you need to stop immediately.

- Limit your exposure to toxins, heavy metals and chemical solvents.

- If you have amalgam fillings have them removed and replaced with non-metal ones.

- Eat flaxseeds (linseed) and sweet potatoes and yams to lengthen luteal phase and naturally increase progesterone levels.

- Try to limit the time spent in front of a computer and/or the TV to 20 hours per week maximum.

Testimonial

A Healthy Pregnancy Following a Miscarriage

I am very thankful to Sarah Dobbyn for helping me to get ready for a pregnancy. I experienced a miscarriage before I met Sarah and did not receive much help from my physician on how to increase the chances of another pregnancy. Sarah's advice on changing my diet was the best thing ever. I went on a strict one-month detox program: no sugar, alcohol, caffeine, eating mainly organic foods and allowing mental relaxation (getting rid of stress in my life). The good news: after that month I got immediately pregnant and I am now in week 18 of my pregnancy (June 2007), feel great and so far it is going well. In addition, based on Sarah's advice I got my thyroid tested and got diagnosed with a thyroid disease which I am treated for – never thought of it before!

I can't thank Sarah enough for sharing her knowledge with me. I hope this book reaches all women going through the hard time of trying to get pregnant. It's just not talked about!

Sonja S, New York, USA, aged 34

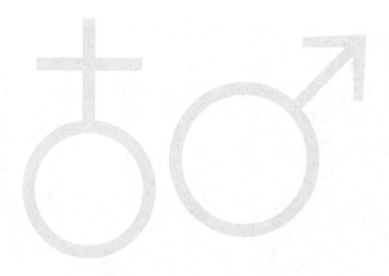

Chapter 27

Polycystic Ovary Syndrome (PCOS)

Polycystic Ovary Syndrome is a serious disorder affecting millions of women; it can significantly impair fertility and increase the risk of miscarriage.[1] The classic symptoms are abnormal periods (irregular or no menstruation), acne, oily skin, weight gain, male pattern baldness, excess body and facial hair, diabetes/insulin resistance, high blood pressure, mood swings and changes in libido. An ultrasound scan or laparoscopic examination normally reveals enlarged ovaries that are full of cysts – fluid-filled structures a bit like blisters – that form on the ovaries' surface from follicles that do not develop and dissolve normally in the menstrual cycle.

According to a 1988 report in the *Lancet*, 10 per cent of women of reproductive age have PCOS[2] but may be unaware of it if they have no symptoms, are misdiagnosed with stress or PMS, or their symptoms are dismissed by doctors as being merely cosmetic concerns.

Causes of PCOS

Hormonal Imbalance

PCOS is a complex, multi-system endocrine and metabolic disorder. Since it is characterized by an imbalance in the sex hormones as well as in insulin levels, it is extremely difficult to know whether the hormone imbalance came first – or whether it is PCOS itself that has led to a serious upset in the finely tuned balance of hormones. Medical and nutritional writers are divided on this 'chicken or egg' issue. What is clear, however, is that PCOS is on the rise and it mirrors the massive increases in obesity, diabetes and insulin resistance, as well as the all-pervasive endocrine-damaging environmental pollutants and chemical additives in food that affect women today.

Dietary Factors: Insulin and Obesity

The distressing symptoms of PCOS mostly stem from excess androgens – the 'male' hormones (testosterone, both in free form and overall levels, DHEA and androstendione) in the bloodstream.

Insulin levels regulate levels of blood glucose. A diet loaded with high glycaemic foods such as sugar, refined carbohydrates, sodas and alcohol causes insulin levels to rise significantly. If this high glycaemic diet is continued for an extended period of time, insulin levels will remain elevated. As previously mentioned in Chapter 3, there are insulin receptors on the ovaries. When high levels of insulin are detected by the ovarian receptors, this alters certain enzymes leading the ovaries to release more androgens rather than the usual balance of oestrogens. The higher levels of androgens then trigger the pancreas to release higher levels of insulin, a vicious cycle that leads of course to more androgens being released by the ovaries. Insulin is the fat-storing hormone, so this high insulin/high androgens circuit is the major cause of the rapid weight gain and inability to lose weight experienced by women with PCOS. Also excess androgens stop the ovaries from releasing eggs, causing irregular or non-existent periods.

The good news is that hormones can be brought into balance by diet, and insulin levels can be controlled. The authors of two excellent, specialist books on PCOS, *The PCOS Diet*[3] and *PCOS and Your Fertility*[4], Colette Harris and Theresa Cheung, have a very reassuring message for women with PCOS. They state that 70 per cent of women with PCOS conceive naturally. That means that you may have challenges, but it is a far from impossible feat, and, based on mounting research, there is a great deal you can do with diet and lifestyle changes to maximize your chances of conceiving and having a full-term healthy pregnancy.[5]

Magnesium Deficiency

Some 50–70 per cent of all PCOS sufferers either have impaired glucose tolerance, insulin resistance or full diabetes. Groundbreaking research into the cause of insulin resistance and the cluster of insulin–glucose imbalances known as metabolic syndrome X was published in 1992 by Professor Lawrence Resnick from Cornell University Medical School. Dr Resnick's team found out that low magnesium levels inside the cell was a key factor leading to insulin resistance[6], diabetes and high blood pressure. They found that, when the levels of magnesium were low inside the cell, and, correspondingly, levels of calcium were high, the metabolic functioning was adversely affected in a number of ways, all of which are tremendously relevant to women with PCOS.

It is my strong suspicion that a magnesium deficiency could be one of the main causes of PCOS and I hope further research will be undertaken in this area. In the meantime, in light of the universal fertility-enhancing benefits of magnesium, I recommend all women with PCOS to take this as a supplement.

Genetic Factors

It does appear that PCOS can run in families and genetics have been cited as a likely culprit.[7] If you are not aware of any family members having PCOS, but are aware of a family tendency to insulin resistance/type 2 diabetes/'apple' body shape fat distribution, then there may be more of a genetic susceptibility to PCOS, especially if you eat a high-sugar and refined-carbohydrate rich diet, which is also likely to be deficient in magnesium. But, remember, genetics are not destiny and PCOS is not your inevitable fate if you eat a wholefood, low-glycaemic diet.

PCOS, Body Weight and Fertility

As discussed in Chapter 9, being under or overweight can impair fertility. The good news is that, although PCOS combined with being overweight increases the risk of infertility, this can be reversed by weight loss.[8]

Losing as little as 5–10 per cent of your weight can be sufficient to break the vicious cycle of insulin overload and PCOS, to stimulate ovulation and normalize periods.[9]

Losing weight with PCOS can be difficult. You can help yourself by trying to stay unstressed. Stress management is purely individual and I am sure you do not need any trite suggestions from me about meditation or aromatherapy baths with candles. You may unwind by hitting a punch bag, or by getting a manicure or stroking a kitten. Acupuncture is one of the best ways to restore harmony in the hormonal mayhem that is characterized by PCOS. The point is that, whatever you know works for you, remember to do it – regularly!

Women under stress are more likely to have higher testosterone levels and lower oestrogen, thus making all the symptoms of PCOS worse.

What to Eat to Heal PCOS

Following the general principles of the Fertility Diet will bring much relief from the symptoms of PCOS. There are, however, certain aspects I would like to emphasize.

Avoid All High Glycaemic Foods

If you have PCOS there is no room for cheating. You must avoid all high-glycaemic foods as your highest priority. The glycaemic index (GI) refers to the ability of carbohydrates to raise blood sugar; foods with a low GI raise blood sugar more slowly than foods with a high GI. The higher the GI of a food, the more insulin is released, so high GI foods stimulate the highest insulin release and all women with PCOS should steer well clear of them. These include candies, cakes, cookies, honey, sweets, white flour (including white bread and pasta), white rice and rice cakes, and white sugar, all packaged and junk foods, and breakfast cereals containing sugar. The high glycaemic vegetables to steer clear of are: cooked carrots, parsnips, peas, potatoes (including crisps and French fries) and cooked sweetcorn. In their raw state these vegetables have higher fibre which is destroyed in the cooking process. The fibre slows down the release of sugar into the bloodstream, so you may eat raw carrots, parsnip and sweetcorn in moderation. Raw potatoes are never recommended. All tropical fruits should be avoided for as long as you have PCOS symptoms: bananas, mango, papaya and pineapple all contain very high amounts of sugar, as do dried fruits such as dates, figs, raisins and apricots.

However, a low glycaemic index diet can control the symptoms of PCOS and help weight loss.[10] Eat your heart out on all the fruit and vegetables (save for the high glycaemic ones mentioned above), nuts and seeds you want. These, together with wholegrains are the richest sources of magnesium. So brown rice, oats, quinoa, wholegrains, wholewheat bread and wholewheat pasta are also on the menu (but don't go crazy on wheat products if you suspect a gluten intolerance). If you can find fish from pure sources (i.e. no PCBs or heavy metals as are found in the bigger ocean fish, or colourants like farmed fish) and free-range organic eggs, these are also OK in moderation (about three times a week). Other sources of concentrated proteins such as meat and diary, while low on the glycaemic index, are not recommended for the reasons set out earlier in this book.

Buckwheat

A special note on buckwheat, which can be found in the form of bran, flour, grits, groats and kasha (my favourite). Buckwheat, particularly its bran, contains a compound called d-chiro-inositol, which is naturally produced by our bodies in response to insulin and has a key role in insulin receptivity. So stock up on buckwheat bran, and find ways to incorporate it regularly in your diet.

Cinnamon

For anyone with PCOS, insulin resistance or diabetes, cinnamon needs to become your new best friend. It promotes insulin sensitivity at the cellular level and helps regulate blood sugar. Try it in hot drinks, sprinkled on fruit, in healthy desserts (see the Recipes section), on oatmeal – anywhere you can incorporate it.

How to Beat Sugar Cravings

It's official: biochemically, the effect of eating high-carbohydrate foods is to trigger brain chemicals with the same mood-elevating effects as cocaine.[11] So, for me to tell you just to stop eating them, even with the powerful motivation of wanting to beat PCOS and have a baby, is not very helpful without a few nutritional tricks given to support you.

The supplemental amino acid l-glutamine, which I take myself two to three times a day to treat a sweet tooth, reduces cravings for sugar, carbohydrates and alcohol. The supplement 5-HTP (5-hydroxytryptophan) also helps address carbohydrate cravings that are caused by feeling stressed out and low on serotonin. Enjoy healthy, low-glycaemic sweeteners such as xylitol and agave nectar, which is a low-glycaemic, high-mineral nectar that comes from the agave cactus, which grows in Arizona, Mexico, Greece and other countries with warm climates. It tastes like a cross between maple syrup and honey and can be used wherever you need (or want!) a sweet liquid syrup. It is delicious stirred into herbal teas, flax seed and fruit puddings, on wholegrain or buckwheat pancakes, as well as in fruit and nut-milk smoothies. You can even bake with it. See the Recipes section for further suggestions and how to use this yummy nectar.

Avoid High-glycaemic Drinks

Beer scores 120 on the glycaemic index; pure cane sugar comes in at only 100! All alcohol has high levels of sugar with zero fibre or fat to slow its absorption into the bloodstream and must not be consumed. Beer, spirits and cocktails are worse than wine. Red wine is, perhaps, the best, lowest sugar of a very bad lot, but, if you have PCOS, a single glass could be sufficient to send your insulin into overdrive and worsen all your symptoms (and just one glass per week will reduce your fertility by one third, remember). It's just not worth it.

Packaged fruit juice is little more than sugar water and should not be drunk. Freshly squeezed juice is nutritionally far better, but still pure fruit juice without the fibre of the whole fruit is going to cause a big insulin spike. If you enjoy fruit juice in the morning, I recommend blending whole fruits (peeled if necessary, of course) together with some mineral water into a delicious fruit smoothie.

Avoid Caffeine

All caffeinated beverages stimulate insulin release – sorry, but, as you know from Chapter 5, caffeine is also a great contraceptive. Switch to herbal or rooibos tea, herbal/grain coffees or decaf tea or coffee, which has been decaffeinated naturally. Note, however, that all decaffeinated tea and coffee still contains small traces of caffeine, which will be causing some increase in insulin, so these are not as beneficial as caffeine-free drinks. Diet colas are off-limits both for their caffeine content and for their aspartame content, which causes prolactin levels to rise; prolactin is a hormone that is already too high in 60 per cent of PCOS sufferers and interferes with ovulation. If you are used to drinking caffeine to get you going in the morning or to deal with the fatigue that is so common with PCOS, then my nutritional tip is to take the supplemental amino acid l-tyrosine – nature's stimulator – in the morning. Do not take this later in the day or it can interfere with sleep.

Helpful Supplements

Alpha-lipoic Acid

Alpha-lipoic Acid (ALA) has been shown to lower chronically high levels of glucose and insulin. It generally appears to help with glucose metabolism, since it is a vital nutrient for the production of energy at the cellular level. Interestingly, many diabetics and or those with hyper insulinism/syndrome x are deficient in ALA.[12] For those with PCOS it will also help improve insulin sensitivity, reduce insulin resistance, and help the body metabolize glucose from food, which will contribute to maintaining a healthy weight.

Chromium

Chromium has a number of benefits for the PCOS sufferer, the majority of whom will be insulin resistant. Chromium is needed for the metabolism of glucose and, without it, insulin is less effective in controlling blood sugar levels. Chromium is the major nutrient in so called Glucose Tolerant Factor, and acts as a transport mechanism to enable insulin to work more quickly and effectively. It enhances insulin receptivity and a number of studies have shown it to be exceptionally effective in helping to prevent and reverse type 2 non-insulin-dependent diabetes. In one study of both types of diabetes, researchers found that a chromium supplement enabled 75 per cent of the participants to reduce their medicine by as much as 30 per cent.[13] All of this is good news for women with PCOS, the majority of whom will be insulin resistant.

Even better, chromium has been the most widely researched mineral in regard to its effectiveness as an aid to weight loss. With sufficient chromium levels you store less fat and use more calories to build muscle. One study showed that people who took chromium picolinate over a ten-week period lost an average of 1.9 kg (4.2 lb) of fat while those on a placebo lost only 0.2 kg (0.4 lb).[14] A further 1998 study reported in Current Therapeutic Research found that individuals who took chromium supplements had an average weight loss of 2.8 kg (6.2 lb) of body fat, whereas those taking placebos lost 1.5 kg (3.4 lb). No lean body mass, i.e. muscle tissue, was lost. Many women with PCOS have frustrating weight gain that appears immune to dieting. Chromium will help – it has the positive attributes of gradually lowering body fat, accompanied by sustained energy levels and, most importantly, diminished cravings and reduced hunger.

Signs of a chromium deficiency include high cholesterol, fatigue, overweight and premature ageing.

Good food sources of chromium include apples, raw carrots, green vegetables, rye bread, sea vegetables and wholewheat bread. Be patient, however, chromium does not work overnight. Its effect builds up slowly and it may be a month or more before you notice any difference.

Essential Fatty Acids

Together with fibre, consumption of fat is the other way to slow the release of sugar into the bloodstream. But, as I hope has become clear by now, not all fats are created equal. Saturated animal fats, such as from meat and dairy products, block weight loss and cause inflammation thanks to the arachidonic acid content. On the other hand, 'good fats' – the omega 3 fats from plant sources as well as from fish oils – can help both with weight loss and in balancing blood sugar.

I would single out flax seeds in particular. They are not just the richest source of omega 3 fats (27 times more than salmon), they help to stabilize blood sugar. One of my favourite breakfasts is a fruit and flax pudding, which I make by blending any fruit, a small amount of water, and flax seeds I have soaked overnight in mineral water. This is a lot more sustaining than a pure fruit breakfast, since the flax moderates the release of the glucose from the fruit.

L-Carnitine

This amino acid assists in the transportation of fats to the mitochondria, the cells' power stations, for conversion into energy. Particularly when taken on an empty stomach it can help break down body fat. It is also a fertility enhancer – see Chapter 17.

Magnesium

As mentioned above, magnesium plays a key role in the proper regulation of blood sugar and insulin in the body. I highly recommend daily supplementation for women with PCOS. The best food sources are leafy dark vegetables, sea vegetables and wholegrains. Raw cacao – raw chocolate – is also loaded with magnesium and many other healing phytonutrients, which I enjoy from time to time in smoothies – see Recipes (it is a great aphrodisiac too). I hesitate to recommend this as a magnesium source for women with PCOS, however, because of its caffeine content that will trigger insulin release. This is perhaps a food to have strictly in small amounts, until you are satisfied that your PCOS is healed and that your glucose/insulin metabolism is working well.

N-acetyl-cysteine (NAC)

An important precursor to the cellular antioxidant glutathione, NAC has been found to improve insulin sensitivity in women with PCOS at doses of 1.8 g per day for normal weight women and 3 g per day for obese patients.[15]

Vanadium

This trace mineral has been shown in a number of studies to enhance insulin sensitivity particularly in the liver[16] and has been used in the treatment of diabetes. If you decide to take this as a supplement then it is important to find one derived from organic compounds; there are concerns over the potential toxicity of the inorganic/synthetic forms. The richest food source is dill seeds. But it is also found in parsley and many vegetables, grains and cereals as well as lobsters.

Zinc

The fertility wonder mineral also helps support insulin sensitivity, so is recommended for women with PCOS.

Herbs

The details and benefits of the following herbs in balancing hormones, regulating periods and boosting fertility have been set out in Chapter 16, so I only need say they are excellent for women with PCOS: black cohosh, dong quai, false unicorn root (*Chamaelirium luteum*), motherwort, red raspberry leaf, saw palmetto and (true) unicorn root.

I have, however, come across research on a few more herbs, which, while not of general applicability to women with fertility issues, have been found to be useful in the treatment of PCOS specifically and I would invite you to discuss them with your herbalist/homeopath to ascertain whether they would be of benefit to you.

Extracts of *Peony lactiflora* (White Peony) and *Glycyrrhisa uralensis* (Liquorice)

There have been three studies showing that a combination of these herbs in a 50/50 mixture can result in a complete healing of PCOS.[17] Peony and liquorice together normalize adrenal function, balance hormones and reduce testosterone levels. It is recommended to consult a herbalist to obtain these herbs so that you can be personally advised on the appropriate dose for you, especially since liquorice should only be taken to regularize menstrual cycles and must not be taken when pregnant/actively trying to conceive.

Fenugreek
Fenugreek appears to lower blood sugar levels by slowing down glucose absorption in the intestines and improving glucose tolerance (use of sugar once absorbed).[18] Note, however, that this should not be taken during pregnancy.

Japanese Herbs
Research on each of the herbs sairei-to, shkuyaku-kanzo-to (TJ 68) and unkei-to from Japan has found them to help women with PCOS, irregular cycles and infertility.[19]

Shatawari
This Ayurvedic (traditional Indian medicine) herb is said to help restore normal menstrual cycles by balancing hormones.

Unicorn root
So-called 'true' unicorn root, this North American herb is a remedy to heal menstrual problems; in particular it is good for restarting periods that have stopped.

Common-sense Caution

As I keep emphasizing, the details of the various medicinal herbs in the Fertility Diet are provided for your information, so that you are aware of natural (but powerful) alternatives to the pharmaceuticals your doctor will suggest. Because of their potency and strong impact on hormones and health in general, I do not encourage the self-prescribing of herbs, and would urge anyone interested in exploring Mother Nature's medicine chest to contact a qualified herbalist, doctor of Chinese medicine, naturopathic doctor or homeopath for appropriate advice.

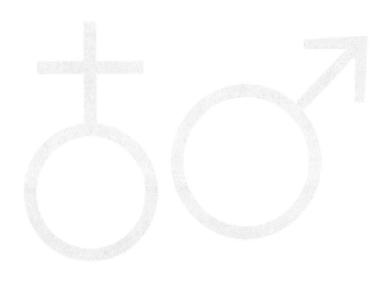

Fertility Action Plan

- Keep your insulin levels in check by eating only low glycaemic/low-sugar foods and using cinnamon as a spice in any sweet foods.

- Try to maintain a healthy body weight, losing weight if necessary.

- Take magnesium and chromium supplements.

- Make an appointment with a herbalist to see what herbs could be beneficial for you.

Chapter 28
Endometriosis

Endometriosis is a painful condition in which tissue from the lining of the uterus (the endometrium) is found outside the uterus where it does not belong, usually in the pelvis or the abdomen or, in rare cases, even in the lungs, brain and spinal cord. These rogue endometrial implants are hormonally responsive, and shed internally during menstruation. Unlike normal endometrial tissue lining the uterus, however, the blood has no way to exit the body and so accumulates in the area of the implant causing painful inflammation, scarring and adhesions that can literally tie up organs with sticky blood.

The typical symptoms of endometriosis are debilitating, crampy pain during periods, painful intercourse, and painful bowel movements, in particular during menstruation. Infertility is another symptom of this disorder.

Endometriosis is estimated to affect two out of every ten women worldwide. It is, in fact, the second most-common condition recognized by reproductive endocrinologists and is found equally amongst all ethnic groups of women.

Why Does It Affect Fertility?

As many as 50 per cent of women with fertility problems have endometriosis. Not all women with endometriosis are infertile, however; it is estimated some 30–40 per cent of them may have difficulty conceiving. This is a catch-22 situation, since pregnancy itself is one of the best treatments for the condition – the cessation of menstruation during pregnancy, and breastfeeding, cause the implants to shrivel up and die.

Endometriosis damages fertility in a number of ways:

- The implants or adhesions may cause blockages in the Fallopian tubes.
- The implants themselves are not just hormonally responsive, they are hormonally active and generate their own oestrogen from the adrenal glands by an enzyme pathway called the aromatase pathway. This leads to further hormone imbalance, in particular oestrogen dominance.
- The implants trigger the release of cytokines – inflammatory immune cells that are toxic to any implanting embryo.
- High levels of inflammatory prostaglandins (hormone precursors), which are caused both by the endometrial implants and a diet heavy in meat and dairy products, cause contractions in the Fallopian tubes, which leads to the egg being expelled too quickly.
- Endometriosis leads to abnormal ovulation: too many follicles begin to develop, but do not mature; then unruptured follicle syndrome, where a follicle develops

but is not released from the ovary into the Fallopian tubes; or also infrequent ovulation.
• Endometriosis is also linked to early miscarriage.

What Causes Endometriosis?

There are a number of theories as to what may cause or contribute to the development of endometriosis.

'Retrograde Menstruation'

One common theory behind endometriosis, developed in the 1920s by Dr Sampson, is that it is caused by a back flux of menstrual fluid through the Fallopian tubes and into the pelvic cavity.[1] This seems plausible, since most endometrial implants are found in close proximity to the opening of the Fallopian tubes on the outer surfaces of the ovaries and uterus and in the base of the pelvis. It is normal for women to have some refluxed endometrial fluid in their pelvic cavity. However, a number of factors can lead to an increase in the normal reflux of menstrual blood:

1. Intercourse during menstruation: one study of 500 women investigating a link between sexual activity and endometriosis, found that women who had sex during their period had an increased rate of endometriosis as well as a higher risk of infertility caused by Fallopian tube abnormalities.[2]

2. Consumption of meat and dairy products: meat and diary products contain arachidonic acid, which triggers the release of an inflammatory prostaglandin called PG2. Not only does this prostaglandin exacerbate any existing endometriosis causing great inflammation and pain, an imbalance in prostaglandins (i.e. more inflammatory than anti-inflammatory) may actually allow excess amounts of endometrial fragments to reflux up the Fallopian tubes by increasing uterine spasm and dilating the Fallopian tubes' diameter.[3]

3. Long-term use of tampons: Research suggests a link between the use of tampons for more than fourteen years and endometriosis.[4]

4. Women who have a blockage preventing blood from flowing out of the vagina, such as a congenital defect or even an imperforated hymen (i.e. they are a virgin), may have higher volumes of refluxed endometrial fluid and a greater probability of endometriosis.[5]

Since some refluxed endometrial fluid is perfectly normal during menstruation but only an average of 20 per cent of women get endometriosis, it is clear that this is only part of the causation and not the sole explanation. It does not account for how endometriosis has been found in men (see below), although, of course, this is very rare! Nor does it explain how endometrial implants could be found in the lungs and spinal cord, some distance from the uterus. It appears to me that whether refluxed endometrial fragments turn into full-blown endometriosis is dependent upon excess oestrogen/hormone imbalance, inflammation/imbalance in prostaglandins, as well as the immune system being under par.

Congenital Defect

Another theory for the occurrence of endometriosis has been developed by David Redwine, MD of the St Charles Medical Center in Bend, Oregon. He suggests that endometriosis is in fact a type of minor birth defect, whereby cells that were destined to become part of the female reproductive organs as the foetus developed in the mother's womb actually failed to make it to their appropriate location, getting left behind and ending up in areas of the pelvic cavity outside the uterus. They then lie dormant until such time as the endometriosis sufferer hits puberty, when the rogue tissues 'wake-up' again under stimulation from rising hormone levels. In other words, it is a condition you are born with. Dr Redwine believes that endometriosis is constant in amount, not growing, so is thus effectively curable by the surgical removal of all implants.

Circulation of Endometrial Fragments by the Lymph

Yet another theory proposes that endometrial fragments can pass into the lymph during menstruation, since the uterus has a very rich network of lymphatic vessels, and this explains how tissues from the endometrium can be found at some distance from the uterus and pelvic cavity, such as the lungs and joints, having been deposited there by the flow of the lymph. While this may explain how the fragments could migrate in the body, it does not really answer why the lymph, as part of the body's sewage system, does not simply dump them in the intestines for excretion along with other wastes, or why the immune system does not break down the endometrial tissue in the lymph or elsewhere (outside the uterus).

Excess Oestrogen Triggering Cellular Change

It has been found that the cells on the surfaces of tissues (epithelial cells) have the astonishing ability to metamorphose into other types of cell! This is the only possible explanation for endometriosis being found in men. For example, in Australia, three men were found to have endometrial implants in their bladders after they had been taking oestrogenic drugs for prostate cancer.[6] Of course, in men this is a medical rarity and requires a massive hormonal imbalance in the form of excess oestrogen.

For the usual endometriosis in women other researchers think that the cells lining the pelvic cavity have altered to become endometrial cells and they then respond to hormonal signals in the same way as normal endometrial cells lining the uterus.[7] This is regarded as an immune system issue, but it seems an excess of oestrogen may play a role here too.

Exposure to Environmental Toxins: Dioxins and PCBs

One thing all endometriosis sufferers have in common is excessively high oestrogen levels. This hormone imbalance can be caused by exposure to such toxins as dioxin, PCBs (from plastics) and other xenoestrogens (fake/chemical oestrogens) such as those found in pesticides and plastics, which in turn leads to endometriosis.[8] As early as 1985 Canadian researchers had found that exposure to PCBs caused endometriosis in monkeys.[9] Later research has confirmed that monkeys exposed to dioxins all get endometriosis; the higher the concentration of dioxin, the more severe the endometriosis.[10] This research is compelling evidence of the role played by environmental pollutants in the development of endometriosis since the disorder is extremely rare among monkeys and apes. What is very worrying is that the endometriosis in the monkeys did not develop until years after the exposure – as many as ten years. In our polluted world, dioxins (a by-product of the manufacturing industry, which is blown by the wind on to all crops, including organic crops) are found in almost all foods, but in concentrated amounts in animal fat (i.e. meat and dairy). This means that many women may be walking around with a potential endometriosis time bomb and unaware of this causal connection, since we do not live in the controlled environment of a laboratory. Even more terrifying, the dose of dioxins added to the monkeys' water, which caused endometriosis, was minuscule. As Dr Elizabeth Vliet so eloquently put it in her book *It's my Ovaries, Stupid!*[11]: 'similar to you spitting once into an Olympic size swimming pool and trying to measure the effects of your saliva'. The dosage given to the monkeys that caused the severest endometriosis, is less than half the amount most women will encounter in daily life. There is now research on human females showing the link between dioxin exposure and endometriosis.[12]

To minimize your exposure to further dioxins, it is important to eat organic food as far as possible and to avoid, yet again, meat and dairy products which have the highest levels of dioxins, even if they are organically produced. Since dioxins are chlorinated hydrocarbons that are found in bleached feminine hygiene products, it is also important to switch to non-bleached natural varieties of sanitary napkins and tampons and to avoid all other chlorine-bleached paper products. It is also imperative to detoxify your system to remove these environmental pollutants, which is possible by, for example, green juice fasting with supplemental liquid zeolite (see Chapter 18).

Exposure to Radiation/Electromagnetic Fields

Research concerning 500 American office workers found that women who worked with computer monitors/visual display units (VDUs) were three-and-a-half times more likely to have endometriosis than women who did not. If you must work with a computer then either attach a protective screen to the monitor, which shields against electromagnetic radiation, or invest in a flat-screen monitor which is also better. Try to take all breaks away from the computer and, of course, turn it off when it is not in use.

Prostaglandin Imbalance: Consumption of Meat and Dairy Products

Women with endometriosis have been found to have an imbalance in prostaglandins, with an excess of inflammatory prostaglandins (PGE2) and too few anti-inflammatory prostaglandins. This adversely affects ovulation, fertilization, embryo development and the functioning of the Fallopian tubes. Diet has a big influence on the ratio of prostaglandins. The arachidonic acid found in meat and dairy products increases inflammatory prostaglandins, and thus pain. On the other hand, the consumption of plant fats, such as evening primrose oil, flax seed, pumpkin seeds, as well as fish oils, reduces inflammation in the body by enhancing the production of anti-inflammatory prostaglandins.

Eliminating meat and dairy products from the diet is an essential step to alleviating endometriosis and to enhancing fertility.

Other Contributory Factors

Alcohol

Research has also found that women with endometriosis tended to consume more alcohol than women who did not drink.[13] A study which established reduced fertility with even moderate consumption of alcohol also noted endometriosis was often a factor.[14]

Caffeine

Women who drank between five and seven grams of caffeine per month – the equivalent of two cups of coffee or four cups of tea per day – have been shown to have a significantly increased risk of endometriosis.[15] The Physicians Committee for Responsible Medicine also confirms high caffeine consumption is linked to the disorder.[16]

Lack of Exercise

One study from Harvard Medical School found that women who had exercised more than seven hours a week before their mid-twenties, had one-fifth the average risk of developing endometriosis.[17] The Physicians Committee for Responsible Medicine have also advised that women who exercise more than two hours per week have half the risk of endometriosis as those who do not.[18] Furthermore, regular exercise has also been found to decrease the rate of oestrogen production in the body.[19]

Healing Endometriosis Through Diet

Eating to Reduce Oestrogen Levels/Balance Hormones

Fibre helps remove excess oestrogen from the body. Eating a low-fibre diet of refined foods will be causing oestrogen to accumulate in your system, creating the hormonal environment which endometriosis needs to flourish. By massively increasing your intake of fibre in the form of fresh fruit and vegetables, and in particular flax seeds (which have the added anti-oestrogen benefits described below), you will be enabling your body to eliminate excess oestrogen through the bowels.

Eat foods that have certain mild plant oestrogens in which help to reduce oestrogen levels by a process called 'competitive inhibition': these are alfalfa, apples, barley, carrots, cherries, citrus fruit, flax seeds, oats and plums.

Eating bitter foods such as chicory, cabbages and radicchio also helps to balance the hormones, according to the principles of traditional Chinese medicine.

Sweet potatoes and yams are the foods with the highest amount of natural progesterone, and so are strongly recommended. I suggest you eat these daily if you like them. They are also a wonderful food to prevent miscarriage.

Eliminate Meat and Dairy Products

Meat and dairy products are the first items that should be removed from the diet. The arachidonic acid contained in the fat of meat and diary is pro-inflammatory, stimulates the release of the pain-inducing prostaglandin PG2 and worsens endometriosis. Since the implants also themselves cause PG2 release and inflammation this leads to acute pain. Secondly, meat and dairy products are the most fattening foods you can eat: 1 lb of meat equals 2,000 calories; 1 lb of cheese adds up to 1,600 calories. Compare that to green vegetables (100 calories per pound) or fruit (250 calories), foods that keep you slim. Fat cells release estrone, the back-up form of oestrogen. The more body fat you have, the higher your general oestrogen levels will be. Focusing on low-calorie, nutritionally dense foods will enable your body weight to normalize, and any excess fat to slowly be burned away – naturally bringing your oestrogen levels down.

Eat Anti-inflammatory Foods

In contrast to meat and dairy products, which worsen pain and inflammation, certain foods reduce the inflammation caused by endometrial implants and the associated pain. These are good plant fats: flax seeds and flax seed oil, hemp seeds, leafy dark-green vegetables, pumpkin seeds, walnuts, as well as fish oils (from a pure source) which contain linoleic acid, thus stimulating the anti-inflammatory prostaglandin PG3.

Other organic vegetable oils such as safflower, sesame

seed, sunflower and, again, walnut and flax seeds when eaten raw, such as in salad dressings, contain linoleic acid, which is also anti-inflammatory, as is evening primrose oil, which contains gamma-linoleic acid. These good fats have been found to reduce the size of endometrial implants.

Flax seeds should be consumed every day by anyone suffering from endometriosis for all their fertility and health-enhancing advantages.

Supplements to Heal Endometriosis

A general magic formula for increasing progesterone levels (to balance too high oestrogen levels) includes vitamin B6, magnesium, vitamin E and evening primrose oil. It is recommended that all women with endometriosis take these micronutrients. Full details of the micronutrients described below are included in Chapter 16. What follows is just the briefest summary of the most helpful for endometriosis.

Magnesium

Magnesium is a key mineral for alleviating pain, spasms and cramping. Magnesium soothes the central nervous system, and is critical in the prevention of miscarriage.

Vitamins B1, B6 and B12

B vitamins help the body in getting rid of excess oestrogen. B6 is one of the best vitamins for balancing all hormonal levels. Vitamins B1, B6 and B12 in combination inhibit inflammation and pain.

Vitamin E

Apart from all its other amazing fertility-enhancing benefits, vitamin E inhibits inflammation in the body, so helps in the healing of endometriosis.

Zinc

This superstar fertility mineral is also another powerful anti-inflammatory micronutrient, which supports good immunity and assists the essential fatty acids to be metabolized into the anti-inflammatory prostaglandins.

L-Phenylalanine

This amino acid, naturally found in high cacao chocolate, is an essential component in the manufacture of dopamine and pain-relieving endorphins by the brain. It is recommended for reducing all the pain associated with endometriosis.

Probiotics

Possibly as a result of inflammation in the intestines, most women with endometriosis have an imbalance of the good bacteria in the colon. Taking supplemental acidophilus or bifidus, or the remedy triphala (from Ayurvedic, i.e. East Indian, traditional medicine) will help, as will the consumption of healthy fermented foods like sauerkraut or fermented drinks like rejuvelac or kambucha (see Chapter 15 for more information on these fertility drinks).

Herbs to Heal Endometriosis

Please refer to Chapter 16 for full details on these herbs.

Dong Quai

This is a general uterine tonic and is the principle herb recommended for endometriosis by herbalists; it supports proper ovulation.

Marigold (*Calendula officinalis*)

This herb lessens menstrual bleeding, reduces muscle spasm and helps with lymphatic drainage. It is prescribed by herbalists for cases of menstrual disorders with impaired immune function or when there is dull, congestive pain with heavy bleeding.

Vitex/Wild Chasteberry

This potent herb directly affects the pituitary and helps regulate hormonal balance.

Healing Endometriosis by Fasting

Apart from the elimination of meat and dairy products and the massive increase in good plant fats in the diet, my top tip for endometriosis sufferers is to fast, while taking supplemental proteolytic enzymes. During a fast, by a process known as autolysis, the body, in its infinite wisdom, consumes diseased and dying cells and toxic residues, and miraculously spares essential organs, lean tissue and muscles. The body turns all its systems and enzymes, which are normally fully engaged in the process of digesting food, towards the elimination of all superfluous and waste material. Even tumours and uterine fibroids have been found to disintegrate while fasting. Although I can find no research directly on this, by using common sense, it is obvious that endometrial implants and adhesions will be regarded as rubbish by the body and broken down during a fast. Proteolytic enzymes, i.e. protein-digesting enzymes, such as a brand called Vitalzym, enhance this process. The full scoop on the fertility-enhancing benefits of fasting is set out in Chapter 18.

Other Helpful Therapies

Finally, a number of complementary therapies have been found to be helpful in alleviating the symptoms of endometriosis: Chinese medicine/acupuncture; colon cleansing (keeping the colon clear supports could immune function and reduces the possibility of inflammation in the body – Chapter 19 deals with colon cleansing); and hydrotherapy (the alternate use of hot and cold water on the pelvic region is meant to ease blood congestion and pain from endometriosis).

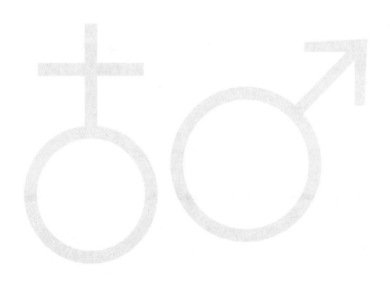

Fertility Action Plan

- Eliminate meat and dairy products as soon as possible to avoid exposure to dioxins, as well as to correct any imbalance in prostaglandins.

- Follow the Fertility Diet guidelines, in particular avoiding alcohol and caffeine.

- Get regular exercise.

- Take supplements of vitamin B6, vitamin E and magnesium.

- Make an appointment with a herbalist to find out which herbs would be most beneficial to you.

Testimonial

Two Beautiful Babies, Despite Endometriosis

At the age of eighteen after a laparoscopy I was diagnosed with severe endometriosis. I was told by the doctors and medical professionals just how difficult it could prove for me to conceive naturally. Of course, I was devastated. After ten years and four further operations – laparoscopies – I had met and married the man of my dreams and it was time to try and start a family. I had discussed my problems with Sarah Dobbyn and her advice was stop smoking and drinking, to eat healthily and, where possible, organically and to take some particular vitamins and supplements.

I took Sarah's advice to heart, and worked hard at my diet and exercise. Happily, after only four months of trying, I discovered I was pregnant. We were delighted, overjoyed and also relieved. Our first daughter was born, a happy and healthy 7 lb 12 oz.

When it came time to try for a second child, I followed the same advice that Sarah had given me previously. This time, much to our complete surprise, it took even less time; just one month later I was pregnant with our second daughter. She was born, a happy and healthy 7 lb 11 oz. After following Sarah's diet and supplement tips through both pregnancies, which were happily uneventful, I can honestly say there isn't a day that goes by that I don't thank my lucky stars – and Sarah's advice – for my 'miracle' babies.

Charlotte A, Cayman Islands, British West Indies, aged 34

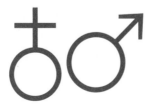

Chapter 29
Uterine Fibroids

The incidence of uterine fibroids is astonishingly high; they affect between 25 and 40 per cent of all women of childbearing age.[1] It is further estimated that 40 per cent of all American women will have a benign uterine fibroid by the time they reach menopause.[2] Particularly at risk are women with African ethnicity, including Afro-Americans and Afro-Caribbean nationals, who have a 50 per cent likelihood of having fibroids, compared with white Caucasians where the chances are around 30 per cent overall.[3] Most alarming of all, fibroids are responsible for 33 per cent of all gynaecological hospital admissions and are the leading cause of hysterectomy.[4] Indeed, all too frequently, hysterectomy is presented to women with fibroids as the only solution to bringing an end to their misery – one that, of course, deprives them of all possibility of having a baby.

So what exactly are fibroids – also called 'leiomyomata' or 'myomata' – of the uterus? They are tumours, usually benign (fewer than 1 per cent turn out to be malignant) that grow from the smooth muscle tissue of the uterus, but are encapsulated in another band of tissue. They grow independently of the uterus: some on the outer wall (subserous fibroids); some inside the uterine cavity (submucosal fibroids) – which can even then be expelled by the body following violent cramping – a so-called aborting submucus myoma; others are found actually inside the uterine wall and are called intramural fibroids; finally, others, known as pedunculated fibroids are attached to the uterus by a stalk. They can be as small as a pea or as large as a beach ball. The medical fraternity seem to like to equate them with different fruit (from lemon to watermelon) or, with some ironic insensitivity if fibroids are the cause behind your infertility, with various stages of pregnancy – such as 'twelve weeks in size'.

Fibroids can cause big problems with fertility. According to a guideline from the American College of Obstetricians and Gynecologists, a woman with a fibroid equating to a twelve-week pregnancy is a candidate for a hysterectomy even if she has no other symptoms![5]

All types of fibroids cause similar distressing symptoms: painful periods – in particular abdominal cramps; heavy menstrual bleeding/prolonged heavy bleeding – including between periods; chronic vaginal discharge; painful intercourse; frequent or uncomfortable urination and bladder infections; incontinence; constipation; backache; and a feeling of fullness or pressure in the lower abdomen. Some woman are lucky enough to have no symptoms at all, and their fibroids are only discovered during a routine gynaecological examination, when the doctor detects abnormal lumps in the uterus. Fibroids interfere with fertility by blocking an egg from implanting, or competing for space with a growing foetus, thereby triggering miscarriage or, later, causing delivery complications.

What Causes Fibroids?

Hormonal imbalance appears to be the root cause of the appearance of fibroids. It is well established that the hormone oestrogen stimulates the growth of the fibroid, so that women who are showing oestrogen dominance (i.e. their oestrogen levels are excessive in relation to their levels of progesterone, testosterone and other hormones such as DHEA) are far more likely to have large and rapidly growing fibroids than women with balanced levels of oestrogen. Fibroids have receptor sites for both oestrogen and progesterone and grow excessively during periods of exceptionally high oestrogen levels, such as during pregnancy or perimenopause. After menopause, when oestrogen levels naturally fall, fibroids also become smaller. There is contradictory research on whether higher levels of progesterone cause fibroids to shrink or grow. However, what does appear to be key is the balance of oestrogen to progesterone levels relative to each other.

Apart from the role played by a poor diet in contributing to hormone imbalance, many holistic practitioners also view fibroids as Nature's way of isolating toxins from food (as well as environmental poisons) that have accumulated in the uterus area and cannot be eliminated through the usual excretory organs, in order to protect the body from their harmful affects. Practitioners of traditional Chinese medicine see it as a condition of mucus congestion in the uterus – a build-up of toxic sludge that the body is having difficulty removing.

A Psycho-spiritual Cause?

According to the well-known medical intuitive Carolyn Myss, fibroid tumours represent creativity that has never been given an outlet or 'birthed', including fantasy images of the self that have never been expressed, as well as creative secrets of other selves. She sees fibroids as resulting when life energy is poured into dead ends – such as jobs or relationships which have been outgrown.[6] Dr Christiane Northrup invites her patients with fibroids to mediate on their relationships with other people and how they express their creativity.[7] If you are in a dead-end job or an unfulfilling relationship, or have a sense that your creativity is blocked or stifled, and you *do* have fibroids, then this hypothesis is one you may wish to explore more deeply. In essence, when your energy is unstuck and flowing creatively, the fibroid can also dissolve along with whatever mental or emotional blocks were holding you back. Dr Northrup had a patient, scheduled for a hysterectomy, who prayed about her fibroids daily. Six weeks later every trace of them was gone and the surgery was cancelled!

Treatment of Fibroids

The answer of conventional medicine in the treatment of fibroids is an array of aggressive surgical interventions. The least severe, in that they at least preserve the uterus and the possibility of pregnancy, are:

1. A myomectomy when the fibroid itself is removed.
2. Cryomyolysis in which the fibroid is destroyed by a probelike instrument that freezes the fibroid's interior.
3. Electromyolysis, which destroys the fibroid's interior by passing an electrical current through it.
4. Laser myolysis which zaps the fibroid with a laser.
5. Uterine artery embolization, which cuts off the blood supply to the tumour.

None of these procedures is without risk or severe pain, and none of them prevents the fibroids from returning if the underlying dietary and lifestyle reasons causing the hormone imbalance that lead to fibroids are not addressed. The most radical solution to fibroids, as previously mentioned, are full and partial hysterectomies. These may put an end to fibroids – but at the cost of terminating fertility.

There is another answer!

A Dietary Solution to Cure Fibroids

If you are a fibroid sufferer, then most likely your immediate concern is 'menorrhagia' – extremely heavy menstrual bleeding – which can last literally all month, together with the passing of large blood clots. It can be like living with a never-ending nightmare period. To remedy this you need to take the herb vitex (wild chasteberry) at a dosage of around 1,200 mg per day, at once. This is the best herb for balancing hormones (see Chapter 16 for more details). Dr Allan Warshowsky, MD, a practising obstetrician and gynaecologist, and author of one of the best books I have found on fibroids, *Healing Fibroids, A Doctor's Guide to a Natural Cure*, also prescribes the herbs yarrow and shepherd's purse to stop bleeding, sometimes almost immediately. He states that these herbs help to heal fibroids by encouraging hormone balance, toning organs and glands, eliminating toxicity and easing congestion in the uterus.[8] Also see Chapter 8 for further details.

Another cure to stop heavy uterine bleeding recommended by the Weston A. Price Foundation involves taking extremely high doses of vitamin A in the form of cod liver oil, since most women with menorrhagia are vitamin A deficient. Initially a high dose of 90,000 iu (that's about 4–5 full tablespoons of cod liver oil) should do the trick, followed by a maintenance dose of 30,000 iu every day (about 1½ tablespoons of cod liver oil). The Weston Price website reports bleeding being cut in half immediately and then stopping within three days on this cod liver oil protocol.[9] On study following seventy-one women with heavy menstrual bleeding found they had significantly lower blood levels of vitamin A compared with women without fibroids. It found 90 per cent of the women had normal levels of bleedings after two weeks of vitamin A therapy.[10] Another study from South Africa found that 50,000 iu of vitamin A reduced bleeding significantly, apparently because of the role of vitamin A in stimulating the production of progesterone.[11]

Food Cure for Fibroids

If you follow all the principles of the Fertility Diet set out in previous chapters, you should notice that your fibroids will shrink and ultimately disappear, and you will have fewer and fewer symptoms as your hormones balance and your fertility increases. Dr Christiane Northrup, who has many years clinical experience, says she normally suggests a three-month trial of a high-fibre, wholefoods diet that eliminates refined sugar and flour products and dairy food.

Following a diet rich in fruit, vegetables and other wholefoods, a woman with fibroids will often experience decreased bleeding, lessened bloating and a decrease in her fibroids.

Supplements

Proteolytic Enzymes

As mentioned at the beginning of this chapter, fibroids are a type of tumour. All tumours, whether benign or malignant, are surrounded by something called a fibrin cloak (a form of blood protein), which is almost like an attempt by the body to wall off the rogue tissue filled with toxins. Fibrin cloaks are a bit like the 'invisibility shields' used by bad guy alien spaceships on *Star Trek*. The downside is, therefore, that tumours are 'invisible' to the immune system. Proteolytic enzymes are the one supplement I would urge women with fibroids (or indeed any one with any kind of tumour or cancer) to get, because they are able to break down the fibrin cloak around (hiding) a tumour, thereby stimulating the body's killer cells (and the anti-cancer macrophages), and overall increasing the body's anti-tumour capacity twelvefold![12]

There are no studies yet to prove this with particular reference to fibroids. However, there is considerable research on the anti-tumour capacity of proteolytic enzymes in general. For instance, German research in the field of breast fibrosis and benign breast fibromas can show 85 per cent of patients have no symptoms after six weeks of enzyme therapy;[13] it seems obvious to me that enzymes are the place to start if you have fibroids and want to dissolve them.

There is no downside to proteolytic enzymes whatsoever: they stimulate the immune system, promote healthy tissue regeneration, remove toxins and waste from the body and are as potent as anti-inflammatory drugs – but with no side effects, except possibly for a mild diarrhoea if you take too many capsules at once.

Proteolytic enzymes need to be taken separately from meals, or they will only serve to help digest your food better, which is a waste of relatively expensive enzymes. From time to time, whenever I want to detox generally, I use an excellent brand of proteolytic enzymes called Vitalzym (as a way to keep my lymph and blood system generally clean). It is best to start out slowly, taking only one capsule three times a day, and building up over time to a medicinal dose of ten capsules three times a day. If you take too many you might get diarrhoea, in which case reduce the dose again. (I would be fascinated to know if my hypothesis about these enzymes destroying fibroids is correct – so please let me know your experiences by contacting me at the details given at the end of the book.)

A full description of the reproductive healing qualities of the following other important micronutrients and herbs is given in Chapter 16. The paragraphs which follow only highlight the key benefits for women with fibroids.

Vitamin A/Beta-carotenes

These promote hormonal balance and normalize bleeding. In high doses they stop bleeding (as mentioned above). They are antioxidants and help detoxify the system.

B Vitamins

Critical for the optimal metabolism of oestrogen and the removal of excess oestrogen from the body. They support a healthy nervous system and counteract the effect of stress, which also appears to play a role in the onset and growth of fibroids.

Vitamin C and Bioflavonoids
Well known for their antioxidant and anti-inflammatory properties, they reduce menstrual blood flow. They help by strengthening capillaries, making them less likely to rupture under the pressure of a growing fibroid. One study showed fourteen out of sixteen women who took 200 mg of vitamin C three times a day experienced reduced bleeding.[14] Together with bioflavonoids it supports hormonal balance needed by women prone to fibroids.

Vitamin E and Selenium
Vitamin E works synergistically with the mineral selenium. It has been dubbed the 'sex vitamin' since it affects so many aspects of the reproductive system. It appears to benefit the pituitary gland – one of the master endocrine glands – and is therefore critical for proper hormone balance. It prevents excess blood clotting and vitamin E can help women with fibroids have normal menstrual blood flow.

Essential Fatty Acids (EFAs)
These fats cannot be manufactured by the body and must be consumed through food or supplements such as fish oils, flax oil, evening primrose oil, borage oil and DHA. They help women with fibroids in a number of ways – they promote hormonal balance, enhance anti-inflammatory factors as well as relieving uterine cramps. Borage oil is particularly good to heal inflammation and cramping. Evening primrose oil is one of the best to optimize hormone levels in general.

Ginseng
There are two types – Gingseng root or Panax, and Siberian gingseng. Panax ginseng will help restore vitality to those completely run down and depleted by fibroids. It is a toner and energizer – but is not recommended for those who may already be highly strung or anxious since it can exacerbate these feelings. It is best taken in the morning, so as not to disturb good sleep. This type of ginseng

should only be taken in the short term; longer-term use can actually cause menstrual abnormalities due to its over stimulating effect.

Siberian ginseng is more important for its role in toning the adrenals and thereby balancing hormones – it may be taken longer term, but should be used in the morning to avoid any possible side effect of insomnia.

Glutathione
A powerful antioxidant that occurs naturally within each cell. It is able to remove toxins found in the fat surrounding organs and glands including the reproductive organs. There is some doubt as to whether supplements of glutathione actually work as well as the natural form the body produces. It is recommended therefore to take the supplement N-Acetyl-Cysteine – a precursor to glutathione, together with vitamin C.

Indole-3-carbinol (I3C)
This compound, found naturally in cruciferous vegetables, is destroyed in the cooking process. I3C assists the liver in the removal of all the 'bad' oestrogen metabolites (called 16 OH and 4 OH oestrogens), which increase the risk for fibroids and all hormone-related illnesses, including cancer of breast, ovary and uterus.

Magnesium
The best supplement to relieve the cramps that are symptomatic of fibroids. This mineral also plays a key role in facilitating the liver's detoxification of hormones including surplus oestrogen.

Methione, Choline and Inosistol
The so-called lipotropic factors are used along with the B vitamins to lower oestrogen levels and relieve symptoms. A dosage of 1,000 mg of each per day is recommended by Dr Christiane Northrup for women with fibroids.[15]

Spirulina

Highly nutritious algae that also contains tumour necrosis factor, a.k.a. tumour-destroying molecules. I recommend taking it daily for everyone trying to conceive, but in particular women with fibroids. Spirulina is something of an acquired taste in its powdered form. I like to add it to delicious smoothies of fresh almond milk, with maca, mesquite and a little agave nectar – yum. It can also be found in capsules.

Zinc

Fertility superstar mineral that both prevents and treats fibroids by optimizing the production and balance of hormones.

Medicinal Herbs

Please see Chapter 16 for a full description of the healing properties of these herbs.

Chamomile

Chamomile tea is a uterine toner and also has a calming effect that counteracts the stress that contributes to fibroid growth.

Dong Quai

One of the best herbs for balancing hormones, especially beneficial for restoring complete gynaecological health when used in combination with vitex (wild chasteberry).

Liquorice Root

The key ingredient in liquorice – glycyrrhizin – helps to normalize oestrogen levels by suppressing levels that are too high and increasing those which are too low. It is a good general anti-inflammatory, toner and energizer for the whole body, in particular the adrenal glands. This should not be taken once you are pregnant, however.

Red Raspberry

This herb reduces menstrual flow (especially when taken in combination with yarrow and shepherd's purse) and relieves cramping in women with fibroids. It assists with all manner of gynaecological problems such as fibroids, by strengthening and toning the uterus. Its use should be stopped once you are pregnant.

Sarsparilla

This herb contains progesterone-like compounds that help to balance out high oestrogen levels. It also tones reproductive organs and glands and increases libido!

Saw Palmetto

Saw Palmetto eases uterine cramps and tones the uterus. Some healers claim that long-term use causes the breasts to enlarge.

Shepherd's Purse

A remedy to stop excessive bleeding. For best, fastest results, take together with yarrow and red raspberry leaf.

Squaw Vine (*Mitchella repens*)

This is good when combined with red raspberry for relieving cramping, pelvic congestion and balancing hormones.

Vitex/Wild Chasteberry

Vitex is my number one recommended herb for women with fibroids, owing to its ability to balance and normalize all sex hormone levels. As a tonic for the entire reproductive system, it actually directly affects the pituitary, increasing the levels of luteinizing hormones (necessary for ovulation to take place) and consequently also increasing progesterone levels. A number of studies have shown that this herb can actually shrink fibroid tumours. Very good to be taken in combination with dong quai as well.

Yarrow

A herb that can be used to stop excessive bleeding, particularly when taken together with shepherd's purse and red raspberry leaf.

Food to Avoid

Basically, all the Fertility Diet no-nos are off the list if you want to get rid of fibroids. Soya, meat, dairy, wheat, gluten, sugar, junk food, fried foods and alcohol are the worst offenders.

Unless your fibroids are at a size that they are life threatening or are causing serious damage to neighbouring organs, change your diet to improve your condition. By following the recommendations in this chapter, in particular under the guidance of a competent herbalist or practitioner of Traditional Chinese Medicine, you will be able to reduce or eliminate fibroids to the point where they no longer have any impact on your fertility or ability to carry a baby to term. Farewell to fibroids!

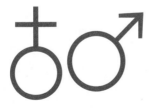

Fertility Action Plan

- Take 4–5 tablespoons of cod liver oil to stop excessive bleeding.

- Take supplements of enzymes (away from meal times).

- Make an appointment to see a herbalist to find out which herbs will be most helpful.

Chapter 30

Changing Your Mind – Reversing Tubal Ligation

According to some estimates, approximately one million American women every year have a bilateral tubal ligation (BTL) – the surgical disconnection of the Fallopian tubes from the ovaries by cutting, clipping, tying or cauterizing the tubes – as a means of permanent birth control. It is estimated that 10,000 later change their minds and have the surgery reversed. Statistics vary as to the percentage of women whose tubes can be successfully reopened. I have read that as many as 90 per cent of reversals are successful, but other sources put the figure closer to only 50 per cent; the outcome depends a great deal on the way in which the BTL was carried out initially, the age of the woman, her general reproductive health and, of course, the skill of the surgeon.

Women over 40, in particular, who have had a BTL may be encouraged to have IVF instead of a reversal. But the chances of conceiving are much higher with a reversal (approximately 65 per cent of couples conceive in the first year after the reversal surgery) compared to IVF (an average of only a 15 per cent chance of having a baby).

Few books on fertility seem to address the unique position of a woman who has reversed a BTL and is trying to have a baby, and nowhere are there any dietary recommendations. Following the Fertility Diet will surely your chances of conception.

Hormonal Impact of Tubal Ligation

One of the best-kept secrets in the gynaecological world is the hormonal impact of having your tubes tied. If you are reading this as someone who has had a BTL, I am certain you were reassured that, apart from rendering you infertile, there would be no adverse hormonal changes after the operation. Yet British medical literature had already noted as early as 1951 that 31 per cent of women had abnormal uterine bleeding after a tubal ligation and 16.5 per cent ultimately had a hysterectomy due to new bleeding problems.[1] Further medical studies in the 1970s also found hysterectomy rates were far higher among women with BTL than in women who had not. Dr Elizabeth Vliet observes that this is because the disruption in ovarian function caused by BTL led to abnormal bleeding or other gynaecological problems, which are then being solved by means of hysterectomy.[2]

In Europe, so called post-tubal ligation syndrome is well documented. The typical symptoms indicate a disruption in ovarian function (namely PMS), lower levels of 17-beta estradiol – the metabolically active form of oestrogen, higher levels of progesterone, less regular ovulation, and perimenopausal type symptoms such as irregular cycles, lighter menstrual flow, mood swings, insomnia, more PMS, cramping and even hot flushes.[3]

A plausible theory as to why tubal ligation would hinder

the ovaries and reduce the amount of estradiol being released has been advanced by an Australian gynaecologist called Dr John Cattanach. He notes that the ligations are done at the narrowest part of the Fallopian tubes – the isthmus – at which point the main artery connecting each ovary to the uterus is so close it is 'almost certainly occluded, or at least interrupted, by most of the usual forms of tubal ligation'.[4] Any damage to these arteries of course means less blood flow and higher pressure in the artery, less oxygen being delivered to the ovary and, in turn, decreased hormone production.

How to Boost Fertility Following a Reversal of Tubal Ligation

If Dr Cattanach's hypothesis, set out above, is right, then the gloomy news is that any damage to the ovarian branches of the uterine artery are unlikely to be healed just because your Fallopian tubes are reconnected. It is in fact possible that the subsequent surgery in the key isthmus area could cause further microscopic damage to the arteries, further interrupting blood flow and reducing hormone levels.

Apart from following the general principles of the Fertility Diet to maximize your chances of conceiving, an organic wholefoods plant-based diet will balance hormone levels and support vibrant good health. However, I would like to make certain specific recommendations to women who have had BTL and have had or are considering a reversal.

Acupuncture

Acupuncture treatments are a very effective way to restore full functioning to your ovaries, Fallopian tubes and uterus. The painless insertion of needles will help to restore 'chi' energy and stimulate blood flow to your reproductive organs. Acupuncture also is excellent for dissolving decongestion in the body, so will help detoxify the whole uterus area, and it is a wonderful complimentary therapy to a fertility diet.

Avoid Phytoestrogens

Since post-tubal ligation syndrome is characterized by too little oestrogen, the last thing you need is a diet high in phytoestrogens, which will occupy your oestrogen receptors and prevent any circulating oestrogen you do have from influencing your cells. The worst offenders here are all soya products, the grain millet and the supplement red clover, all of which should all be carefully avoided by anyone with a possible oestrogen deficiency.

Boron

As mentioned previously in Chapter 16, the mineral boron is more effective than hormone replacement therapy in raising levels of estradiol. Indeed, in one study, women given boron supplementation doubled the levels of estradiol found in their blood. It is thought that boron raises estradiol because it boosts the amount of steroid hormones found in the bloodstream. Boron is found in a number of fruit and vegetables: apples, cabbage, grapes, leafy greens, peaches, pears and raisins. It is also found in almonds and hazelnuts.

Dong Quai

Dong quai balances hormones and enhances fertility in women. It is also a blood thinner which, of course, helps keep blood pressure lower, including in the arteries between uterus and ovaries!

Juice Fasting

Fasting on fresh organic fruit and vegetable juices may be of particular benefit to women trying to conceive after a BTL reversal. By a process known as autolysis, the body's metabolic enzymes, which are usually deployed in the digestion of food, are able instead to begin a 'clean-up' operation in the body, removing diseased and dying cells and waste products in the blood. This process is enhanced if proteolytic enzymes (protein digesting enzymes) are taken as a supplement while fasting. I particularly like a brand called Vitalzym. This is the only natural process by which the body can start to deal with and dissolve any blockages in arteries – and will thus heal any obstruction in the uterine arteries and even the Fallopian tubes themselves. See Chapter 18 for full details on how fasting can massively increase your fertility.

Magnesium

Apart from the many fertility-enhancing properties of magnesium set out in Chapter 16, this mineral is key for the health of your blood vessels – including those running from the uterus to the ovaries. It is a vasodilator, it expands blood vessels by improving the function of the cells lining them, making them more flexible. This is a key mineral – it can also be found in leafy greens, nuts, seeds, wholegrains and raw cacao (raw chocolate) – since this will help to optimize the performance of the uterine arteries and mitigate any damage caused to them by surgery.

Vitex (Wild Chasteberry)

This is the best overall herbal tonic for restoring perfect hormonal balance. It functions at the level of the pituitary gland, and will even out levels of oestrogen to progesterone.

Zinc

Zinc is the number one fertility-boosting mineral and will help women trying to conceive after a BTL reversal since it is necessary for the production of oestrogen in the ovaries. It also protects against chromosomal damage that can reduce fertility, particularly in older women.

The Mental–Emotional Connection

I must once again emphasize the huge impact your thoughts and feelings have on your hormones. If you have been berating yourself with guilt and regret for having the BTL in the first place (when, no doubt, your circumstances were very different and you had excellent reasons for making that choice), you will be prompting your adrenals to release the stress hormones adrenalin and cortisol, which suppress fertility and upset hormonal balance. Any techniques you can find to help you to forgive yourself, and to ask your body to forgive you, as well as visualizing health and wholeness in this area, will be very beneficial. Try to find a counsellor or spiritual advisor who can help you deal with any unresolved feelings concerning the original ligation surgery.

A further fascinating fact to cheer you up: according to Dr Allan Warshowsky, a practising obstetrician and gynaecologist for more than twenty years, if one Fallopian tube is not functioning, the remaining 'good' Fallopian tube can reach all the way across the abdominal cavity to grab the egg as it appears from the ovary on the opposite side of the body.[5] Amazing, eh? So, given half a chance, literally, your body will try to help you conceive. I wish you the best of luck.

Remember that you have numbers on your side: 65 per cent of couples conceive within twelve months following a reversal of BTL. If your body is taking a little longer to get on the programme, the suggestions in this chapter should at least increase your chances of having a baby the good old-fashioned way. Good luck.

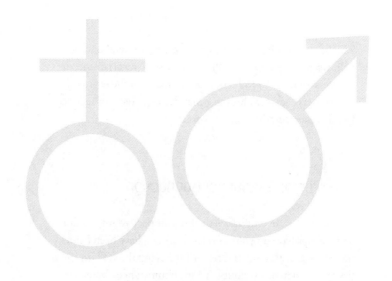

Fertility Action Plan

- Make an appointment to see an acupuncturist to help restore energy to the uterus area.

- Take supplements of boron, zinc and magnesium.

- Take the herbs vitex/wild chasteberry and Dong quai to restore hormonal balance.

- Avoid all foods with phytoestrogens – in particular soya, millet and supplements of red clover.

Chapter 31
Low Sperm Count and Sperm Abnormalities

The man's role in the fertility equation depends, of course, entirely upon both the quantity and quality of his sperm. The international average sperm count is 60 million per millilitre and the usual range per ejaculation is 60–100 million per ml (with a usual volume of 3–4 ml); however, anything above 20 million is considered normal. Compare these figures, though, to a man eating organic food all the time, such as an organic farmer in Denmark with an astonishing average sperm count of 363 million per millilitre, and you start to get the picture as to how much diet can boost your little swimmers.

The widespread decline in eating fresh, wholefoods over the past fifty years – as refined, processed and junk foods have become so readily and cheaply available – together with an ever-increasing bombardment of heavy metals and environmental toxins for most men in the Western world, has taken its toll upon sperm. Research shows that average sperm count in the USA has decreased by 30 per cent since the 1950s. The already lower than average sperm count dropped by a staggering 50 per cent in the period 1982 to 1992 alone.[1] In Europe sperm counts dropped by 3.1 per cent each year from 1971 to 1990.[2]

The number of sperm in seminal fluid is only half the picture for male fertility. The sperm also need to be normal in shape and size (morphology) and they need to have good motility, i.e. to be moving forwards. Unfortunately, an ever-increasing number of abnormalities in sperm quality, motility and development are also becoming apparent.[3]

In Chinese medicine the energy expended in ejaculating is referred to as 'jing', which translates as 'essence'. Non-ejaculatory sex is recommended – unless trying to procreate – in order to preserve this precious elixir.

The production of sperm in the testes, the male nursery organs, is a complex and lengthy process, which can take up to ninety days to complete. So their health and number will be significantly affected by all diet and lifestyle choices made by the man during this time. This is why preparing for conception ought to be a joint project for couples, and ought to commence at least three months ahead of any planned pregnancy to ensure that the sperm, which will provide 50 per cent of the DNA of your future baby, is of the highest possible quality.

Take a little investigation into the factors that cause low sperm count or damage to sperm during the long manufacturing process, and it starts to become clear why the number of infertile men is increasing every year.

How to Commit Spermicide

Smoke

Smoking cigarettes causes both a lower sperm count and a decrease in sperm motility. Studies on smoking show that chemicals in tobacco smoke damage the DNA in sperm and deplete the antioxidant vitamins C and E (see below), which help to protect the sperm from free radical damage. The damaged DNA caused by paternal smoking in turn leads to an increase in the likelihood of miscarriage, stillbirth, birth defects and even of a 70 per cent increase in subsequent childhood cancers.[4] The bottom line is that it is a choice is between a cigarette or a healthy baby – what do you really crave more?

Alcohol

Yes, I am the party pooper. There is now clear evidence that drinking alcohol causes a decrease in sperm count, an increase in abnormal sperm and a lower percentage of motile sperm.[6] Alcohol adversely affects a man's fertility by interfering with the way testosterone is produced and released by the testes.[7] It causes higher levels of female hormones, which extinguish libido, lower sperm count and reduce sperm potency and production. No wonder that 80 per cent of chronic alcoholic men are sterile and that drinking alcohol is a common cause of impotence.[8]

Any sperm produced while alcohol is being consumed will be less healthy and effective.[9] Alcohol is also well known to be a mutagen, i.e. it causes cell mutations.

Alcohol also blocks the absorption of the essential male fertility mineral, zinc, which is essential for the manufacture of healthy sperm by the testes.

Ideally, since it takes between 70 and 90 days for sperm to mature, alcohol should be avoided by men for at least this amount of time prior to planned conception. Once junior is safely on the way, you can hit the bottle (in moderation, of course) if you want to.

Caffeinated Beverages

The more coffee men drink, the more they are likely to have low sperm count and problems with sperm motility or abnormality.[10] Research also shows an increase in miscarriages, stillbirths and premature births of the babies fathered by men who drank caffeine even when their female partner didn't. This is attributed to caffeine's negative impact on the production of sperm.[11] Caffeine also has a diuretic effect, meaning vital fertility nutrients and minerals such as zinc and calcium needed for conception and producing healthy sperm, are thus peed away down the toilet in higher quantities.

So I'm afraid, guys, that it really will matter if you drink caffeinated tea and coffee in the three months prior to trying to conceive, when you will be manufacturing sperm. Try to find organic decaffeinated and caffeine-free beverages that are palatable to you – remember it is only for as long as it takes for the stork to call at your house – then you can head to the nearest Starbucks.

Stress

Men under pressure have lower sperm count and far more abnormal sperm with decreased motility.[12] In one study involving 150 men, stress caused by a death in the family, separation or divorce slowed their sperm adversely enough to affect their ability to conceive.[13] Men on death row – probably the most stressful place of all – have been found to have sperm counts close to zero.

Assisted conception treatments can, of course, be very stressful experiences. A study from 1999, which evaluated the link between psychological stress and sperm quality in forty men in couples undergoing IVF, found that increased stress lead to a significant deterioration in sperm quality. [14]

Stress can impact badly on sperm production and quality. However, once the stressful event is over, sperm count will be restored to previous high levels and healthy quality.

Avoiding as much stress as possible while trying to conceive is recommended, as is finding a way or ways to manage your stress; prioritize whatever works to help you unwind and relax no matter what is going on in your life in order to keep your sperm healthy and abundant.

Heat

Sperm need to keep cool. They require up to three degrees below normal body temperature to develop; it is no accident that the testes are located outside the body. Research from the University of Virginia found that overheating of the testes – from the frequent use of saunas and hot tubs – can result in a lower sperm count.[15] In one of the hundreds of books on fertility I have studied, I read an account about a couple whose infertility issues were cured when the man abandoned his leisurely evening soak in the hot tub in favour of a quick lukewarm shower!

Tight Underwear and Trousers

Into the heated debate comes the issue of whether boxers or briefs are best for keeping the genitalia cool. Unbelievably, there is serious research on this issue! If you wear tight briefs or pants, your testes will be held closer to your body and their temperature will inevitable be higher than if they are well ventilated. So let it all hang out, guys, and stay cool!

Significant prolonged elevations in the temperature of the testicles can adversely affect sperm count.

Mobile Phones

We have known for a while that the electromagnetism from mobile phones can kill off brain cells, but researchers at the Cleveland Clinic in Ohio have now found that the electro-magnetic fields generated by mobile phone handsets are also interfering with sperm production. In a study following 361 male infertility patients, they found that the men who were heavy users of mobile phones had significantly lower sperm counts than those who did not use them. In fact, the research indicated both the quantity and quality of a man's sperm declines in direction proportion to the time he spends on his mobile phone. The most significant effects were seen among men who spoke on their mobile phone more than four hours a day. They had sperm counts 40 per cent lower than men who had never used a mobile phone. Smaller falls in sperm count were found among men who used the phone less often.

In light of this compelling research, my strong advice to any man who would like to father a baby in the near future is to communicate on a landline or by email from a desktop computer. It appears that the radiation from having a mobile phone used in the proximity of your body is likely to damage your sperm significantly.

Illicit Drugs

Marijuana damages the DNA of sperm, increasing the possibility of infertility, miscarriage and birth defects. Cocaine decreases sperm count. Won't an even bigger high be witnessing the birth of your healthy baby? Forget the drugs.

Lubricants

Even non-spermicidal lubricants can kill sperm. The most fruitful approach, literally, is to take time for foreplay and intimacy, so that both partners' own natural lubricants can be secreted, just as nature intended. Saliva may also diminish sperm function. Options that should be OK include vegetable oil, pure water or, according to some sources, egg whites. Yes, I know this sounds messy and disgusting, and you could just end up with a sheet omelette, but the protein in the egg white can actually act like a little sperm snack – nourishing them on their journey.

Echinacea, Ginkgo Biloba and St John's Wort

Heavy use of the herbal supplements echinacea (to boost immunity); ginkgo biloba (to enhance circulation and memory); and St John's Wort (a natural antidepressant) may cause infertility in men and should be avoided. Research has found that these herbs reduce sperm's ability to penetrate the egg, lower sperm viability and damage sperm DNA.

'The greater the use of cell phones, the greater the decrease in these four parameters: sperm count, motility, viability and morphology.' Dr Ashok Argawal at the American Society for Reproductive Medicine Conference in New Orleans, 23 October 2006

Non-organic Foods

Many animal studies have shown how pesticides interfere with fertility, and there is no reason to believe the same is not true in humans. Choose organic foods whenever your circumstances or budget permit to maximize your sperm count.

Supplements to Boost Sperm Count and Quality

Vitamin B12

Vitamin B12 helps to maintain fertility since (in combination with folic acid) it is needed for the production of DNA and RNA, which ensure cells – including the 4 million daily sperm cells on the production line in the testicles – reproduce perfectly. Research has shown it is very important in increasing male fertility: Men with low sperm counts who were given vitamin B12 on a daily basis showed significant increases in sperm count; 25 per cent of the men improved their sperm count by 500 per cent! One very good source of vitamin B12 is to be found in blue-green algae (available in capsules from health stores); this is a wonderful natural source of the vitamin. B12 supplements can also be taken, and B12 injections are available.

Vitamin C

Vitamin C works like a miracle drug on sperm count, motility, viability and in preventing agglutination (the clumping up of the sperm together). See the information on vitamin C in Chapter 16.

Vitamin E

Vitamin E has been shown to make sperm more fertile and able to penetrate the ova, and to correct sub-fertility caused by free radicals damaging sperm or interfering with sperm production in the testes. A 1996 Israeli study found that taking 300 mg of vitamin E twice per day improved fertilization rates for men with fertility issues.[16]

Vitamin E is also recommended for couples with unexplained infertility, since research has shown that giving vitamin E to both partners leads to a significant increase in fertility.[17]

Food sources of vitamin E include nuts, oily fish (such as tuna, sardines, mackerel, salmon), sesame seeds, and unrefined oils such as olive oil.

L-Arginine

The head of the sperm contains a very high amount of the amino acid l-arginine. If men are deprived of l-arginine for even just a few days their sperm will not mature correctly.[18] Supplementing with l-arginine increases sperm count, sperm quality and helps sperm motility.[19] Other research showed that l-arginine supplements made sperm counts double and led to an increase in the number of pregnancies achieved.[20] Good sources of l-arginine are fish and nuts.

L-Carnitine

L-carnitine is another important amino acid for men, since it is critical for normal functioning of sperm cells. The higher the level of l-carnitine found in sperm cells, the better the sperm both in terms of sperm count and motility.[21] L-carnitine supplements will prevent abnormal sperm being produced and will increase sperm count.[22] Since l-carnitine (in combination with alpha-lipoic acid and co-enzyme Q10) is generally anti-ageing as well as a supportive of fat burning, there are many reasons to take this supplement.

Selenium

A lack of selenium in the diet has been found to cause infertility in men. The depletion of this key DNA-protecting mineral from soil, means men averagely consume 50 per cent less of this than they did 25 years ago. Supplementation with selenium improves sperm count. Selenium is essential both for sperm formation and for optimum testosterone production. One study from a team at the Glasgow Royal Infirmary in Scotland found that a selenium supplementation programme raised fertility from 15.5 per cent to 35.1 per cent in sub-fertile men.[23] In another study sperm donors with low sperm counts were also found to have correspondingly low selenium levels.[24]

Selenium can be found in avocados, sesame seeds, shellfish, sunflower seeds, tuna and wholegrains.

Zinc

Research has now confirmed that a zinc deficiency can cause low sperm count, chromosome changes in sperm and low testosterone levels in men.[25] Fortunately, this can be reversed when sufficient amounts of the mineral are taken.

Men lose around 9 per cent of their daily zinc intake with each ejaculation, so it is important that men have adequate zinc; supplementation is the best way to ensure this.

For couples undergoing IVF the fertilized egg can only be reimplanted once there has been adequate cell division, which will be dependent on both the sperm and ova having adequate levels of zinc.

Zinc is found in almonds, carrots, leafy greens, oats, pumpkin seeds, rye and wholewheat. Also shellfish (especially oysters) and sea vegetables. If you are taking zinc in supplement form, the recommended daily dose is 15 mg.

Seeds for your Seed

Bee Pollen

Bee pollen is a highly nutritious food and one of the most potent fertility tonics for men and women. See Chapter 13 for further information and how to use it. One cautionary note, though: a small percentage of men are allergic to bee products; if you do not know if you are, start off with barely a pinch of the bee pollen granules.

Pumpkin Seeds

For men, pumpkin seeds are one of the best fertility foods. They are very rich in unsaturated essential fatty acids, organic iron and pangamic acid (vitamin B15), all of which are vital for a healthy prostate gland. They are rich in zinc, a deficiency that is linked with low sperm count, decreased sperm motility and potency.

Besides having amazing fertility health benefits, zinc is a key mineral in protecting the prostate.

Sunflower Seeds

Like pumpkin seeds, sunflower seeds are one of the best fertility foods for men. They are very rich in unsaturated essential fatty acids, organic iron and pangamic acid (vitamin B15), all of which are vital for a healthy prostate gland. Like pumpkin seeds they are also rich in zinc, with all it male fertility benefits.

Herbs to Improve Sperm/Male Fertility

Horny Goat Weed (*Acertanthus sagittatum or Epimedium sagittatum*)

Also known by the Chinese name Yin-Yang-Huo, this is the superstar of fertility herbs for men. It is a male aphrodisiac and increases both sperm count and density. According to Chinese folklore, this herb was discovered in China by a goatherd who noticed his male goats became sexually aroused after eating this plant. In Chinese medicine this is regarded as the best herb for enhancing male potency.

Ho Shu Wu (*Polygonum multiflorum*)

This rejuvenating herb root also boosts sperm count. It is even reputed to preserve natural hair colour and prevent greying. Not bad, eh?

Saw Palmetto

This herb is known to increase sperm count. It safely tones and strengthens the entire male reproductive system enhancing male hormones where necessary.

Frequency of Sex for Maximum Sperm Count/Conception

If you are an organic farmer, or you know from tests that you have a very high sperm count, having sex every day when your partner is ovulating will obviously maximize your chances of conception. If, on the other hand, you do not know your sperm count, and maybe you have been drinking beer and coffee, using a mobile phone and even smoking, spacing sex – having intercourse every 36–48 hours – is the general advice to conserve sperm, and help them to build up their numbers so as to increase the chances of conceiving a baby. Sperm can live up to five days in fertile cervical fluid, so there is no need to worry that skipping a day or two will cause you to miss the moment. Sperm banks and IVF clinics ask men who are going to give sperm samples to abstain from sex (and, of course, masturbation) for 2–3 days beforehand. It will not be helpful to hold off longer than five days, however, since sperm age quite quickly and after 5–7 days they will be starting to die off and are not able swim so well anymore.

The Good News

I will conclude with some good news. For men, age does not appear to matter. Everyone knows Charlie Chaplin become a dad again in his seventies. Larry King and Donald Trump have become fathers again in their sixties. So, providing you are following the advice in this chapter, taking care of your sperm, and avoiding the obvious spermicides, you will still be able to father babies in your dotage. One other interesting factoid – it seems your sperm really want to impregnate your partner. Contrary to the standard belief that your sperm race towards the egg in mortal competition with each other, researchers have discovered that the spermatozoa collaborate, forming teams to help the champion, and often joining together to create a 'love train' so as to reach the target egg faster.[26] Ahhhh! Bet you did not know that!

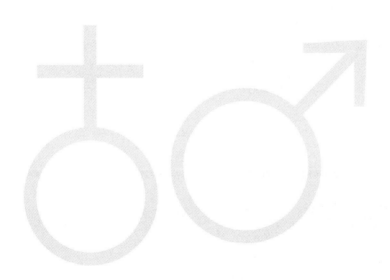

Fertility Action Plan

- Follow the Fertility Diet guidelines – in particular give up alcohol and caffeine.

- Stop smoking.

- Take supplements of vitamin C, vitamin B12, vitamin E and zinc.

- Take supplemental amino acids L-arginine and L-carnitine.

- Eat as many seeds as possible, as well as bee pollen granules.

- Visit a herbalist to explore which herbs will be best for you.

Chapter 32
Erectile Dysfunction

There is a commonly held belief that an inability to perform sexually is 'all in the mind'; this is very misleading when there are a number of physiological and nutritional reasons for 'impotency'. (Really, this is a dreadful label, much better expressed by the phrase 'erectile dysfunction', which makes it organ specific and not equivalent to an entire body defect.)

The causes are divided between circulation, i.e. 'internal plumbing' issues, and other factors such as smoking, drinking, prescription medications, stress, mineral deficiencies and diabetes. In a small number of cases, erectile dysfunction can be attributed to a disorder in the pituitary–hypothalamus axis.

Approximately 51 per cent of healthy American men between the ages of 40 and 70 report occasional to frequent problems with erections – this amounts to 18 million men in the USA alone.[1]

Circulation

Men are used to being bombarded with the message that they must take care of their arteries if they are to enjoy cardiovascular health, but few realize the undeniable importance of good blood circulation if they are to maintain sexual vigour. The blood vessels in the male genitalia are incredibly small and are adversely affected by all the factors that lead to a general hardening and narrowing of the arteries.

A high-fat diet interferes with having and maintaining an erection: eating animal fat clogs the arteries that transport blood to the penis for an erection in the same way that it clogs the arteries to the heart. Arterial blockages are a significant cause of impotence in men.

Several studies have confirmed that eating fatty meals may impair sexual performance and lower sex hormones in men since it causes testosterone to plunge. A study conducted by Professor Wayne Meikle at the University of Utah School of Medicine, found that blood testosterone levels went down by a whopping 50 per cent in a group of eight men after they consumed fatty milk shakes containing 57 per cent of their calories as fat, 9 per cent in protein and 34 per cent in carbohydrates. In contrast, when the men drank a low-fat shake, in which 73 per cent of the calories came from carbohydrates, 25 per cent from protein and 1 per cent from fat, there was no adverse impact on testosterone levels. Professor Meikle observed, 'We looked only at the immediate result of one high fat meal; though it could be hypothesised that after some time a high-fat diet could weaken a man's sex drive.'

The other serious downside concerning fat for men is that fatty foods lead to obesity and men with higher body fat levels have higher oestrogen and lower testosterone levels.

Alcohol

The consumption of alcohol, as discussed in Chapter 5, is one major culprit in a man's inability to achieve an erection, no matter how fired up his libido may feel after a boozy night out (as many a disappointed lady can confirm). The fact is that alcohol undermines sexual performance because it leads to a reduction of sex hormones in men (and women too).

Just one or two drinks can have an adverse impact on a man's ability to perform.

Smoking

Smoking constricts blood vessels. As mentioned at the beginning of this chapter, this means *all* blood vessels. Yes, even those tiny ones in your genitals. One study from the Queen's University in Kingston found that 81 per cent of men who had problems with erections were smokers, compared to the overall total of 58 per cent of men in the population at large (or rather, at small). Even more compelling evidence comes from a study of 4,400 Vietnam veterans which found that there was a 50 per cent higher rate of impotency among current smokers compared with non-smokers, including former smokers.[2]

Prescription Drugs

An alarming number of regularly prescribed drugs cause erectile dysfunction as a side effect. There are far too many to list here unfortunately – see Chapter 11 for more information. If you are concerned that a medication may be affecting your virility you could look it up in any of the comprehensive encyclopaedias of medicine that are available, or ask your physician.

A common-sense caution: under no circumstances should

you abandon taking any medication without consulting your physician first.

Diabetes

The founder members of the organization Impotents Anonymous (yes, apparently it exists) state that, as at 1998, approximately 80 per cent of the estimated 13 million diabetic men in the USA suffer from premature hardening of the arteries, especially to those of the penis.[3] The restricted blood supply not only impairs the engorgement process but can lead to permanent nerve damage.

All the side effects of type 2 diabetes including impotency can be alleviated by following a low-glycaemic diet. In a United Press International news story, Associate Professor Somasundaram Addanki, a biochemist and nutritionist at Ohio State University, recounted how he cured six years of diabetic impotency by cutting sugar, white flour products and fatty foods from his diet.

A diet low in sugar and refined carbohydrates such as the Fertility Diet will also act as a preventative measure against the onset of type 2 diabetes.

Stress

Some men will become temporarily impotent when under a lot of stress. Stress can also exhaust supplies of the B vitamins, in particular vitamin B6 (pyridoxine), leading to problems with erections.

Pituitary–Hypothalamus Axis Malfunction

One other cause of erectile dysfunction is problems with the hormonal axis between the hypothalamus and the pituitary endocrine glands. In one study measuring the serum testosterone levels of 105 patients suffering from impotence, it was found that 37 of them had previously undiagnosed hypothalamus–pituitary axis disorders.[4]

The Nutritional Answer to Erectile Dysfunction

Apart from eliminating the artery clogging, fatty foods such as meat and dairy products, alcohol and cigarettes, the following nutrients will assist with curing or preventing any problems with having an erection.

B Vitamins
B vitamins are essential for good nervous system health, especially in times of stress, and help maintain testosterone levels, sperm count and sexual drive. Vitamins B5 (pantothenic acid), B3 (niacin) and B6 (pyridoxine) are especially recommended.

Calcium and Magnesium
Calcium is necessary for good hormonal health and is known to be important in sexual performance. Calcium must, however, be balanced with adequate magnesium levels (a mineral in which it is estimated 75 per cent of all Americans are deficient).[5] Magnesium dilates the arteries, increasing blood flow to all areas of the body including the genitals. It is a natural calcium channel blocker namely it blocks excess calcium without any of the unpleasant side effects of the typical calcium channel blockers prescribed for hypertension. The two minerals at healthy levels work synergistically and will maximize hormonal health and sexual performance. Recommended foods rich in calcium are leafy greens, nuts and sesame seeds. Recommended foods as sources of magnesium are leafy greens, raw cacao powder, very dark (and low-sugar) chocolate and wholegrains.

Cordyceps
Yes, this really may be fungal Viagra! Try it and see . . .

Garlic

A very powerful aphrodisiac, garlic stimulates and invigorates all hormonal secretions. In India men even rub garlic on their genitalia to assist with erections.

Horny Goat Weed

Another excellent herb for virility.

Saw palmetto

An excellent herb for potency and sex drive.

Tyrosine

This amino acid is a precursor to the lusty neurotransmitter dopamine. It is so energizing, however, that you will need to reduce or eliminate any caffeine (if you are still having tea and coffee – in which case, shame on you) or you may become wired.

Yohimbe

Probably the best herb for treating erectile dysfunction.

Zinc

Yes, the star fertility mineral for both men and women plays a key role in sexual potency in men. A study from the Wayne State University School of Medicine, in Detroit, Michigan, found the testes to be very sensitive to zinc. Zinc foods were restricted in the diet of five healthy men aged 51 to 65 for a six-month period. Four of the men showed lowered sperm count – in three of them to the point of technical sterility. All of the men had a reduction in testosterone levels and diminished sexual drive. Once the participants returned to normal eating with additional zinc supplements of 30 mg per day (double the usual maximum dose) their sperm count, testosterone and libido all returned to healthy levels.

Dr Ananda Prasad, the professor leading the study, recommends that, once organic and psychological causes of impotency have been ruled out, plasma zinc levels should be checked. A protocol of 20–30 mg of zinc daily is suggested if a deficiency exists.[6] The usual maximum daily amount is 15 mg for maintenance. Foods rich in zinc include: carrots, nuts, oysters, seaweeds and seeds.

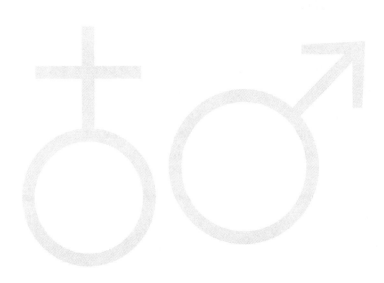

Fertility Action Plan

- If you smoke you need to stop immediately.

- Cut out alcohol and saturated fats found in meat and dairy products.

- Take supplements of B vitamins, calcium, magnesium, garlic capsules and zinc.

- Try the amazing cordyceps, the herbs yohimbe and horny goatweed. Seek additional advice from a herbalist.

Chapter 33
The Thyroid and Infertility

One easily overlooked cause of infertility is an underactive or overactive thyroid gland. The butterfly-shaped thyroid gland is located in the neck, in the region of your Adam's apple. It affects every cell in the body by producing hormones which are necessary for metabolism, growth, nerves, muscle and circulation. You probably know already that the thyroid gland is the body's metabolic motor and thermostat, regulating the speed at which the body functions and the rate at which energy and heat are generated. What you may not know is that the thyroid gland also regulates ovarian function and fertility. There are thyroid receptors on the ovary and ovarian hormone receptors on the thyroid. Through the miraculous bio-feedback communication system of the body, the thyroid gland, reproductive glands, and the hypothalamus and pituitary in the brain are in constant communication with each other. Your thyroid is a key player in determining whether now is a good time for your body to have a baby.

The body, in its wisdom, will prevent conception when it detects thyroid hormones are not at optimal levels for the development of a perfectly healthy baby.

Thyroid hormones not only play a key role in our own brain functioning and mental health, they are also crucial for foetal brain development during pregnancy. If adequate and balanced amounts of thyroid hormones and the mineral iodine are not present in the mother, permanent brain damage can be caused to the baby – ranging from severe retardation to less obvious learning and neurological challenges. Untreated and unrecognized hypothyroidism (underactive thyroid) doubles the risk of miscarriage, stillbirths and premature births as well as tripling the risk of birth defects.[1]

Since 90 per cent of thyroid problems affect women and appear to be more damaging to the fertility of women than of men, this chapter is slanted towards women's reproductive health. Of course, if you are one of the rare men with a thyroid that is not functioning properly, this will also adversely impact your fertility and the nutritional guidelines later in this chapter will also be relevant to you.

Even mild, so-called sub-clinical, thyroid disorders can cause menstrual problems and general infertility.

Symptoms of Thyroid Disorders

Hypothyroidism and Infertility

Classic symptoms of a sluggish thyroid are feeling tired and lethargic all the time, feeling cold especially having colds hands and feet (are you regularly wearing socks to bed?), the inability to lose weight and weight gain, depression, menstrual problems such as PMS and excessive bleeding, reduced libido, low blood pressure, poor concentration and memory, headaches and dry, coarse or thick skin.

When the thyroid gland is underactive, namely T4 and T3 levels are too low, the pituitary will raise levels of the hormone prolactin – which is normally only elevated in breastfeeding women. High prolactin disrupts normal menstrual cycles, leading to irregular cycles, no ovulation and generally decreased levels of sex hormones such as oestrogen and progesterone.

But it gets worse. The body tries to rectify there being fewer sex hormones released by lowering the amount of a hormone-binding protein called SHBG, so that more hormones are free to circulate in the body. Now hormone levels can again become unbalanced: there can be chronic excess oestrogen (which will cause heavy bleeding) or excess androgens (male hormones) causing excess body hair, weight gain, loss of head hair and polycystic ovaries. All this highly abnormal feedback to the pituitary throws off the proper release of the gonadotrophin hormones needed for ovulation – follicle stimulating hormone (FSH) and luteneizing hormones (LH). The end to this sad tale can be described less technically – infertility, no baby.

Hyperthyroidism and Infertility

If your thyroid is overactive everything in the body speeds up and will ultimately leave you feeling exhausted – 'tired but wired' as one author puts it.[2] The typical symptoms are feeling anxious and irritable, having insomnia, feeling hot all the time and sweating, menstrual irregularities such as no period and very light blood flow, palpitations and a racing pulse, high blood pressure, staring eyes and a swollen neck – a goitre – from the enlarged gland.

When the hypothalamus and pituitary register T3 and T4 levels are too high – namely, when the thyroid is overactive, this leads to an elevation of FSH and LH, and thus a disruption in normal ovarian cycles. In itself, this can cause ovulation to cease and lead directly to infertility. Women with hyperthyroid also have very scanty menstrual blood flow so that too little endometrial lining is built up to sustain a pregnancy by allowing an embryo to implant. If they do conceive, the chances of miscarrying are therefore greatly increased.

Foods to Optimize Thyroid Function

In respect of thyroid, this is one area where I cannot assert that food will always provide a complete cure, particularly if the thyroid disease is an autoimmune disease. What I can promise, however, is that thyroid function (and thus fertility and overall hormonal balance) *can* be significantly improved and managed through diet, to the point where, in sub-clinical cases, of hypo or hyperthyroid, the symptoms/dysfunction will no longer exist.

Foods/Supplements for Hypothyroidism

Calcarea Carbonica

This homeopathic remedy is thought to increase thyroid function. Best taken under the guidance of a qualified homeopath.

Cayenne Pepper

This condiment is very useful for improving hypothyroid conditions, or for those who want to lose weight. It increases the body's metabolic rate, according to some studies by as much as 25 per cent.

Cayenne enhances circulation by dilating capillaries, and lowers blood pressure; it is also a natural pain reliever and is meant to be exceptionally effective in the treatment of both cluster headaches and arthritis.

Apart from the addition of cayenne to any spicy meals you are preparing, another way to add cayenne into your diet is through a cleansing lemonade drink. Devised by Stanley Burroughs in his well known Master Cleanse, the basic recipe is the juice of one lemon, one teaspoon of organic maple syrup and one pinch of cayenne in eight ounces of hot or cold water. I drink this lemonade nearly every day, it tastes delicious and is a wonderful tonic. Made with hot water, it is perfect for getting a warm, tingly feeling in cold weather, or for staving off the slightest hint of a cold or flu.

Coconut

Most people are so brainwashed by the propaganda defaming the wonderful health-giving coconut, that they are oblivious to its metabolic stimulating qualities. Certainly, coconut fat is saturated, but it is, in fact, a medium chained fat, not a short chained fat like some animal fats, so actually facilitates the breakdown of body fat, rather than the clogging of arteries. Coconut in all its forms (except dried desiccated coconut with sugar added), and the fresher the better, is great for those whose thyroid is under par.

Pure Water

Pure drinking water is important for everyone trying to conceive. For those with hypothyroid you must particularly avoid drinking water containing fluoride or chlorine like tap water.

Radish

One of the most potent thyroid tonics is the humble radish. Who would have guessed that, beneath that innocuous red and white exterior, lurked a vegetable able to normalize the production of T4 or thyroxine as well as another thyroid hormone, calcitonin, in the thyroid gland. They raise levels if too little is being produced and lower them if they are too high. Calcitonin regulates the amount of calcium released into the bloodstream and affects the amount of calcium deposited in the bones during bone formation. In Russia, radishes have been used by physicians to treat both hyperthyroidism and hypothyroidism for decades.[3]

Sea Vegetables/Iodine

Iodine is the key mineral needed for functioning of the thyroid. Kelp as a supplement is a good source of iodine. All seaweeds and algaes are rich in iodine. The nori seaweed used in sushi is loaded with iodine. You should be aware, however, that an excess of iodine can itself trigger thyroid problems. A healthy level would be about 500 mcg per day.

Iodine is best taken with other minerals to ensure a good balance. Zinc and selenium are especially good for the thyroid.

Thyroid Glandular Supplements

Natural desiccated thyroid extracts are available on prescription from naturopathic doctors and homeopaths. The natural compound 'Armor Thyroid' has been recommended by some authors.

Tyrosine

The amino acid tyrosine can be taken as a supplement to stimulate the thyroid. It is, after all, together with iodine, the raw material from which the hormones T3 and T4 are made. Tyrosine is water soluble and is safe even in doses tested up to 7 g – whatever your body does not need will be excreted out in your urine. I recommend a dose of 1–2 g taken in the morning. If taken later in the day, it could interfere with sleep. Good vegetarian sources of tyrosine include almonds, avocados, beans, pumpkin and sesame seeds. It is also found in eggs and fish. If you are taking it as a supplement it is better to avoid caffeine, since, in combination, you could find yourself overstimulated and feeling wired or anxious instead.

Zeolite

This mineral from Asia usually comes in a liquid form under the brand name Natural Cellular Defence. Its extraordinary ability to remove the heavy metals and toxins from the body which interfere with thyroid function, as well as to boost immunity, make it a good choice for anyone with hypothyroid, especially if this has been caused by Hashimoto's syndrome.

Key nutrients to support a sluggish thyroid are: zinc, vitamins B, C and E.

A Diet to Manage Hyperthyroidism

1. Foods to Avoid
a) Stimulants
If you have an overactive thyroid, the first thing to cut out are any dietary stimulants such as caffeine – including chocolate, soft drinks, alcohol and tobacco. All of which I hope you are steering clear of anyway because of their disastrous impact on your fertility.

b) Foods and products containing iodine
Apart from avoiding iodized salt, sea salt, seaweed and all forms of algae, it is important to know iodine is also found in some asthma and cough medications, vitamin pills and sun lotions.

c) Foods containing tyrosine
Tyrosine is an amino acid that is a precursor to T3 and T4. If you are hyperthyroid you should avoid foods rich in tyrosine: pork meat has the highest amounts, followed by other types of meat, dairy products and fish. Consume almonds, avocados, beans, pumpkin and sesame seeds in very moderate amounts. There is minimal tyrosine to be found in all other fruit, vegetables, cereals, grains and plant oils.

d) Medicines
Note that cough and cold medicines containing decongestants are too stimulating for those with hyperthyroid.

2. Foods to Counteract Hyperthyroid
a) Goitrogenic foods
These vegetables interfere with the iodine utilization and the thyroid enzyme TPO and prevent the conversion of T4 into T3 and thus suppress thyroid. They are, therefore, ideal foods for anyone with hyperthyroid and should be eaten as much as possible: cabbage, kale, broccoli, Brussels sprouts, mustard greens, pears, peaches, peanuts, pine nuts, swede/rutabaga and turnips. The goitrogenic factor is reduced or eliminated by cooking, so

try to eat these foods raw or as lightly steamed as possible.

b) Tempeh

The one exception I might make to my clear no soya for fertility rule is that, for those suffering from hyperthyroid, a fermented form of soya, in very moderate amounts, could be beneficial because of the disruption caused by soya to the thyroid gland in converting T4 to T3. The isoflavones in soya lead to underactivity in the thyroid gland and could work as a medicine for those with hyperthyroid.

c) Thyme

The herb thyme, in very high amounts, has been shown to reduce thyroid activity – and should be used as much as possible.

d) Radish

The only vegetable I have found that is a natural thyroid regulator increasing or suppressing thyroid function as necessary. For hyperthyroid it will reduce the amount of T3 and T4 being released. Try to eat as much radish as you can.

e) Zeolite

This mineral from Asia usually comes in a liquid form under the brand name Natural Cellular Defence. Its extraordinary ability to remove heavy metals and toxins from the body, as well as to boost immunity, make it a good choice for anyone with hyperthyroid, especially if this has been caused by Grave's Disease.

Other Tips for Hyperthyroid Sufferers

Rather than grazing throughout the day – i.e. eating small amounts at regular intervals, which boosts thyroid – it will help calm your metabolism if you eat only two or three well-spaced meals a day (as much as you want of course) and avoid snacks in between.

Over-exercising (if you have the energy) will also rev up the thyroid, so you may like to reduce your gym habits – especially if you are exercising more than an hour a day. The recommended amount to sustain good health is 30–45 minutes five times a week.

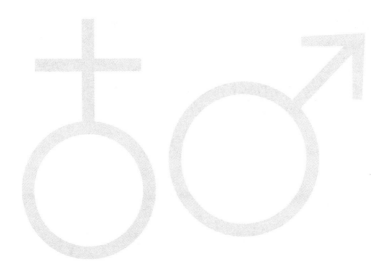

Fertility Action Plan

- For hypothyroidism eat cayenne pepper, coconut products, seaweeds and radishes. Drink plenty of water.

- Supplements for hypo-thryroid include iodine and the amino acid tyrosine.

- For hyper-thyroidism avoid all foods rich in iodine and tyrosine, these include seaweeds, meat, dairy products and fish.

- For hyper-thyroidism eat plenty of cabbage and broccoli and other goitogenic vegetables. Also eat radishes and the herb thyme.

Part VII:
Sex – Conceiving the Old-Fashioned Way

Chapter 34

Ovulation and the Miracle of Conception

As I researched into what foods and lifestyle factors block fertility, I began to wonder how anyone is having a baby naturally at all these days. Classic wisdom on fertility also states that there is only a 24–36-hour window of opportunity around ovulation when conception can take place. A meagre window of time that is extended only by the fact that sperm can survive up to five days in fertile cervical mucus, so that, providing one of the little swimmers is hanging out at the top of a Fallopian tube at the time an egg is released, you can conceive, even if it is a few days since you had sex.

Luckily for all couples trying to have a baby, the traditional view of ovulation as occurring only mid-cycle on approximately day fourteen turns out to be wrong! Groundbreaking research lead by Dr Roger Pierson and Dr Angela Baerwald and their team at the University of Saskatchewan, Canada, published in *Fertility and Sterility* in July 2003[1] found that 100 per cent of women have more than one hormonal surge a month, each with the potential to trigger ovulation. These scientists were the first to track ovulation and follicle development patterns in women using advanced uterine ultrasound technology. Being able to track what goes on in the ovaries with high resolution 3-D imaging totally overturned what was previously known about ovulation, which had been based on measuring hormone levels in the urine and the bloodstream. As Dr Pierson put it, 'this study shows we have not fully understood the basic biological processes that occur during menstrual cycles; we are literally going to have to rewrite medical textbooks'.[2]

The Canadian scientists found that all women have *more than one* 'wave' or peak period during the menstrual cycle when the follicles in the woman's ovaries prepare to release an egg. This information is a bit hard to digest, since it contradicts everything you may have known or been told about your menstrual cycle. Yes, 100 per cent of women have more than one ovulatory wave or time when they can potentially conceive each month. For 60 per cent of women there is one surge before ovulation itself, when a follicle grows to 10 mm, i.e. a size capable of being released; and in the remaining 40 per cent of women there are two of these surges – each leading to a follicle developing to 10 mm or larger, before the big event of ovulation itself. According to Dr Pierson this means that 40 per cent of women *could be fertile at almost any time in their menstrual cycle!* How is that for good news? It is my opinion that this research is not widely known enough. In researching this book, I must have read approximately 400 books on fertility, the endocrine system, nutrition, ageing and related subjects. Only in one of them – published in 2004[3] – did I find a brief reference to this important study, even though the information is, at the time of writing, now over four years old.

This information explains a lot – how it is that some women have conceived during their period, while breast-feeding, even on the contraceptive pill (many of which tail off hormone doses at the end of the cycle, at the supposedly infertile time!). Indeed, I once read about a tribe in Africa, where, for religious reasons, sex may *only* take place during menstruation. Well, there was obviously a lot of cheating going on – or these women were ovulating during their periods –since this tribe is not extinct!

Research from the US National Institute of Environmental Health Sciences (NIEHS) in North Carolina shows that two-thirds of healthy, fertile women will ovulate on a day other than on day fourteen of the cycle, the traditional day it is supposed to occur.

So, the good news is that you should not be totally fixated on having sex only at the 'right time' since up to three possible times to get pregnant exist each month. Indeed, having sex at the 'wrong' time could do the trick. The bad news is that, since ovulation can occur at any time in the cycle, it is good to become a bit of a hormone detective, to know when after either one or two 'false start' waves, you are actually ovulating/tend to ovulate each month.

How to Tell You are Ovulating

The female body gives many clues as to when ovulation is occurring or about to take place. One of the key indicators is the presence of slippery, stretchy cervical mucus, that looks a bit like globby egg white. On non-fertile days cervical mucus is dry, crumbly, non-stretchy, indeed may not be there at all. The cervix itself alters position. Exactly at ovulation it is low in the uterus and open. On other days it is higher up in the uterine cavity and 'closed'.

There is only one way to notice these changes. Go to the bathroom, wash your hands, insert a finger into your vagina and feel where your cervix is – you will begin to be able to perceive the difference in position. You also can collect cervical mucus on your index finger and test its quality by bringing the index finger against the thumb to see if it stretches and to test its texture. As you begin to pay attention to your mucus, something you may never even have thought much about before, you will be able to notice conspicuous differences throughout your monthly cycle. Whether ovulation has occurred can also be seen by charting body temperature every morning. The shift to progesterone release after ovulation causes a spike in temperature. Unfortunately, taking your temperature every morning does not give you advance warning of ovulation so you could miss the key time, but at least it lets you know you are ovulating each month. Furthermore, if you have been monitoring your temperature for a number of months and observe a consistent thermal shift to a higher temperature on, say, day 12, 13 or 14 (counting day 1 as the first day of your period), you know that, in the following month, day 11, 12, 13, or whichever is the day before the temperature rise, is likely to be the most auspicious day to try baby making.

An entire branch of fertility education called 'Natural Fertility Awareness' has been developed, which is all about monitoring these key signs of ovulation, which I have set out only in a very summarized form in the paragraph above. I highly recommend a book entitled *Taking Charge of Your Fertility* by Toni Weschler, which sets out a very lucid account of how to monitor and chart temperature, position of the cervix and cervical fluid (complete with graphic pictures of mucus, which are simultaneously icky and fascinating!), all of which will help you know exactly when is the best time to have sex.

Some women know they are ovulating because they experience a dull ache or pain just as the ovary is about to release an egg (mittelschmerz is the jargon term); they may have breast tenderness, a lift in libido, or even one-night insomnia. It is worth noting that, in animals, the urge to mate coincides exactly with ovulation. Certainly it is nature's way to trigger a rise in libido at the most optimal time for woman, and this hormonal signal could well be detected through pheromones smelt by your partner – so any sudden friskiness you feel is worth capitalizing on, even if it is not on 'timetable'.

My own favourite way to keep track of ovulation is

through the use of a mini microscope. This is usually a lip-stick-sized microscope, widely available to purchase online (even on Amazon) for about £10–20; it shows changes in saliva, indicating ovulation is approaching or taking place. Just before ovulation, the surge in oestrogen is accompanied by an increase in electrolytes (or salts) in body fluids such as cervical mucus or saliva. When a drop of saliva is placed on the lens of the mini microscope and allowed to dry, a 'ferning' pattern can be seen in the saliva (magnified fifty times) from about three days prior to ovulation and around two days after ovulation. The fern shapes (basically the dried electrolyte/salts) become clearer and clearer showing the height of their clarity at ovulation/peak fertility. Outside this fertile period all that can be seen in the dried saliva droplet is a chaotic 'dots' pattern. These microscopes have an accuracy of 98 per cent so are perfect for women with irregular cycles too. They can, of course, later also be used for family planning by avoiding sex whenever the ferning pattern can be seen.

The microscopes are all pretty similar: some have higher magnification; some are backlit for easy viewing; some have focusing adjustment possibilities; and some have detachable slides so you can compare previous days' results. The test is also easy to perform. Just take a drop of your saliva, preferably first thing in the morning before eating or drinking anything or at least 2 hours away from food/drink, by either putting a drop on your finger or by spitting directly on to the lens. Make sure that the saliva sample is not foamy/with air bubbles. Wait for the drop to dry (about as long as it takes to clean your teeth in the morning!) then view, remembering to clean the lens carefully afterwards to avoid an incorrect reading the following day. Of course cervical mucus could be tested instead if you really wanted to since it also shows the fern/dots patterns – but this is not quite as convenient and certainly cannot be tested anywhere!

Of course there are many other ovulation-testing devices that require peeing on a test stick to check for levels of luteinizing hormones – which peak exactly on ovulation. These ovulation predictor kits can be quite expensive. They work well for women with regular cycles, but may not be quite so reliable for women with irregular cycles, or conditions such as PCOS.

One final tip: many fertility experts believe that ovulation is most likely to occur at 4 p.m. in the afternoon[4] not at night. So, if it is at all possible to have afternoon hanky panky, that could also help. Have fun!

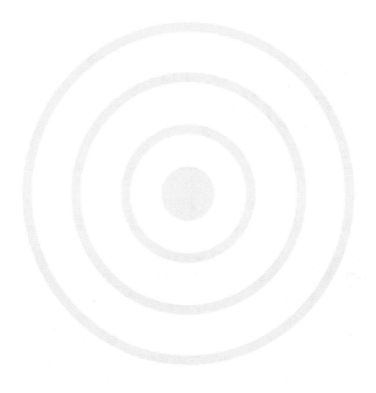

Chapter 35
Hitting the Target – Fertility Sex

No amount of advice on eating organic produce or taking supplements is going to help you have a baby in the traditional way, unless you and your beloved are having regular sex, timed around ovulation. But when it comes to baby making (as opposed to purely recreational love making) certain positions are much more likely to lead to conception than others, and some pleasurable activities could actually impair your chances of procreation.

The Law of the Universe

To conceive a baby, you need to remember one universal law: that of gravity. You have got to be frolicking in such a way that places the sperm as close as possible to the opening of the cervix, to give them a few inches head start on their voyage to rendezvous with an egg in the Fallopian tube. The best position to have sex for conception is the old-fashioned favourite: the missionary position (man on top) since the vagina naturally slopes downwards when a woman is lying on her back, so that sperm can literally 'go with the flow'. If the woman also places a pillow under her bottom to raise her hips higher then her torso, this will help her partner to penetrate more deeply and bring his penis closer to the target area.

The second-best sexual position for optimal chances of conceiving, according to a number of fertility experts, is so-called 'doggie style', i.e. where the man enters the woman from behind, particularly if she sticks her buttocks in the air, i.e. higher than her head, since this angle will also encourage sperm to swim in the right direction.

Of course any positions that work contrary to gravity will cause sperm to run out of the vagina and hinder conception. So making love with the woman on top, or standing or sitting up, bending over, swinging from the chandeliers, and just about every pose in the *Kama Sutra*, while being tremendously good fun if you are flexible enough, will impair a likely conception. The spooning position is also not optimal for the same reason, unless you can engineer some crafty angle to put the woman lower than the man at the same time.

However, I can give you some consolatory news if I have now put a dampener on your love life preferences: having reviewed all the experts' advice, it is obvious that it is only the position you are in as the man ejaculates that counts. It appears logical to me that you can get up to any shenanigans you like (subject to the paragraphs that follow) prior to the man's orgasm, but as that moment approaches you need to 'finish off' with the man on top in the missionary or doggie position.

A friend of mine and his wife experienced secondary

infertility for some four despairing years after their first daughter was born. They went the assisted conception treatment route – 'motor cycle couriers have carried my sperm all over London . . . ' he told me with a wry smile – but all in vain. He then volunteered the secret behind the birth of their two youngest children: 'My wife read somewhere that putting her legs up against the wall after sex helped you to conceive.' Well, it worked superbly for them – they conceived their second child the very same month they tried this. It makes sense as it keeps the sperm inside the woman as long as possible in a direction flowing towards the Fallopian tubes. A pillow under your hips and lying still for a while would work well too. But do not worry ladies, you do not have to lie like this all night: the fastest sperm can reach the egg in five minutes, the slower within forty-five minutes1 – so lying still for around half an hour with your pelvis elevated somehow after you have had sex should give your partner's sperm all the time they need even to dawdle to their destination.

For the best chance of conceiving, do not jump out of bed to go to the bathroom the very moment after the last gasp of pleasure has been uttered. Lie in a position that helps the sperm make their way to the egg.

Variety is the Spice of Life?

Since the writing of this chapter is embarrassing me, vaguely aware as I am that my mother is likely to be reading this some day (hi, Mum), I will digress with a little anecdote. One of most intriguing pieces of legislation I learned while practising law in the Cayman Islands was that, under the Cayman Penal Code (that's penal, not penile, folks), any sexual act not for procreation constituted an 'unnatural act' and was therefore illegal! This meant, of course, that having anal or oral sex was illegal. There is no record of anyone ever being prosecuted in the Cayman Islands for these heinous 'crimes', but it nevertheless gave my friends and me a kick to know we could commit a criminal offence in our bedrooms every day of the week if we wanted and never be found out!

The Victorian moralistic legislators, while trying to keep a tiny British colony in the Caribbean well populated, were actually on to something: neither anal nor oral sex are recommended when you are trying to have a baby.

The problem with anal sex is that it can introduce fertility-damaging bacteria and thus infections into the vagina through faecal matter on the penis. If this is your, er, cup of tea, then only practise this type of sex wearing a condom that is removed and discarded before the penis is placed inside the vagina. I am still unconvinced this is entirely the answer if you are trying to have a baby, however, given that condoms normally have some kind of spermicide, which could affect any sperm subsequently ejaculated.

As to oral sex, a number of brave researchers have looked into the question of whether oral sex (of the fellatio kind) could be a risk factor for decreased fertility. The theory is that, since sperm cells are foreign to a woman's body, if she swallows her partner's semen she could sensitize her immune system against his sperm and start producing antibodies against it, which would subsequently attack it when it innocently enters the vagina, thus leading to infertility.[2] The results of the studies on oral sex and infertility have been mixed[3] (imagine the data-collection difficulties!) but it does look like blow jobs are not such a good idea when you are trying for a baby. I will give you one potential remedy however – ladies, spit, don't swallow. As far as I am aware, there is no research on this! By the way, since sperm are unique to each man, any antibodies developed to a previous partner's sperm would not attack the sperm of your present bedfellow.

Girls Just Want To Have Fun Too!

While it is biologically obvious that if a man does not have an orgasm there cannot be any conception, there is also evidence that when a woman has an orgasm as well the chances of conceiving significantly increase. There appear to be a number of theories behind this: one study found that, when a woman climaxes any time between one and forty-five minutes after her partner ejaculates, she retains significantly more sperm than she does after non-orgasmic sex.[4] Research also indicates that the strong muscular contractions of a woman's orgasm create a kind of vacuum that pulls sperm from the vagina to the cervix where they are better placed to reach the egg.[5] Another hypothesis is that orgasm is the sophisticated means by which a woman's body chooses which sperm should impregnate her.[6] I have also read that increased levels of the hormone oxytosin released during orgasm increase fertility.

Seriously, guys, I am not just telling you this in order to become a folk heroine among women. Women who enjoy a satisfying sex life have been found to have more regular and more ovulatory menstrual cycles than women who do not.[7] Just to soothe the male ego a little, celibate women who enjoyed sexual 'self help' (masturbation) did not, according to a small study carried out by the Athena Institute for Women's Wellness, have as many regular ovulatory cycles as women enjoying real-life sex with a man.[8] Although the scientists did not say why, I wonder to what extent the sense of smell and pheromones play a key role in enhancing fertility, such that if you are single and celibate, even if you are having regular periods, nature will be carefully conserving your eggs by not releasing one each month with ovulation, if there is no signal from the nose that a hot man is in your bed. The good news is that other research shows women spontaneously ovulate when they fall in love.[9] Isn't the cosmos amazing?

Quality not Quantity

There is evidence that sex every day or more than once a day can lead to a lowered sperm count in men who are borderline on the normal range or have low sperm count. So, unless you know for a fact that you have a ridiculously high sperm count, it might be better to aim for sex every other day during the woman's fertile time. Of course men, if you are also squandering your precious semen through daily masturbation, this could lead to lower sperm count, so restraint and cold showers, please – use it where it matters.

Slip Sliding Away

No matter what the packaging says, artificial lubricants, such as KY jelly, may kill sperm. The most fruitful approach, literally, is to take time for foreplay and intimacy, so that both partners' own natural lubricants can be secreted, just as nature intended. If you think you do need lubrication do not use saliva, which contains bacteria that might diminish sperm function. Your best bets would be pure water, or, according to some sources, egg whites. Yes, I know this sounds messy and disgusting, and you could just end up with omelette between the sheets, but I gather that the protein in the egg white actually nourishes sperm on their journey, like giving them a little picnic. It could be worth a crack! In Chinese medicine bananas (when eaten of course!) increase the 'yin fluids' that should help things flow smoothly too.

Final Thoughts

To conclude, there is still much that science does not know about the miracle of conception and the magic X-factor of loving energy being exchanged between two people. Since all women have at least two ovulatory waves as I mentioned in the previous chapter, and appear to ovulate spontaneously when they are in love, being too fixated on having sex only when the ovulation predictor kit tells you is a good time might be precluding you from conceiving. On the other hand, making love whenever you feel like it, as an expression of your mutual physical, mental, emotional and spiritual connection, with a view to creating a baby out of the surplus of that love energy, might be all that is required for the mystery we call Life to bless you with a child. Who knows? Have fun trying for a baby anyway.

Part VIII:
Getting Started on the Fertility Diet

Chapter 36
The Fertility Diet Protocol

Making changes in the diet is never easy. Our eating habits become so ingrained, usually from childhood. The stakes generally have to be very high to motivate us to eat differently – for some people, their very life has to hang in the balance before they will stop ingesting substances that are destroying their health. In this instance a life, a new life, really does hang in the balance. No one can advise you on how to get the necessary psychological leverage on yourself to transform what you eat, except yourself. You need to find a way to keep your baby goals always at the forefront of your mind when making food and drink choices, thereby making your commitment to your health and fertility a priority over any gastronomic temptation. Only when you are gazing into the eyes of your newborn, healthy baby will the sacrifices seem worthwhile.

Ideally, you should aim to follow the Fertility Diet Protocol for at least four months before even trying to conceive to give your future baby the best possible start in life.

Most people cannot leap from the extreme of a cooked food junkavore to a 50 per cent-plus raw food organic vegan overnight. The suggestions outlined in this book could represent a nutritional revolution to some people used to eating a lot of non-organic, convenience, packaged or microwave foods. The key is to start wherever you are at and do the best you can to make positive changes – eliminating some things and introducing others. Please also remember one thing: nutritional (particularly mineral) deficiencies are what cause cravings for sugar, fat or junk, or a tendency to overeat. When you focus first on massively increasing the amount of high nutrient food (such as spinach, broccoli, parsley or sunflower seeds) in your diet, then some of the urges to eat less healthy items will begin to fall away without any willpower on your part.

Addressing Contraceptive Addictions: Cigarettes, Alcohol and Caffeine

If you smoke, cut down first to only those best cigarettes of the day and then give them up entirely as soon as possible – this really is a non-negotiable step for anyone who wants a baby.

If you are used to drinking alcohol every day start by picking a manageable numbers of days a week you will not touch a drop. Once you are down to one day a week, reduce to 'only on very special occasions', then go teetotal. The longer you continue to drink alcohol, the longer you will wait to conceive – please decide what matters to you most.

Caffeine is relatively easy to give up by switching immediately to decaffeinated tea and coffee (where the caffeine has been removed by water filtering or some natural method). Dependent upon how much caffeine you used to consume, you may get a headache, which, it is my theory, lasts the same number of days as the number of daily caffeinated drinks you would normally have. Thus a three coffees a day person might averagely have some kind of headache for three days. Once you are used to decaffeinated tea and coffee (which still contains 3 per cent caffeine) change to herbal teas instead of black teas and acquire a taste for organic 'grain coffee' often made from barley and chicory – there are some good ones out there!

Wholefoods, Come On Down!

Breaking free of junk, convenience and takeaway foods requires some self-discipline and good recipes! Start with as many fresh-foods-only days as you can, until all you are eating is items purchased from the periphery of the supermarket – fruit, vegetables, free-range eggs and organic lean chicken, fish and meat (if you are still eating animal product, despite the fertility disadvantages as explained in Chapter 4).

Ditching the Dairy

When trying to eliminate dairy for the first time, start by replacing butter with vegan, non-hydrogenated margarine, which is organic and free of trans fats. My favourite is made from organic cold-pressed plant oil sources. Soya margarines are definitely not recommended.

At first drinking (decaffeinated) tea and coffee without milk is very strange. Just make your hot drinks a lot weaker than you normally do; after a while you will be so used to the pure taste of your decaf coffee and tea that putting milk in them will be unthinkable. Herbal teas do not require any milk, so letting caffeine and dairy go at the same time is a good idea.

For breakfast cereals delicious homemade almond or other nut milks are the answer. Almond, oat and rice milks can be bought in the supermarket but do not taste anything like as nice as fresh nut milks made at home (see Recipes section).

Dairy-free home baking of cakes, desserts, cookies (all sweetened with xylitol, of course) and pies is easy. Use almond or oat milk instead of cow's milk and vegan margarine instead of butter – just check the latter is suitable for baking. Coconut oil always works well as the fat in cakes and muffins. My colleagues, friends and family gobble up my dairy-free, wheat-free baked goodies with no complaints!

Retreat from Wheat

To avoid wheat I bake using different mixtures of oat, spelt and millet flour depending on the recipe. It is easy to make oat flour – just put your porridge/oatmeal whole oats in a coffee grinder or food processor and, after a minute of blending, you will have instant oat flour! There are also some excellent organic breakfast cereals made from Kamut, spelt and grains other than wheat.

Go For It!

If you have an 'all or nothing' kind of temperament or if you are very impatient to have a baby and are able to let go of all your destructive, contraceptive eating habits overnight then this is the way to go! For most people, however, the shock to the system would be too much, so evolve at your own pace to an improved, fertility-enhancing diet: set yourself goals and commit to a time frame in which you eliminate the 'bad' things and introduce the good. Good luck!

The Fertility Diet Protocol

Step 1 – Today:
Eliminate Immediately (NO EXCUSES)
- Tobacco
- Recreational drugs
- Aspartame, artificial sweeteners and 'diet' food stuffs.
- Genetically modified foods – the Frankenstein foods

Note on Step 1:

These are the contraceptive substances and food that has no nutritional value and/or could be causing serious harm to your fertility long term.

Step 2 – First Month:
Set Goals to Eliminate Completely Within One Month

- Alcohol: beer, wine, spirits
- Caffeinated coffee
- Caffeinated black tea
- Chemically decaffeinated, non-organic coffee
- Chemically decaffeinated, non-organic tea
- Soya beans, soya milk, tofu and all other soya products
- Non-organic meat
- Non-organic non-dairy products
- Non-organic free-range eggs
- Junk foods
- Junk drinks: sodas and tonic water
- Any packaged and convenience foods containing artificial chemicals and additives
- Peas
- Rhubarb
- Microwaved (i.e. dead) foods

Note on Step 2:

These are all foods or drinks that may have some nutritional merit, yet contain substances like caffeine, alcohol, pesticides, artificial chemicals or other compounds which inhibit conception. Some of you may be able to stop eating/drinking these things immediately. Others, dependent upon your own addictions, habits or preferences may need to take the entire month to wean yourself off – but, remember, the sooner the better in terms of getting and staying pregnant/impregnating your partner.

Step 3 – Second Month:
Reduce Significantly/Totally Eliminate as Much as Possible

- Refined sugar and sweets
- Refined flour and processed baked goods
- White rice
- All dairy produce (all cow's and goat's milk, yogurts, cheeses and butter; even if organic)
- All meat (even if organic)
- All fish and shellfish
- Non-organic honey and molasses
- All heated oils
- All fried foods except vegetable stir fries
- Organic decaffeinated (water or natural process) coffee and tea
- Non-organic vegetable oils

Note on Step 3:

Having cut out the worst contraceptive food offenders in Steps 1 and 2, during this stage you can take your health and fertility to the next level by removing all the highest gly-caemic foods (which accelerate ageing and deplete minerals), and the harmful cooked fats that upset cell membranes. This is the time to cut out all meat, fish and dairy products, which for the reasons described in Chapter 4 can interfere with fertility. Fish is included on this list since it is so diffi-cult to find seafood from uncontaminated sources without fertility-destroying mercury or PCBs. If you are wary about following a vegetarian diet, and are *certain* you have a pure source of fish, like freshwater trout from a pristine lake or river, or Alaskan wild salmon, then you may continue to include fish in your diet; otherwise, it is not worth the risk.

Most naturally decaffeinated teas and coffees, including organic ones, still contain around 3 per cent caffeine – it is time to let them go as well.

Step 4 – Third Month Onwards:
Consume Sparingly/in Moderation

- Free-range eggs
- Non-organic fruits you can peel

- Non-organic vegetables you can peel
- Non-organic or roasted nuts
- Non-organic or roasted seeds
- Packaged/bottled fruit and vegetable juices
- Wholewheat cereals and pasta
- Stir-fried vegetables
- Cooked, starchy (high glycaemic) vegetables: carrots, parsnip, Swedes, sweetcorn and white potatoes.
- High-glycaemic fruits: bananas, dates, dried apricots, mango, papaya, pineapple and raisins.
- Agave nectar and raw honey

Note on Step 4:

Step 4 is the final tweaking phase which leads you to full implementation of the Fertility Diet. At this time you begin to limit significantly the amount of high-glycaemic or non-organic fruits and vegetables and ration the amount of wheat consumed.

If you buy any non-organic fruit or vegetables, choose ones with thick skins that can be peeled before eating, like citrus fruit and sweet potatoes. The most heavily sprayed crops, which I recommend you never eat unless you can find them as certified organic, are (in order of highest pesticide levels): strawberries, green and red bell peppers, spinach, cherries, peaches, cantaloupe melon, celery, apples, apricots, green beans and cucumber. To help remove pesticide residue from any non-organic vegetables, spray them with apple cider vinegar, leave for a couple of minutes, then wash before eating/cooking.

I have included eggs on the Step 4 list. Eggs, providing they are organic and free-range, appear to be neutral for fertility. I could find nothing to suggest they would significantly enhance your chances of conceiving (although they do have a good range of amino acids), but equally no evidence that free-range eggs would be harmful for fertility either. With apologies to all the hard-core vegans out there I have now offended, I leave it entirely up to you whether you include free-range eggs or not in your diet. Factory-farm eggs will contain hormones and antibiotics and should already have been eliminated from your diet during Step 2.

Eat All You Want from Day One!

- Organic, low glycaemic fruits
- Organic non-starchy (low glycaemic) vegetables
- Organic raw nuts
- Organic raw seeds (especially sunflower seeds)
- Organic cold-pressed flax, hemp, olive, sesame, coconut, sunflower and almond oils
- Organic herbs
- Organic spices
- Himalayan crystal salt
- Sea vegetables and seaweeds (especially spirulina and blue-green algae)
- Xylitol
- Non-wheat grains, especially quinoa, millet, oats, buck-wheat, amaranth, spelt and brown rice
- Beans – all kinds, including chickpeas
- Pulses – lentils
- Pure/mineral water
- Hemp protein
- Mesquite meal
- Caffeine-free organic herbal teas
- Caffeine-free organic grain or dandelion coffee
- Raw (i.e. unprocessed in any form) coconut
- Appropriate daily doses of food-derived supplements: green powdered superfood mixes, blue-green algae, spirulina, brewer's yeast, bee pollen granules and maca.

Note on the Fertility Foods:

It is likely you are eating some of these wonderful foods already – just aim to eat more and more of them, until the good stuff is crowding out the more dubious elements of your present diet. Try the ones you have never had before, like quinoa, millet, hemp protein, maca and mesquite meal.

Aim to increase the nutritional quality of every meal: add spirulina, maca and mesquite to fruit smoothies; spinach and dandelion to soups or sauces; keep a pot of sunflower or sesame seeds with your condiments and sprinkle them on every salad and in every sandwich; eat quinoa instead of rice or pasta. Go a little crazy with the bee pollen granules, fresh chopped parsley and alfalfa sprouts – see how many meals you can sprinkle them on! When you approach cooking with the mentality of making it like a game to earn nutritional gold stars, it is amazing how many easy ways you can find to incorporate fertility power foods in your life.

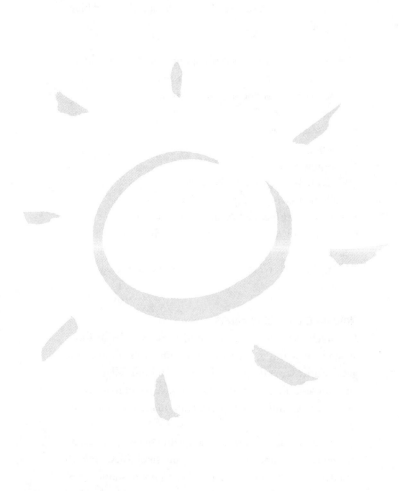

Testimonial

Over 35? On the Pill a Long Time? Or Breastfeeding a First Baby? No Problem!

My husband and I decided to try for a baby in May 2003 and I had expected to have to wait about a year, given the fact that I had been on the pill for over 15 years and that I was by then 36 – and meant to be over the fertility hill. In fact we had to wait only 21 days before finding out I was expecting our beautiful daughter, Virginia, who was born in February 2004 when I was 37.

I have always had a very healthy diet and cook almost all our meals from scratch so I did not have to specifically change our diet much in order to conceive. As a rule, I try to buy organic food as much as possible, although it took me a bit of time to source vegetables in my area that did not come from Tesco. I do not smoke or drink fizzy drinks. At the time I conceived I was already drinking very little coffee, sticking mainly to herbal teas.

I was still breastfeeding Virginia when my second baby was conceived – also very easily, despite the 'obstacles' of my age, as well as breastfeeding itself, which is meant to be a powerful contraceptive! I had turned 38 (almost 39) when I had a gorgeous, healthy son Alexander, who was born on Christmas Day 2005. Both births were natural births with no pain relief other than gas and air. I breastfed both of them until they were each a year and three months. The only change to my diet since Alexander was born has been an increase in my coffee intake. They are healthy, happy children and I continue to maintain a similar diet to ours for them.

Alison C, Perthshire, Scotland, aged 40

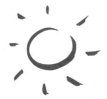

Chapter 37

Recipes for Fertility

Over the years I have bought hundreds of diet, health and nutri-tion-type books. In many instances, as I tucked into a nice fat book with anticipation of great learning, I would be very disap-pointed to find only a scant couple of chapters covered the author's theories/research and that most of the book was padded out with esoteric recipes, which I knew I was unlikely to try. Do not worry, this is not one of *those* books. I would like to set out a few basic principles of preparing food when following the Fertility Diet. The easiest way for me to do this is to take you into my own kitchen, and guide you through some of my favourite recipes and reveal much of what I might be eating on a typical day. This will also appeal to the nosiness of those who like to know what these would be health/fertility-guru authors actually eat.

If you want more elaborate recipes, then look out for one of the excellent raw food vegan or normal vegan/dairy-free vegetarian cookbooks and just adapt any recipe you like to make it Fertility Diet-compatible (like eliminating soya). I have listed my favourite cookbooks in the Bibliography section.

Fab Fertility Breakfasts

Fertility Diet breakfasts are easy. You will mainly be enjoying fresh fruit, smoothies, flax and fruit puddings, raw nuts and seeds, nut milks and organic cereals (not wheat-based).

Sarah's pre-breakfast-breakfast: three steps for outstanding health and fertility. Before eating my main breakfast each morning, I take 3 things that are my nutritional 'insurance policy' for the day.

Part 1 – Himalayan Mineral Infusion

To make this sole solution (see also Chapter 13), first of all I prepare the base solution by spooning around 5–6 tablespoons of Himalayan crystal salt into a glass jar filled with water. What you are aiming at is that the water is so saturated with this magic salt that you can see the pink salt crystals still at the bottom – so depending on the size of your glass jar, keep adding crystal salt until it cannot dissolve completely in the water (of course, shake it with the lid on, to see if solids are settling). First thing each morning I put 3 tablespoons of the sole brine solution from its jar into a large (500 ml) glass of water to dilute it down, and drink it all in one go – or sometimes pausing just to take my blue-green algae, spirulina or brewer's yeast supplements at the same time. It tastes a little bit salty of course, but is quite manageable. Just to be clear – always dilute the sole solution! This drink immediately rehydrates my body and gets all bio-electrical circuits firing. The sole contains traces of all minerals needed for fertility and is a complete health tonic.

Part 2 – Green Superfood Drink plus Home-made Mega Green Powder

The second step is to flood my body with cleansing chlorophyll and health-enhancing superfoods by drinking a superfood green drink. I mix one tablespoon of the green powder in with my second 500 ml of water for the morning. All right, I will admit this tastes quite horrid, so, unless you are masochistic, it is best to drink this without pausing for breath. But, with one glass putting the nutritional equivalent of fifteen plates of salad inside me (and eating this much greenery in one day is just *not* going to happen), as well as setting off an explosion of nutrients in my grateful body, its well worth the negotiation with the taste buds. Green superfood powders of freeze-dried wheatgrass/barley grass, herbs, seaweeds and other nutrient-dense goodies can be bought in all health-food stores.

Recently, I have boosted my green superfood drink with my own home-made mega-powder of dandelions, rosemary, sage, thyme and parsley. No folks, this is not hard to make. I gather heaps of dandelions (yes, those weed things) plus the herbs from my organic garden, and, after washing them, put them in my dehydrator to dry out. If you are not a kitchen-gadget freak like me and do not own a dehydrator, then leaving them out in sunshine for about 2–3 days or in the airing cupboard at home should do the trick. When all the leaves are dry and crispy, I grind them up into a powder (I have a gadget for this as well – but your coffee grinder or food processor will do the job too). Now I will let you into a secret. The combination of a regular superfood powder drink with a tablespoon of my own predominantly dandelion powder, although tasting a bit yucky, makes you totally high within half an hour of drinking it! Really, you will be on the healthiest 'trip' of your life. My body loves it! It gives me an absolute buzz, well worth tolerating the disgusting taste while I chug it down fast.

One caution: build up to two tablespoons of any green superfoods very slowly. If you started with this amount right away, then (depending on how healthy your diet was previously) you could make yourself completely nauseous, since it could be too much hypernutrition for your body to handle at once.

Part 3 – Lovely Lemon 'Tea'

The third part of my early morning ritual involves drinking the juice from one whole organic lemon in hot water (cooled from boiling). Sometimes I add xylitol to sweeten, otherwise, in winter, a pinch of cayenne pepper to warm me up and speed up my metabolism. This lemon tea sends a 'wake up, clean out' call to your liver and your intestines. When I have whole root ginger in the house I make a ginger lemon tea with two tablespoons grated ginger, organic lemon juice and mineral water. I place all the ingredients into a saucepan and bring to a boil with the peel of the lemon in the pan too. This is because most of the powerful phytonutrients in lemons are in the peel and pith. I discard the peel of course before drinking. You can only use the peel if your lemon is organic. Do not boil yourself some brew with pesticides!

I know my pre-breakfast breakfast sounds like a lot but I can prepare and drink my mineral infusion, superfood drink and lemon/lemon-ginger tea inside about five minutes. I then feel on top of the world and ridiculously smug; no matter what nutritional transgressions I may commit later in the day, I have woken my body up and boosted my fertility with the best combination of rapidly absorbable nutrients, and already consumed almost an entire 1.5 litre bottle of mineral water.

Main Breakfasts

Fertility Fruit Smoothie, a.k.a. 100 per cent pulp juice

Ingredients for 1 serving:

1 large organic citrus fruit (orange, grapefruit or 2 tangerines) OR 1 cup of organic berries (strawberries, raspberries, blackberries, blackcurrants)

1–2 cups mineral water

¼ teaspoon MSM powder

Optional: 1 tsp soaked flax seeds (see recipe below).

Preparation:

Place fruit into a high-speed blender and add enough water to cover fruit. Spoon in MSM (do not exceed ¼ teaspoon) and blend until all lumps have disappeared (around 20 seconds to 2 minutes depending on blender). Enjoy!

Nutritional Notes:

Unlike packaged pasteurized fruit juice, this smoothie allows you to enjoy a fresh juice, with all the vitamins, minerals and enzymes still intact. You will have consumed 100 per cent of your daily dose of vitamin C in a natural form – great for women's fertility and even more so for men as a sperm wonder tonic. You will also be getting the full fibre of the fruit which ordinary juicing removes. Adding MSM to the juice injects an anti-ageing boost, since vitamin C and MSM collaborate to keep your cell membranes very happy. Finally, a blender jug is a lot easier to clean than messing around cleaning all the component parts of a juicer! I make this 100 per cent pulp juice every morning after my pre-breakfast-breakfast and use it to wash down any other morning supplements I want to take.

Nut Milks

Ingredients for 4 servings:

½lb of almonds (or hazelnuts, brazils, walnuts)
¾ litre mineral water
2 dates or 2 tsp agave nectar or 2 tsp xylitol (optional)
1 pinch Himalayan crystal salt

Preparation:

So how do you milk a nut? I am sure you are eager to know. Easy! Put the almonds in a bowl or glass jug and cover with water. Leave overnight to soak. The next morning tip all the soaked almonds and the soak water into a blender. Add optional sweetener (dates, agave nectar or xylitol) and 1 pinch of salt (preferably the wonderful, mineral loaded, Himalayan crystal salt). Blend for as long as is necessary for your blender to thoroughly puree the nuts and water into a smoothie. More water produces a skimmed milk consistency, less water can bring you right down to a double cream viscosity and if you actually want to make almond cream just add much less water!

This mixture now needs to be strained. Your options are to pour it through a fine mesh sieve over a bowl squishing the pulp with a spoon, or to put it into a mesh 'sprout' or 'seed' bag, and squeeze the 'milk' out. I take option two – and this always reminds me of squeezing an udder (not that I have ever done so!). Someone once told me that you can use a clean nylon stocking as an effective seed bag for this process but the idea does not appeal to me (not to mention what chemicals could be inadvertently added from the stocking!). Once the fluid is strained you can use this unbelievably delicious milk in any way you would use regular cow's milk. It is a fantastic base for a fertility smoothie. Almond milk, of all types of nut milks, contains the most fertility nutrients.

But what to do with the almond nut pulp you now have it in your sieve/mesh bag? Well, waste not, want not! Into the dehydrator at 40°C it goes and after about five hours – voila! dried almond nut 'flour' which you can add to any recipe as a part substitute for wheat or other grain flour. The almond meal can also be dried out in the oven on the lowest possible setting and will be ready in about one hour or less (depending on how low your oven heats). This flour is high in protein and minerals and a great addition to any baking recipe.

Almond Aphrodisiac Smoothie

Remember, drinking this smoothie could make you late for work. Only prepare it when you may have time to enjoy the consequences . . .

Ingredients for 2 servings:

500ml almond milk (as above)

1 tbsp maca*

1 tbsp mesquite*

2 tbsp raw cacao powder (note: contains a small amount of caffeine)*

1 tsp spirulina powder

2 tbsp agave nectar

1 pinch Himalayan crystal salt

* You will find these unusual fertility ingredients in your local health-food shop or on online.

Preparation:
Place all ingredients in a blender and blend until smooth and lump free. That's it. Serve to your beloved with a flower from the garden (on the side of course). You will not believe how orgasmic this smoothie tastes, my mouth is watering as I type. It is also amazingly filling and you will not be hungry, er, for food that is, for many hours.

General tips for sensational ultra-healthy smoothies:
Belonging to the 'bung-it-in' School of Cookery as I do, I am reluctant to inhibit your own culinary creativity with dictatorial sounding recipes. Luckily, smoothie making is an art, not a science, so you may adjust the ingredients in any smoothie up, down, in or out, to please yourself.

Preparation:
Pour a base fluid of about 500 ml mineral water OR nut milk (recipe above) into your blender jug. To this you can add any of the following, pretty much in any amount or combination you like – I list quantities below only for general guidance:
1 cup fresh or frozen, raw, organic fruit
3 tbsp soaked flax seeds
1 tbsp sunflower seeds
1 tbsp sesame seeds
1 tsp spirulina (dodgy taste vanishes in most smoothies)
1 pinch Himalayan crystal salt
1 tbsp maca
1 tbsp mesquite
2 tbsp hemp protein powder
2 tsp bee pollen (if you are not allergic)
2 tbsp raw cacao powder (contains caffeine – exercise moderation)
1 tbsp of superfood green powder (tastes very strong!)
1 tbsp coconut oil
1 tbsp flax oil
aloe vera leaf filet
1–2 tbsp agave nectar
2 tsp xylitol
2–3 dates

Blend your selected ingredients and enjoy. No, do not add them all, silly, that would be overkill. Everything on this list will be contributing in some way to optimal health and fertility.

Coconut-spice Porridge

Ingredients for 2 servings:

1 cup old-fashioned, organic whole oats
2 cups organic coconut milk
1 cup water
Spices (optional): ½ tsp cinnamon, nutmeg, ground cardamom, cloves
2 tsp agave nectar or xylitol
1 pinch Himalayan crystal salt

Preparation:

Put all the ingredients in a saucepan, bring to the boil, simmer for about 5 minutes until the porridge thickens. Serve. Soaked flax seeds (see recipe below), sunflower seeds and sesame seeds can be sprinkled on the top of this delicious porridge.

Nutritional Notes:

Oats are a fertility-friendly food, being high in fibre, low in gluten and moderate on the glycaemic index. Made with high-protein coconut milk for a change instead of the usual 3 cups of water (or cow's milk), and with warming, blood-sugar regulating spices, and topped with seeds, this porridge is a yummy, highly nutritious breakfast for a cold morning, and takes no longer than regular porridge to make.

Coconut Rice Pudding (Gluten and Dairy Free!)

Instead of porridge, you can make a gluten-free coconut rice pudding by substituting 1 cup of organic brown rice instead of the 1 cup of oats in the porridge recipe. You will need to simmer the rice for 40 minutes or so for it to be cooked, so this breakfast takes much longer to make. Nutmeg and flax/sesame/sunflower seeds sprinkled on the top of this pudding taste sublime. This can of course also be eaten as a dessert.

Fantastic Flax Seed Recipes

I know very few people who eat flax seeds regularly. Most people do not know what to do with them and they taste very boring just eaten plain. It is great to eat flax seeds at breakfast/in the morning since the fibre gets the bowels moving, they help stabilize blood sugar, while balancing oestrogen levels.

Flax Jelly (Soaked Flax Seeds)
Ingredients:
2 tbsp flax seeds
½ cup mineral water
Optional: dried fruit

Preparation:
Place flax seeds in a glass jar, cover with water. Leave in the fridge overnight. That's it! The following morning the flax seeds will have turned into a mucilaginous gel. By soaking with dried fruit at the same time (these are high glycaemic and should not be eaten too often), you create a sweet compote of fruit and flax.

You can set up a production line: I prepare 5/6 small glass jars with flax and water at a time and put them in the fridge, so that my week's supply of flax has been prepared in 30 seconds of effort. There are then a number of things you can do with the soaked flax seeds:

- Add them to all fruit or nut milk smoothies.
- Create a flax and fruit pudding, by blending flax and fruit together (a ratio of 1 part flax to 3 parts fruit) in a food processor and adding a little xylitol, agave nectar or honey for extra sweetness. (See also recipe for flax and banana pudding, below.)
- Blob them on top of your porridge/coconut porridge.
- If you own a dehydrator you can make flax crackers (see recipes below).

Flax and Banana Pudding.

Ingredients:

1 serving of soaked golden flax seeds – about 5
    tablespoons (as per above recipe)

2 bananas

2 tsp agave nectar or xylitol

1 tsp cinnamon

Preparation:

Place all ingredients in high speed blender or food processor, blend until mixture is smooth. Serve immediately and enjoy.

Nutritional Notes:

Any children you know will gladly eat this banana pudding and it can even be given to your future baby once he/she gets on to solid foods – so think of this as a practice parent recipe. The golden flax seeds look prettier than the brown seeds in this recipe, since it makes the pudding yellow instead of caramel brown, but you can use brown flax seeds if you want. The high omega 3 fat content of the flax seeds mitigates the high-fruit sugar levels of the bananas, and, together with cinnamon, this prevents an insulin spike, and keeps blood sugar stable. This is a great way to get the fertility power of flax into your life. If the pudding mixture is placed on dehydrator sheets and dehydrated over night, you will get wonderful sweet flax crackers. Do *not* bake in the oven, however, as the nutritional value of flax is lost **in temperatures over 118°F**.

Flax Crackers

You need a dehydrator to make this recipe – nothing else will work – sorry!

Ingredients:

Soaked flaxseeds

and

for savoury crackers: crystal salt, herbs, sesame seeds,
    sunflower seeds

for sweet crackers: agave nectar, bananas, dried fruits,
    raisins

Preparation:

According to your preferences add savoury or sweet ingredients to your soaked flax seeds. Rather than prescribe any fixed amounts I would just say make sure 80 per cent of your cracker mixture is flax and 20 per cent is the flavouring. Spread the flax mixture on to the dehydrator sheets and score in grooves with a knife to divide the flax into your desired cracker shapes. Dehydrate at about 40°C/110°F overnight.

Nutrtional Notes:

These health- and fertility-enhancing crackers will keep for a month in an airtight container/the fridge. They might even last longer but none I have made have ever been around uneaten long enough for me to find out.

Fab Fertility Lunches and Dinners

Flax and Sesame Seed Salt

Ingredients:

1 tbsp whole flax seeds

1 tbsp sesame seeds

1 tbsp Himalayan rock crystal salt

Preparation:

Grind the flax seeds and sesame seeds into powder in your coffee grinder (that you are no longer using for its intended purpose of course). In a bowl mix the ground seeds with the salt. Store in a glass jar, sprinkle on all foods you wish to season with salt.

Nutritional Notes:

This recipe brings the extra mineral and vitamin power of flax and sesame seeds to the mineral-packed Himalayan salt. Flax seeds are not only rich in omega 3 essential fatty acids, they are also a very mild phytoestrogen and help women to maintain balanced oestrogen levels. Using this salt every day will go a long way to covering your mineral needs for conception.

Super Soups

Soups are one of the mainstays of every bung-it-in cook's repertoire. I love them because having a soup of some kind available every day means I can quickly heat it up and eat this before my hunger drives me to eat something else not-so healthy I will regret! With a yummy warm bowl of soup inside me as a starter, I can calmly plan healthy lunch and dinner options with my nutritionist's brain, not my appetite, driving my choices.

Usually when vegetables are boiled, particularly for too long, many of the nutrients are lost into the water. The beauty of soups is, you then get to recover these nutrients in the fluid (as well as those in the vegetable stock to begin with) and eat them with the soup!

I learned how to make wonderfully nutritious vegan soups from the Queen of Soups: my mum, who can seemingly turn any ingredients/leftovers/anything in the bottom of the fridge drawer into delicious broths, soups and stews.

Soup Base: Vegetable Stock

Every delicious soup begins with a good foundation of vegetable stock. As you start to follow the Fertility Diet you will be eating a lot of vegetables. Each time you boil or preferably lightly steam, any vegetable do so using mineral water. This is not an extravagance, because you are now going to start to save all your vegetable pot-water as a stock for your soup bases (and indeed for steam frying instead of using vegetable oils – see later). My fridge always contains a glass jug with vegetable water from that day. I will usually add an organic vegetable bouillon cube to my veggie water just to give it some extra oomph.

Basic Vegan Soup

Ingredients:

1 large onion – finely chopped

2 cloves garlic – crushed/finely chopped

1 litre vegetable stock

1 potato or, preferably, sweet potato – chopped up into smallish pieces

1 carrot – chopped

2 tsp herbs: oregano, parsley, rosemary, sage, basil

Any other organic vegetable you like

1 cup millet – optional

½ tsp Himalayan crystal salt

2 sticks celery (optional)

Preparation:

Steam fry the onion and garlic in a large saucepan, by adding a little vegetable stock to the vegetables in the pan, and stirring them over a medium heat until they are translucent. Add 2 tsp of any preferred herbs – fresh and organic if possible, steam fry a further minute. Add the remaining vegetable stock. Next I put in whatever root vegetable I am using to thicken the soup and make it hearty. This is usually sweet potato (a fertility power food), regular potato when I cannot get sweet potatoes, or sometimes swede or butternut squash. I usually have organic carrots in my fridge, so I add one or two to bring some more vitamin A, carotenoids and zinc to the soup. If I want a soup that tastes creamy (and has even more minerals) I will add a cup of millet grains. This is the basic soup. It would taste pretty dull if you added nothing else at this point.

With all soups, both this basic one and the variations described below, you let them come to a boil, then simmer for at least 10–15 minutes. Before serving I use a handheld stick-blender to break down the ingredients as much as I want (sometimes its nice to leave whole pieces) and to thicken the soup – this saves a lot of fuss and bother of transferring it into a blender jug and back again to the saucepan.

For busy working folk, I suggest you invest in a crock pot/slow cooker. Then, before you leave for work, you can throw in all the ingredients and stock/mineral water at once (and maybe a few beans as well). By the time you get home a yummy hot soup will be waiting for you.

I recommend adding as much spinach, broccoli and parsley to soups as you can stand – these really are amazing vegetables in terms of their nutritional content.

I like to make soups in my rice cooker – a trick I discovered during a hurricane in the Cayman Islands! The soup cooks quickly, but there is no risk of it burning if, as usual, I get too absorbed in some writing or garden project and forget about it. Making soup in a rice cooker means you can also keep the soup on the warm setting – ready for when you want it.

From the base recipe you can add pretty much *any* vegetable you like. Here are some examples to create specific soups:

Leek and Potato Soup
Add 2 chopped leeks and 2 more potatoes. Sprinkle on fresh parsley before serving.

Tomato and Basil Soup
1 tin organic chopped tomatoes (or 1 lb fresh tomatoes), 1 tin tomato puree, fresh or dried basil leaves, 1 tbsp xylitol to bring out tomato taste (no idea why sugar does this), 1 tsp apple cider vinegar.

Lentil Soup
1 entire bag of red lentils, 1 further finely chopped medium sized onion. Best to leave out the optional millet when making lentil soup or it will get too thick.

Asparagus Soup
Add 8–12 asparagus spears or 1 tin of asparagus. The herb thyme tastes delicious with asparagus.

Carrot, Coconut and Peanut Soup

Omit the optional millet. To the basic recipe, add 2 lb carrots, 1 whole jar of organic peanut (or almond) butter, 3 inches of ginger root grated, 1 tbsp curry powder, the juice of 1 lemon. Add 1 tin of organic coconut milk at the very end, just before serving. Needless to say this soup is pretty high in calories, but tastes *so* good. My friends and I enjoyed this as our starter for our Christmas meal.

Butternut Squash and Spinach/Dandelion Soup

To the basic soup recipe add 1 butternut squash chopped into 2-inch pieces, plus 1 cup fresh or frozen spinach (and if you want to max out the nutrient content – ½ cup fresh raw dandelions).

Frisky Onion Soup

Omit the potato, carrot and millet from the basic soup recipe. You simply throw 6 chopped onions and 6 finely chopped cloves of garlic into a litre of vegetable stock in a saucepan and bring to the boil. This soup does not need blending. Serve fresh parsley on top (to take away garlic breath!). That is it – this is a complete aphrodisiac soup, and yet, despite being so ridiculously easy to make, tastes yummy.

I hope you get the idea. Whatever soup I have on the go depends upon what vegetables I have left over from a previous meal, and what is in the fridge that needs to be eaten up quickly or be thrown away.

Easy Vegan Meals

Ratatouille

Ingredients for 6 servings:

1 cup vegetable stock

2 tins organic chopped tomatoes/1.5 lb of fresh organic tomatoes (chopped)

1 lb of courgettes (zucchini) cut into round slices
1 lb aubergine (egg plant) – this is optional and slows the
   preparation time down
4 finely chopped cloves of garlic
4–5 spring onions (scallions) – chopped into small pieces
1 red pepper – chopped
1 green pepper – chopped
½ cup fresh parsley or fresh basil
½ tsp cayenne pepper (optional)
½ tsp oregano, fresh or dried
1 bay leaf

Preparation:

If you are including aubergine, then slice it up, layering the slices in a sieve, each layer covered with normal table salt (this is just to remove the bitterness – do not waste precious Himalayan crystal salt with this step), leave for 30 minutes, then rinse all the salt away thoroughly.

Steam fry the chopped spring onions and garlic in vegetable stock until translucent. Add the cayenne, oregano and bay leaf, as well as the prepared aubergines (if you are using them) and the chopped red and green peppers and continue to steam fry a few minutes. Add the courgette slices, then all the tomatoes and tomato puree. Bring to the boil adding more vegetable stock if necessary, then turn down the heat and let simmer for around 30 minutes.

Serve with fresh parsley or fresh basil on the top. Can be eaten as a main dish with rice or quinoa or as a tasty vegetable side dish.

Nutritional Notes:

This easy Mediterranean dish is very low calorie, yet packed with nutrients. The onions and garlic are, of course, powerful aphrodisiacs. The fertility power food parsley is added at the end. It keeps well in the fridge and also freezes well, if you are making it in the quantities of this recipe. Sometimes for a change I will eat it with 1 cup of spinach stirred it at the end to give it even more nutritional clout.

Very Veggie Tomato Sauce

Ingredients for 3–4 servings:

½ cup vegetable stock
1 tin organic tomatoes/1 lb of organic tomatoes (chopped)
1 small tin tomato puree
1 onion
2–3 cloves garlic
1 red bell pepper
1 tsp xylitol
1 tsp balsamic vinegar
½ tsp oregano
Additional selection of any organic non-starchy vegetables
    finely chopped: mushrooms, spinach, asparagus, carrots,
    broccoli, cauliflower, green beans, zucchini
Crystal salt and black pepper to taste
½ cup fresh basil

Preparation:

Steam fry the onion and garlic in vegetable stock, or in the tomato juice from the tinned tomatoes. Next add the oregano and the chopped red pepper and continue to steam fry for a few minutes. Add the tinned or fresh chopped tomatoes, tomato puree, xylitol and vinegar and any additional chopped organic veggies you feel like eating. Bring to the boil, then turn down the heat and simmer for about 20–30 minutes. Add the fresh basil at the very end before serving.

Nutritional Notes:

This easy and versatile vegan tomato-veggie sauce can be eaten with non-wheat pasta, rice or quinoa. You can boil and mash some potato or sweet potato and serve this layered over the sauce in a serving dish, like a shepherd's pie without the meat. You can add more vegetable stock and convert it into a tomato basil soup. On cold days or to boost metabolism it can be converted into an 'arrabiata' version of tomato sauce by the addition of cayenne pepper.

Vegan Chilli
Ingredients for 6 servings:
2 tins kidney beans, drained
½ cup vegetable stock
1 tin organic tomatoes/1 lb of organic tomatoes (chopped)
1 small tin tomato puree
1 onion
2–3 cloves garlic
1 red bell pepper
1 tsp xylitol
1 tsp balsamic vinegar
1 tsp chilli powder
½ tsp cayenne pepper
½ cup fresh parsley
Crystal salt and black pepper to taste

Preparation:
Steam fry the onion and garlic as usual in the vegetable stock or in the tomato juice from the tinned tomatoes. When translucent add the chilli powder and cayenne pepper and the chopped red bell pepper and continue to stream fry a few minutes. Add the tinned or fresh tomatoes, tomato puree, drained kidney beans, xylitol and balsamic vinegar. Bring to the boil, then simmer for around 20–30 minutes to let the flavours merge. You can add more or less chilli powder and cayenne pepper according to your own taste preferences. Sprinkle with fresh parsley before serving. This yummy chilli goes well with brown rice, quinoa or just on its own.

Sesame Spinach
Ingredients for 1 serving:
1 cup frozen organic spinach
¼ cup vegetable stock
2 tbsp sesame seeds
1 clove garlic
1 tbsp grated fresh ginger root
1 tbsp lemon juice or pseudo-soya sauce (see recipe
   below), both optional

Preparation:

Add spinach, ginger and garlic to vegetable stock and cook until spinach in thawed and cooked. Keep stirring, since most of vegetable stock will be absorbed. Before serving stir in sesame seeds. Before learning about the contraceptive qualities of soya sauce I used to add 1 tsp of soya sauce to this before eating. Now I usually add lemon juice. If I want to have a really Asian taste I occasionally make up a soya-sauce substitute using 4 oz (120 ml) of molasses, with 1.5 oz (45 ml) balsamic vinegar and a little extra xylitol. This tastes pretty good and I add 1 tbsp of this NOT_soya sauce to my sesame spinach.

Nutritional Notes:

I am a bit addicted to this recipe at the moment and eat it about three times a week. It is ready in five minutes and is delicious. It is also a fertility power meal – spinach, sesame, ginger and garlic all being fertility power foods and aphrodisiacs. Enjoy.

Hummus

Ingredients:

1 tin chickpeas (or 2 cups cooked chickpeas plus ¼ cup vegetable stock)
3 tbsp tahini (sesame seed puree)
3 cloves garlic – finely chopped
Juice of 1 lemon
¼ cup fresh parsley

Preparation:

Place all the ingredients in a blender or in a food processor – including the water in the tinned chickpeas – and go brsssshhhhhh, for as long as necessary to remove all the lumps. Enjoy on flax seed crackers or as a dip with raw vegetables like baby carrots and celery.

Variations: if you make this with more water you will have a delicious salad dressing.

Add red bell pepper, or extra parsley, or cayenne pepper for changes to the basic hummus recipe. It tastes great, however it is made. Remember chickpeas and garlic are aphrodisiacs!

Quick Quinoa Recipes

Most people do not have a clue what to do with quinoa and have never even tried it. You are in for a treat. You cook it just like rice and it has a pleasant, faintly nutty taste. It is very versatile. You can make a batch of quinoa, have it like rice one day, and then turn the leftovers into a salad or use it to stuff peppers or tomatoes the following day. I love food like this, since I have a life, and do not intend to spend hours on end in the kitchen every day, but want everything I eat to make a massive contribution to my health.

Basic Quinoa

Ingredients for 3 servings:
1 cup quinoa
2½ cups vegetable stock
1 vegetable bouillon cube

Preparation:
Place everything in a rice cooker, stir a little and 15 minutes later– voilà – perfect quinoa. If cooking on a stove top, put everything in a saucepan. After the vegetable stock with added bouillon cube and quinoa comes to the boil, turn the heat down and let it simmer for another 15 minutes or so until all the liquid is absorbed and you are left with a pot of fluffy quinoa. Use quinoa in place of rice with all your favourite dishes.

Nutritional Notes:
Quinoa is a fertility power food, loaded with nutrients – particularly amino acids and minerals – and far better for you than rice. It is an aphrodisiac too.

Quinoa Salad

Ingredients:
3 cups cooked basic quinoa, cooled
1 tin organic sweetcorn – drained
1 tin organic kidney beans – drained and rinsed
3 raw organic tomatoes

1 red bell pepper
¼ cup sunflower seeds
Any other favourite organic salad vegetables: cucumber,
    radishes, celery, avocado, beets, etc.

Preparation:
First drain the sweetcorn from its tin, drain the kidney beans
from their tin and quickly rinse them. Secondly, mix the
quinoa, drained sweetcorn and kidney beans and all the
extra salad vegetables of your choice together in a large bowl
and enjoy. Use crystal salt, pepper and your favourite salad
dressing. I usually just put a little salt and the juice of a
lemon on my quinoa salad. In the summer I make this a lot.
My friends seem to love it too.

Stuffed Quinoa Peppers
Ingredients for 4 servings:
2 cups cooked quinoa
4 large red bell peppers
2 tbsps olive oil
1 onion
2 cloves garlic
1 tsp oregano

Preparation:
Cut the tops off the bell peppers and save the tops (to be
little hats later). Scoop out the seeds inside the peppers and
discard. Steam fry the onion and garlic in the vegetable
stock. Add the quinoa and oregano to the garlic and onion
in the pan and mix well. Spoon the quinoa/onion/garlic
mixture into each of the hollow peppers and replace the cut-
off top on each. Bake the stuffed peppers on a non-stick
baking tin in the oven at 200°C for 20 minutes. Drizzle
with a little olive oil before serving. You could brush the
olive oil on the peppers before roasting, but cooked oils are
not recommended on the Fertility Diet.

Variation: stuffed tomatoes. Prepare in the same way, just
save whatever you scoop out from the inside of the tomato
to add it to the quinoa/onion and garlic stuffing.

Special Treats

There are those times, the wrong time of the month, after a hard week at work, or following a negative pregnancy test, when eating spinach or such like is not really going to hit the emotional spot as a comfort food (although a raw cacao smoothie can be some consolation!). I have two nice recipes up my sleeve for when I want something sweet, emotionally indulging, but reasonably healthy.

Banana Bread (Wheat, Dairy and Sugar Free)

Ingredients for 10 servings:

4 bananas
1 cup water or apple juice
4 cups oat flour
4 tbsp xylitol (or agave nectar)
1 tsp baking soda
2 tsp baking powder
3 tsp spices – your pick: ginger, cinnamon, nutmeg, cloves, all spice, cardamom
½ cup raisins

Preparation:

Blend the bananas and water or juice together in a blender. Mix all the other ingredients together in a separate bowl. Slowly add the liquid banana mixture to the dry ingredients and mix in well with a wooden spoon or using electric beaters.

Pre-heat the oven to 350°F and grease either a bread tin or a muffin tin with coconut oil. Use the bread tin for a traditional-looking banana bread, or muffin tin to make banana bread individual muffins. Bake for 40 minutes.

Variations: My Greek-American friend Clare makes my banana bread but with masses of ginger and spices, and it tastes *really* good. For a ginger-cake version, omit the other spices, use at least 5 tbsp ginger and replace the xylitol/agave nectar with molasses as the sweetener.

Nutritional Notes:

With this yummy recipe you are eating little more than the baked equivalent of a bowl of porridge with banana – yet it tastes as if it must be unhealthy. My small nieces and nephews love this recipe and demand 'cake' for breakfast when they visit me, not suspecting I am only giving them nutritionally the same as one of their normal breakfasts.

Sarah's Insanely Healthy Vegan Scones

Ingredients for about 18 scones:

8 oz non-wheat flour (50 per cent oat, 50 per cent spelt recommended)

3 oz vegan (non-soya) margarine

2 oz xylitol

2 oz raisins

2 tsp baking powder

2 tsp baking soda

⅔ of a litre almond milk (or rice milk)

1 pinch salt

bananas/other fruit/chopped nuts/spices (optional)

Preparation:

Put the flour, baking powder, baking soda and salt into a bowl. Add the vegan margarine, and begin to rub it in, until the fat and the flour is integrated and looks like bread-crumbs. Then add sugar, raisins and any optional ingredients like spices, chopped nuts or chopped bananas to the crumb mixture and stir well. Slowly add the almond milk, keep stirring and dribbling in the milk until the mixture is a thick dough consistency – do not make it too runny. Grease a muffin tin. Spoon a large dollop of the dough mixture in each compartment. Place in a pre-heated oven at 425°F and, within 20 minutes, you will have perfect, delicious scones. Yummy!

Conclusion

This recipe section is not meant to be a comprehensive list of all the delicious fertility-friendly dishes you can eat, rather an account of some of my favourite recipes that are all easy and quick to prepare, full of healthy nutrients, yet very tasty.

I hope I have inspired you to find ways you can adapt your own favourite meals to fit in with the Fertility Diet principles.

Good luck and best baby-making wishes.

Sarah Dobbyn

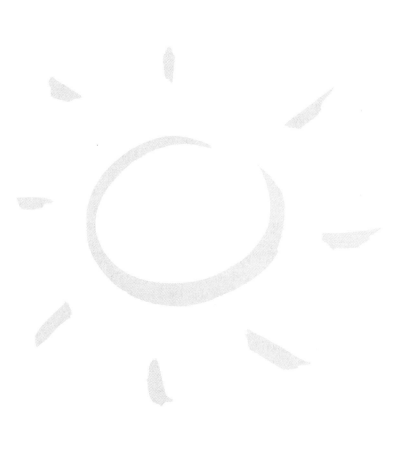

TESTIMONIAL

Over 38 and Long-term Pill Use is No Obstacle to Conceiving Easily!

My baby time clock started to 'tick' when I was 38. Luckily, when it struck, I was with a wonderful man who was also quite happy to have a baby so, one December, five years ago, I said goodbye to my last packet of little anti-baby pills and set to the task of getting pregnant. I had been on the pill for forever and was a little concerned in light of my age about how long, if ever, it would take until I became pregnant. So I spoke to Sarah Dobbyn, who assured me that it definitely was not too late and she made a few suggestions such as to cut out the caffeine and alcohol and to eat more organic fruit and vegetables and generally to get my body into a 'healthy' baby-friendly mode which I did. Lo and behold, 5 months later, there I was pregnant and at age 39 I had the most gorgeous, healthy little bundle of joy to show for it!

I also went for some 'Body Talk' sessions, which were very bizarre and very fascinating. The lady told me that she was 'talking' to my body and that it was aligning itself and preparing me for my pregnancy. The last time I saw her, she had a huge grin on her face, she didn't say too much during our session but, when I left, she gave me an enormous hug and asked me to call her in two weeks or so. Of course, two weeks later, I found out that I was 4 weeks pregnant with my daughter!

Kate A, Cayman Islands, British West Indies, aged 44

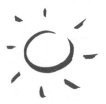

Notes

Introduction

1 Swan, S.H. and Elkin, E.P. (1999) 'Declining semen quality: can the past inform the present?', BioEssays, 21 (7), 614–21.
2 Carlsen, E., et al. (1992) 'Evidence for the decreasing quality of semen during the past 50 years', *British Medical Journal*, 305, pp. 609–13.
3 Ibid.
   Van Waeleghem, K.., et al. (1994) 'Deterioration of sperm quality in young Belgian men during recent decades', *Human Reproduction*, 9 (4), p. 73.
   Auger, J., et al. (1995) 'Decline in semen quality among fertile men in Paris during the past 20 years', *New England Journal of Medicine*, 332 (5), pp. 281–5.
   Irvine, D.S. (1994) 'Failing sperm quality', *British Medical Journal*, 309, p. 476.
4 (1995) 'Pre-conceptual care and pregnancy outcome', *Journal of Nutritional and Environmental Medicine*, 5, pp. 205–8.

Chapter 1

1 Northrup, Christiane (1994) *Women's Bodies, Women's Wisdom; Creating Physical and Emotional Health and Healing*, Bantam Books, p. 379.
2 Quoted in Klatz, Ronald (1998) *Grow Young with HGH*, HarperPerennial, p. 49.
3 Reported by Brant Secunda, a Shaman trained by the Huizol Indians, to Dr Christiane Northrup in (2002) *Women's Bodies, Women's Wisdom*, Bantam Books, p. 419.

4 Baker, Barbara (1994) 'Older women make the grade as oocyte donors', *ObGyn News*, 15 July, p. 49.

5 Quoted in 'The whole person fertility program', p. 50.

6 Chopra, Deepak (1993) *Ageless Body, Timeless Mind: The Quantum Alternative to Growing Old*, Harmony Books, pp. 5, 7.

Chapter 2

1 Paper presented at the 21st annual conference of the European Society of Human Reproduction and Embryology on 21 June 2005.

2 Herkind, A.M., et al. (1996) 'The heritability of human longevity: a population-based study of 2872 Danish twin pairs born 1870–1900', *Human Genetics*, 97, pp. 319–23.

3 Cherniske, Stephen (2003) *The Metabolic Anti-Ageing Plan*, Piatkus, p. 6.

4 Such as Cherniske, *The Metabolic Anti-Ageing Plan*.

5 For information on glyconutrients I recommend the following books:

Mondoa, Emil and Kitel, Mindy (2001) *Sugars that Heal: The New Healing Science of Glyconutrients*, Ballantine Books.

Elkins, M.H., Rita (2003) *Miracle Sugars – the glyconutrient link to disease prevention and improved health*, Woodland Publishing.

Harper's Textbook of Biochemistry, 27th edition, 2006, Lange Medical Books, McGraw Hill; Chapter 46 on glycoproteins, p. 523.

Chapter 3

1 Klatz, Ronald (1998) *Grow Young with HGH*, HarperPerennial, p. 44.

Quoted in ibid., p. 127.

3 Ibid., p. 131.

4 Vliet, Dr Elizabeth (2001) *Women, Weight and Hormones*, M. Evans and Co. Inc., p. 157.

Chapter 4

1 Young, Robert, 'The pH miracle: balance your diet, reclaim your health, p. 90.

2 'Seeds of deception' (2004) Interview with Jeff Smith, *Acres USA* newsletter, February, 34 (2).

3 Smith, Jeffrey (2001) 'Dead babies', *Ecologist*, 5 December.

4 Ibid.

5 Weiss, R.F. (1988) *Herbal Medicine*, AB Arcanum, p. 320.

6 Vliet, *Women, Weight and Hormones*, p. 128; Cassidy, Bingham and Setchell

(1994), 'Biological effects of a diet of soy protein rich in isoflavones on the menstrual cycle of premenopausal women', *American Journal of Clinical Nutrition*, 60 (3), pp. 333–40.

7   Benson, J.E, Engelhart-Fenton, K.A. and Eisenman, P.A. (1996) 'Nutritional aspects of amenorrhea in the female athlete', *International Journal of Sports Nutrition*, 6, pp. 134–5.

8   Abstract of study in *British Journal of Obstetrics and Gynaecology*, November 2004.

9   Nagata, C., Inaba, S., Kawakami, N., Kakizoe, T. and Shimizu, H. (2000) 'Inverse Association of soy product intake with serum androgen and oestrogen concentration in Japanese men', *Nutrition and Cancer*, 36 (1), p. 418.

10 Sher, K.S. and Mayberry, J.F. (1996) *Acta Paediatrica* Supplement, 412, pp. 76–7.

Chapter 5

1   Mendelson, J.M. (1978) 'Effects of alcohol on plasma testosterone and luteinizing hormone levels', *Alcoholism Clinical & Experimental Research*, 2, pp. 225–58.
    Ylikahri, R.., et al. (1974) 'Hangover and testosterone', *British Medical Journal*, 2, p. 445.

2   Wynn, M. and Wynn, A. (1991) *The Case for Preconception Care for Men and Women*, Ab Academic publishers.

3   van Thiel, D.M.. (1974) 'Hypogonadism in alcoholic liver disease: evidence for a double effect', *Gastroenterology*, 67, 1188–99.

4   Hakim, R.., et al. (1998) 'Alcohol and caffeine consumption and decreased fertility', *Fertility and Sterility*, 70, (40), pp. 632–7.
    Quoted in Hendel, Barbara and Ferreira, Peter *Water and Salt, the Essence of Life, the Healing Power of Nature*, p. 38.

5   Streissguth, A.P., et al. (1986) 'Attention, distraction and reaction time at age 7 years and prenatal alcohol exposure', *Neurobehav Toxicol Tratol*, 8 (6), pp. 717–25.

6   Kline, J., et al. (1977) 'Smoking a risk factor for spontaneous abortion', *New England Journal of Medicine*, 297, pp. 793–6.

7   Parazzani, F., et al. (1993) 'Risk factors for unexplained dyspermia in infertile men: a case control study', *Archive of Andrology*, 31 (2), pp. 105–13.

8   Kamen, Betty (1982) 'Nutrition dialogue, let's live', November, 96–7.

9   Stanton, C. and Gray, R. (1995) 'Effects of caffeine consumption on delayed conception', *American Journal of Epidemiology*, 142 (12), pp. 1322–9.
    Hatch, E.E. and Bracken, M.B. (1993) 'Association of delayed conception with caffeine consumption', *American Journal of Epidemiology*, 138, pp. 1082–92.

Boulmar, F., et al. (1997) 'Caffeine intake and delayed conception: a European multi-centre study on infertility and subfecundity', European Study Group on Infertility and Subfecundity, *American Journal of Epidemiology*, 145 (4), pp. 324–34.

10 Navarro-Peran, E., Cabezas-Herrera, J., Garcia-Canovas, F., Durrant, M.C., Thorneley, R.N., Rodriguez-Lopez, J.N. (2005) 'The anti-folate activity of tea catechins', *Cancer Reearch.*, 15 March, 65 (6), pp. 2059–64.

11 Frassetto, L., et al. (2001) 'Diet, evolution and ageing: the pathophysiologic effects of the post-agricultural inversion of the potassium-to-sodium and base-to-chloride ratios in the human diet', *European Journal of Nutrition*, 40 (5), pp. 200–13.

Tucker, K.L. (2003) 'Dietary intake and bone status with ageing', *Current Pharmaceutical Design*, 9 (31), pp. 1–18.

12 Lamberts, S.W. (1997) 'The endocrinology of ageing', *Science*, 278 (5337), pp. 419–24.

13 Robertson, D., et al. (1978) 'Effects of caffeine on plasma rennin activity, catecholamines and blood pressure' *New England Journal of Medicine*, 298 (4), pp. 181–6.

Lane, J.D., et al. 'Caffeine effects on cardiovascular and neuro-endocrine responses to acute psychosocial stress and their relationship to level of habitual caffeine consumption' *Psychosomatic Medicine*, 52 (3), pp. 320–36.

14 Porta, M., et al. (2003) 'Coffee drinking: the rationale for treating it as a potential effect modifier of carcinogenic exposures', *European Journal of Epidemiology*, 18 (4), pp. 289–98.

Kaufmann, W.K., et al. (2003) 'Caffeine and human DNA metabolism: the magic and the mystery', *Mutation Research*, 27 November, 532 (1–2), pp. 85–102.

15 (1989) *Lancet*, 2.

16 (1999) *American Journal of Epidemiology*, 150.

17 (1998) *Digestive Science*, November, 43, 11.

18 (1992) *Los Angeles Times*, 18 November.

Chapter 6

1 Ward, N., et al. (1987) 'Placental element levels in relation to foetal development of obstetrically normal births: a study of 37 elements. Evidence for effects of cadmium, lead and zinc on foetal growth and smoking as a cause of cadmium', *International Journal of Biosocial Research*, 9 (1), pp. 63–81.

2 (1997) 'The Oxford survey in childhood cancers', *British Journal of Cancer*.

3 Campbell, J.M. Harrison (1979) 'Smoking and infertility', *Medical Journal of Australia*, 1, pp. 342–3.

4 Jick, H., et al. (1977) 'Relation between smoking and age of natural menopause', *Lancet*, 1, pp. 1354–5.

5 Powell, D.J. and Fuller, R.W. (1983) 'Marijuana and sex: strange bed partners', *Journal of Psychoactive Drugs*, 53, pp. 315–22.

6 Braken, M.B., et al. (1990) 'Association of cocaine use with sperm concentration, motility and morphology', *Fertility and Sterility* vol. 53, pp. 315–22.

7 Smith, C.G. and Gilbean, P.M. (1985) 'Drug Abuse effects on reproductive hormones', *Endocrine Toxicology*, Raven Press.

Chapter 8

1 I've been surprised to find out not everyone with English as their mother tongue knows what 'mojo' means. Originally an American jazz term, it was widely popularized by the Austin Powers films – and denotes a mixture of libido and general 'joie de vivre'.

2 Engel, Cindy (2002) *Wild Health, How Animals Keep Themselves Well and What we can Learn from Them*, Houghton Mifflin.

3 Giblin, P. T., et al. (1988) 'Effects of stress and characteristic adaptability on semen quality in healthy men', *Fertility and Sterility*, 49, pp. 127–32.
   Lenzi, A., et al. (2003) 'Stress, sexual dysfunctions and male infertility', *Journal of Endocrinological Investigation*, 26 (3); pp. 72–6.

4 Laino, Charlene (1994) 'Stress due to loss of a loved one tied to male infertility', *Medical Tribune*, 1 December, p. 16.

5 Glenville, Marilyn (2000), *Natural Solutions to Infertility*, M Evans and Company, p. 140.

6 Negro-Vilar, A. (1993) *Environmental Health Perspectives* supplements, 101 (2), pp. 59–64.

7 Barnea, E.R.. and Tal, J. (1991) 'Stress-related reproductive failure', *Journal of In Vitro Fertilization and Embryo Transfer*, 8 (1), pp. 15–23.

8 Referred to in Harris, Colette (2004) *PCOS and Your Fertility*, Hay House, Inc.

9 Jakobovits, A.A., et al. (2002) 'Interactions of stress and reproductions', *Zentralbl Gynakol*, 124 (4), pp. 189–93.

10 Menninger, K. (1939) 'Somatic correlations with the unconscious repudiation of femininity in women', *Journal of Nervous and Mental Disease*, 89, p. 514.
   Benedeck, T. and Rubenstein, B. (1939) 'Correlations between ovarian activity and psycho-dynamic processes. The ovulatory phase', *Psychosomatic Medicine*, 1 (2), pp. 245–70.

11 Tessler, Gordon S. (1989) 'The correct nutrition to cope with stress', *Total Health*, June, 11 (3), p. 12.

12 Barbieri, Robert, Domar, Alice and Loughlin, Kevin (2000) *6 Steps to Increased Fertility*, Simon & Schuster, pp. 69–121.
   Domar, Alice D. and Kelly, Alice Lesch (2002) *Conquering Infertility*, Viking.

Chapter 9

1 Bolumar, F., et al. (2000) 'Body mass index and delayed conception: a European multicenter study on infertility and subfecundity', *American Journal of Epidemiology*, 151 (11), pp. 1072–9.

2 Pirke, K., Scheiger, U., Laessle, R.., et al. (1985) 'The influence of diet on the menstrual cycle of healthy young women', *Journal of Clinical Endocrinology & Metabolism*, 60 (6), pp. 1174–79.

3 Grodstein, F., et al. (1994) 'Body mass index and ovulatory infertility', *Epidemiology*, 5 (2), pp. 247–50.

4 Clark, A.M.., et al. (1995) 'Weight loss results in significant improvements in pregnancy and ovulatory rates in annovulatory obese women', *Human Reproduction*, 10, pp. 2705–12.

   Clark, A.M., et al. (1998) 'Weight loss in obese, infertile women results in improvements in reproductive outcome for all forms of fertility treatment', *Hum Reprod*, 66, pp. 1502–5.

5 Crosigiani, P. G., et al. (2003) 'Overweight and obese anovulatory women with polycystic ovaries: parallel improvements and fertility rates induced by diet', *Human Reproduction*, 18 (9), pp. 1928–32.

6 Bray, G., et al. (1997) 'Obesity and reproduction', *Human Reproduction*, 12 (1), pp. 26–32.

7 Kitell, Mary (2004) *Stay Fertile Longer*, Rodale, Inc.

Chapter 10

1 Nevison, J., 'Report on genitourinary infection', available from the UK charity for preconception care, Foresight.

2 Kitell, Mary (2004) *Stay Fertile Longer*, Rodale, Inc.

3 Lee Vliet, Elizabeth (2003) *It's my Ovaries, Stupid!*, Scribner.

4 Fourteen studies detailing the serious consequences of chlamydia causing all the conditions referred to in this paragraph are set out in a booklet entitled 'The adverse affects of genito-urinary infections' distributed by the UK Charity Foresight; also available online at www.foresight-preconception.org.uk.

5 Westrim, L. (1980) 'Incidence, prevalence and trends of acute pelvic inflammatory disease and its consequences to industrialized countries', *American Journal of Obstetrics and Gynecology*, 138, pp. 880–92.

6 Suommen, J., et al. (1983) 'Chronic prostitis, chlamydia, trachomatis and infertility', *Journal of Andology* 6, pp. 405–13.

7 Survey carried out by the UK Royal College of Physicians' Committee on Genito-Urinary Medicine (1987), 'Chlamydial diagnostic surveys in the United Kingdom and Eire: current facilities and perceived needs', *GenitoUrin Medicine*, 63, pp. 371–4.

Chapter 11

1 Perricone, N. (2005) *The Perricone Weight-loss Diet*, Ballantine Books, p. 39.
2 Referred to by Salaman, Maureen Kennedy (1998) *All Your Health Questions Answered Naturally*, MKS, Inc.

Chapter 12

1 Quoted in Hendel, Barbara and Ferreira, Peter, *Water and Salt, the Essence of Life, the Healing Power of Nature*, Natural Resources, p. 37.
2 Ibid. p. 38.
3 From Engel, Cindy, *Wild Health*, p. 180.
4 Quoted in Cousens, Gabriel, *Conscious Eating*, p. 442.
5 Dr Kouchakoff's paper entitled 'The influence of cooking on the blood formula of man' was presented at the International Congress of Microbiology.
6 Willstetter, Dr, *Biliothek verlager*, 123, pp. 437–70; *Nagoya Journal of Medical Science*, 3, pp. 51–73; (1935) *Biochem Zeit*, 275, pp. 216–33; quoted by Santillo, Humbart in *Food Enzymes*, p. 30.

Chapter 13

1 (2001) 'Is organic food healthier?', *Organic Consumers' Association*, 1 October.
2 Ibid.; Staigler, D. (1988) 'The nutritional value of food from conventional and biodynamic agriculture', *IFOAM Bulletin*, 4, pp. 9–12; (2000–2003) 'Organic diets increase fertility', *Food Market Exchange*.
3 Plochberger, K. (1989) 'Feeding experiments – a criterion for quality estimation of biologically and conventional produced foods', *Agriculture, Ecosystems and Environment*, 27, pp. 419–28; Pfeiffer, E.E. (1938), *Soil Fertility, Renewal and Preservation*, trans. F. Heckel, Anthroposophic Press.
4 Abell, A., Ernst, E. and Bonde, J.P. (1994) 'High sperm density among members of the Organic Farmers' Association', *Lancet*, 343 (8911), p. 1498.
5 Carlson, E., et al. (1996) 'Semen quality among members of organic food associations in Zeeland, Denmark', *Lancet*, 347, p. 1844; Juhler, R.K., et al. (1995) 'Human semen quality in relation to dietary pesticide exposure and organic diet', *Archives of Environmental Contamination and Toxicology*.
6 (2005), *Harvard Magazine*, October–November.
7 McKeith, Gillian (2000) *Living Food for Health*, Piatkus Ltd.
8 Cousens, Gabriel (2000) *Conscious Eating*, North Atlantic Books, p. 613.
9 Karmen., Betty, 'Bee pollen: from principles to practice', p. 67.
10 Scheer, James F. (1990) 'Bee pollen: worth its weight in gold', *Health Freedom News*, October, pp. 18–19.

11 McKeith, *Living Food for Health*, Chapter 8.

12 Study cited in Hendel, Barbara and Ferreira, Peter (2003) *Water and Salt, The Essence of Life*, Natural Resources, Inc.

Chapter 14

1 Mars, Briggite (2002) *Sex, Love and Health*, Basic Health Publications Inc., p. 40.

Chapter 16

1 Campbell, T. Colin (2006) *The China Study*, BenBella Books, p. 228.

2 Davis, D.R.., A, Riordan, H.D. (2004) 'Changes in USDA food composition data for 43 garden crops, 1950–1999', *Journal of American College Nutrition*, December, 23 (6), pp. 669–82.

3 Riso, P. , Visioli, F., Gardana, C., et al. (2005) 'Effects of blood orange juice intake on antioxidant bioavailability and on different markers related to oxidative stress', *Journal of Agricultural Food Chemicals*, 23 February, 53 (4), pp. 941–7.

    Heo, H.J. and Lee, C.Y. (2005) 'Strawberry and its anthocyanins reduce oxidative stress-induced apoptosis in PC12 cells', *Journal of Agricultural Food Chemicals.*, 23 March, 53 (6), pp. 1984–9.

    Zhang, Y., Vareed, S.K., Nair M.G. (2005) 'Human tumour cell growth inhibition by non-toxic anthocyanins, the pigments in fruits and vegetables', *Life Science*, 11 February, 76 (13), pp. 1465–72.

4 Serrano, M., Guillen, F., Martinez-Romero, D., Castillo, S. and Valero, D. (2005) 'Chemical constituents and anti-oxidant activity of sweet cherry at different ripening stages', *Journal of Agricultural Food Chemicals.*, 6 April, 53 (7), pp. 2741–5.

5 Giutini, D., Graziani, G., Lecari, B., et al. (2005) 'Changes in carotenoid and ascorbic acid contents in fruits of different tomato genotypes related to the depletion of UV-B radiation', *Journal of Agricultural Food Chemicals.*, 20 April, 53 (8), pp. 3174–81.

    Diaz, D.L.G., Quinlivan, E.P. , Laus, S.M.., et al. (2004), 'Folate biofortification in tomatoes by engineering the pteridine branch of folate synthesis', *Proceedings of the National Academy of Sciences USA*, 21 September, 101 (38), pp. 13720–5.

6 Seneweera, S.P. and Conroy, J.P. (1997) 'Growth, grain yield and quality of rice (Oryza sativa L.) in response to elevated CO_2 and phosphorus nutrition', *Soil Science and Plant Nutrition*, 43, pp. 1131–6.

7 Glenville, Marilyn (2001) *Natural Solutions to Infertility*, M. Evans and Co., p. 99.

8   Ibid., pp. 98–9.

9   Propping, D. and Katzorke, T. (1987) 'Treatment of corpus lustrum, insufficiency', *Zeitschrift Akgemeinmedizin*, vol. 63, pp. 932–3.

10 (1987) *Journal of Urology*, 137, p. 1168.

11 Bradstreet, Karen, *Overcoming Infertility Naturally*, p. 37.

12 Anderson, R.A. and Polansky, M.M.. (1981) 'Dietary chromium deficiency: effect on sperm count and fertility in rats', *Biological Trace Element Research*, 3, pp. 1–5.

13 (1992) Miscarriage Association Newsletter.

14 Saner, G., et al. (1985) 'Hair manganese concentrations in newborns and their mothers', *American Journal of Clinical Nutrition*, 41, pp. 1042–4.

15 Scott, R.., et al. (1998) 'Selenium supplementation in sub-fertile human males', *British Journal of Urology*, 82, pp. 625–9.

16 Krznjavi, H., et al. (1992) 'Selenium and fertility in men', *Trace Elements in Medicine*, 9 (2), pp. 107–8.

17 Davies, S., (1984-1985) 'Zinc nutrition and health', in Bland, E. (ed.) *Yearbook of Nutritional Medicine*, Keats Publishing.

18 Schwabe, J.W.R. and Rhodes, D. (1991) 'Beyond zinc fingers: steroid hormone receptors have a novel structure motif for DNA recognition', *Trends in Biochemical Science*, 16, pp. 291–6.

19 Hurley, L.S. (1991) 'Teratogenic aspects of manganese, zinc and copper nutrition', *Physiological Reviews*, 61, pp. 249–95.

20 Kidd, G.S., et al. (1982) 'The Effects of Pyridoxine on pituitary hormones secretion in amenorhea-galactorrhea syndromes', *Journal of Clinical Endocrinology and Metabolism*, 54 (4), pp. 872–5.

21 (1979) *Medical Aspects of Human Sexuality*, 10 October, 13, p. 134.

22 Reuben, Carolyn and Prestly, Joan (1989) 'Vitamins Against Miscarriage', *East West Magazine*, January, pp. 59–62.

23 Wright, Jonathan (1979) *Dr Wright's Book of Nutritional Therapy*, Rodale Press, p. 10.

24 Tarin, J., et al. (1998) 'The effects of maternal ageing and dietary anti-oxidant supplementation on ovulation, fertilization and embryo development in vitro in the mouse', *Reproduction, Nutrition, Development*, 38 (5), pp. 499–508.

25 Bayer, R. (1960) 'Treatment of infertility with vitamin E', *International Journal of Infertility*, 5, pp. 70–8.

Chapter 17

1   Isadori, A, Monaca, A.L., Capa, M., et al. (1981) 'A study of growth hormone release in man after oral administration of amino acids', *Current Medical Research and Opinion*, 7, pp. 475–81.

2 Holt Jr., L.E. and Albanese, A..A.. (1944) 'Observations on amino acid deficiencies in man', *Transactions of the Association of American Physicians*, 58, p. 143.

3 De Aloysio, D., et al. (1982) 'The clinical use of Arginine aspartate in male infertility', *Alta Europaca Fertlitatis*, 13, pp. 133–67.

4 Gaby, A.R. (1996) *Townsend Letters for Doctors and Patients*, April, p. 20.

5 Costa, M., et al. (1994) 'L-Carnitine in idiopathic asthozoospermis: a multi-centre study', *Andrologia*, 26, pp. 155–9; Vitali, G., et al. (1995) 'Carnitine supplementation in human idiopathic asthenospermia. Clinical results', *Drugs Under Experimental and Clinical Research*, 21, pp. 157–9.

6 Pearson, D. and Haw, S. (1982) *Life Extension: A Practical Scientific Approach*, Warner Books.

Chapter 18

1 Cousens, Gabriel (2000) *Conscious Eating*, North Atlantic Books, Berkeley, p. 230.

2 Buhner, Stephen Howard (2003) *The Fasting Path*, Avery, p. 77.

3 Cousens, *Conscious Eating*, p. 232.

4 Quoted in article on fasting at www.falconblanco.com.

Chapter 19

1 (1993), Burroughs Books.

2 Assisi, Francis C., *Ayurvea's Triphala Emerging as Cancer Fighter* (http://www.indolink.com/display/articles)

3 Quoted in Watson, Brenda (2002) *Renew your life, Improved Digestion and Detoxification*, Renew Life Press, p. 86.

Chapter 20

1 Lopez, N.J., Da, S, Ipinia, J. and Gutierrez, J. (2005) 'Periodontal thereapy reduces the rate of preterm low birth weight in women with pregnancy associated gingivitis', *Journal of Periodontal Research*, November, 76 (11 suppl.), pp. 2144–53.

2 Solan, Matthew (2006) 'Preventing disease by improving your oral health', *Life Extension*, April, pp. 71–5.

3 Hasturk, H., Nunn, M., Warbington, M. and Van Dyke, T.E. (2004) 'Efficacy of a fluoridated hydrogen peroxide based mouthrinse for the treatment of gingivitis: a randomized clinical trial', *Journal of Peridontology*, January, 75 (1), pp. 57–65.

4 Al-Zahrani, M.S., Borawski, E.A. and Bissada, N.E. (2005) 'Periodontics and

three health-enhancing behaviours: maintaining normal weight, engaging in recommended level of exercise and consuming a high-quality diet', *Journal of Periodontology*, 76 (8), pp. 1362–6.

Solan, 'Preventing disease by improving your oral health'.

5 Ibid.

6 A study analyzing vitamin C intake and periodontal disease indicators in 12,419 US adults by Nishida, M, Grossi, S.G., Dunford, R.G., et al. (2000) 'Dietary vitamin C and the risk for periodontal disease', *Journal of Periodontal Research*, August, 71 (8), pp. 1215–23.

7 Stradte, H., Sigusch, B.W. and Glockmann, E. (2005) 'Grapefruit consumption improves vitamin C status in periodontitis patients', *British Dental Journal*, 27 August, 199 (4), pp. 213–17.

8 'The Invisible Toothbrush', article posted on the website of the Weston A. Price foundation – www.westonaprice.org.

9 A study analysing vitamin C intake and periodontal disease indicators in 12,419 US adults by Nishida, M, Grossi, S.G., Dunford, R.G., et al. (2000) 'Dietary vitamin C and the risk for periodontal disease', *Journal of Periodontal Research*, July, 71 (7), pp. 1057–66.

10 Hanioka, T., Tanaka, M., Pjima, M., Shizukuishi, S. and Folkers, K. (1994) 'Effect of the topival application of coenzyme Q10 on adult periodontitis', *Molecular Aspects of Medicine.*, 15 Suppl, pp. 241–8.

11 Gaby, A.R. 'Coenzyme Q10' in Pizzorno, J.E. and Murray, M.T. (eds) (1998) *Textbook of Natural Medicine*, Bastyr University Press.

12 Solan, Matthew (2006) 'Preventing disease by improving your oral health', *Life Extension*, April, pp. 71–5.

13 Soukoulis, S. and Hirsch, R. (2004) *The Effects of Tea Tree Oil-containing Gel on Plaque and Chronic Gingivitis, Australian Dental Journal*, 49 (2), pp. 78–83.

14 Sintes, J.L., Escalante, C., Stewart, B., et al. (1995) 'Enhanced anti-caries efficacy of a 0.243 per cent sodium fluoride/10 per cent xylitol/silica dentifrice; 3 year clinical results', *American Journal of Dentistry*, October, 8 (5), pp. 231–5.

15 Taweboon, S., Thaweboon, B. and Soo-Ampon, S. (2004) 'The effect of chewing gum on mutans streptococci in saliva and dental plaque', *Southeast Asian Journal of Tropical Medicine and Public Health,* December, 35 (4), pp. 1024–7.

16 Wright, Karen (2005) 'Our preferred poison', *Discover*, March, 26 (3), 'Biology and Medicine'.

17 Ziff, S. and Ziff, M. (1987) *Infertility & Birth Defects – is mercury from silver dental fillings an unsuspected cause?* Bio probe, Inc.

18 Stock, A. (1982) 'Die Gefaehlichkeit des quecksilberdampfes' (The dangerousness of mercury vapour'), *Zeitschrift Angewandte Chemie*, 39, pp. 461–6.

Svare, C.W., et al. (1981) 'The effect of dental amalgams on mercury levels in expired air', *Journal of Dental Research*, 60, pp. 1668–71.

Gay, D.D., Cox, R.D. and Reinhardt, J.W. (1979) 'Chewing releases mercury from fillings', *Lancet*, 1 (8123), pp. 985–6.

Stortebecker, P. (1985) *Mercury Poisoning from Dental Amalgam – A Hazard to the Human Brain*, Stortebecker Foundation for research.

Vimy, M.J.and Lorschneider, F.L. (1985) 'Intra-oral air mercury released from dental amalgam', *Journal of Dental Research*, 64, pp. 1069–71.

Vimy, M.J. and Lorschneider, F.L. (1985) 'Serial measurements of intra-oral mercury estimation of daily dose from dental amalgam', *Journal of Dental Research*, 64 (8), pp. 1072–5.

19 (1984) US EPA *Mercury Health Effects Update*. Final Report, EPA 600/8-84-019F, United States Environmental Protection Agency.

20 Ziff, S. and Ziff, M., *Infertility & Birth Defects*.

Chapter 21

1 Binkley, S.A. (1995) *Endocrinology*, HarperCollins College Publishers, p. 384.

2 Cousens, G. (2001) *Depression Free for Life*, Quill, HarperCollins, p. 53.

3 Gamblichter, T., et al. (2002), 'Impact of UVA exposure on psychological parameters and circulating serotonin and melatonin', *Dermatology*, 2 (1), p. 6.

Kripke, D.F. (1998) 'Light treatment for non-seasonal depression: speed, efficacy and combined treatment', *Journal of Affective Disorders*, 49 (2), pp. 109–17.

Kripke, D.F., et al. (1983) 'Bright white light alleviates depression', *Psychiatry Research*, 10 (2), pp. 105–12.

Lam, R.W., et al. (1989) 'Phototherapy for depressive disorders – a review', *Canadian Journal of Psychiatry*, 34 (2), pp. 140–7.

Prasko, J., et al. (2002) 'Bright light therapy and/or imipramine for in patients with recurrent non-seasonal depressions', *Neuroendocrinology Letters*, 23 (2), pp. 109–13.

Rao, M.L., et al. (1990) 'The influence of phototherapy on serotonin and melatonin in nonseasonal depression', *Pharmacopsychiatry*, 23 (3), pp. 155–8.

4 Null, Gary, *The Complete Guide to Health and Nutrition*, Arlington Books.

5 Cousens, Gabriel, *Conscious Eating*, North Atlantic Books, p. 578.

6 Ibid., p. 579.

Chapter 22

1 Merieb, Elaine N. (1998) *Human Anatomy and Physiology*, 4th edition, Addison Wesley Longman.

2 Ayre, E.A. and Pang, S.F. (1994) 'Indomelatonin binding sites in the testis and ovary: Putative melatonin receptors in the gonads', *Biological Signals,* 3, pp. 71–84.

3 Lacey, Louise (1975) *A Feminine Odyssey into Fertility and Contraception,* Coward McCann & Geoghegan.

4 Kippley, John F. (1976) *By the Light of the Silvery Moon: Report #R2,* Couple to Couple League.

De Felice, Joy, R.N. B.S.N., P. H.N. (2000) *The Effects of Light on the Menstrual Cycle.* Also (2000), *Infertility.*

Referred to in Singer, Katie (2004) *The Garden of Fertility: A guide to charting your fertility signals to prevent or achieve pregnancy – naturally – and to gauge your reproductive health,* Avery.

5 Referred to on website www.westonprice.org

Chapter 23

1 Cherniske, Stephen (2003) *The Metabolic Anti-ageing Plan,* Piatkus.

2 Quoted by Kittel, Mary in (2004) *Stay Fertile Longer,* Rodale, Inc., p. 80.

3 Ibid., p. 81.

4 In his book *On the Diseases of Women.*

5 Williams, Christopher (2001) *The Fastest Way to Get Pregnant Naturally,* Hyperion.

6 In ibid., p. 152.

7 Bullen, B.A., et al. (1985) 'Induction of menstrual disorders by stenuous exercise in untrained women', *New England Journal of Medicine,* 312, pp. 1349–53.

Chapter 24

1 Spiegel, K., Leproult, R. and Van Cauter, E., 'Impact of sleep on metabolic and endocrine function', *Lancet,* 199, 354, pp. 1425–9.

2 Van Cauter, E., et al. (2000) 'Age-related changes in slow wave sleep and REM sleep and relationship with growth hormone and cortisol levels in healthy men' *JAMA,* 16 August, 284 (7), pp. 861–8.

3 Ibid.

4 Ibid.

5 Ibid.

6 Malesky, Gale and Kittel, Mary (2001) *The Hormone Connection,* Rodale, p. 285.

7 Walsleben, J. and Baron Faust, R. (2000) *A Woman's Guide to Sleep: Guaranteed solutions for a good night's rest,* Random House.

Chapter 25

1 Cantin, M. and Genest, J. (1986) 'The heart as an endocrine gland', *Scientific American,* 254, pp. 76–81.

2 Berbieri, Robert, Domar, Alice and Loughlin, Kevin (2000) *Six Steps to Increased Fertility,* Harvard Medical School Books, p. 82.

3 Ibid.

Chapter 26

1 Willcox, A.J., et al. (1988) 'Incidence of early loss of pregnancy', *New England Journal of Medicine,* July, 319, (4), pp. 189–94.

2 Such as blood tests to check for chromosomal abnormalities or hormonal imbalances, a procedure called 'cerclage', by which the weakened cervix is stitched where there is a uterine abnormality; and hormone replacement-type treatments where the miscarriage is caused, for example, by levels of progesterone being too low.

3 Hogge, W.A. (2003) 'The clinical use of kayotyping spontaneous abortions', *American Journal of Obstetrics and Gynecology,* August, 189 (2), pp. 397–402.

4 American College of Obstetricians and Gynecologists (2001) 'Management of recurrent early pregnancy loss', *ACPG Practice Bulletin,* February, 24.

5 Foresight '1990–1993 study of preconceptual care and pregnancy outcome'. Results published in a letter (1995) to the Editor of *Journal of Nutritional & Environmental Medicine,* 5, pp. 205–8.

6 American College of Obstericians and Gynecologists (2000) 'Repeated miscarriage', *ACOG Education Pamphlet,* February, Ap 100, Washington DC.

7 Golding, J. (1994) 'The consequences of smoking in pregnancy'. Talk given to a conference on 'Smoking in pregnancy' commission by the UK Health Education Authority, 2 February.

8 Torgerson, D.J., Thomas, R.E. and Reid, D.M. (1997) 'Mothers' and daughters' menopausal ages: is there a link?', *European Journal of Obstetrics, Gynecology & Reproductive Biology,* 74 (1), pp. 63–6.

9 Bernard, P. (1962) Die Wirking des Rauchens auf Frau und Mutter', *Munc. Med AWochenschr,* 104, p. 1826.

   Jick, H., Porter, J. and Morrison, A.S. (1977) 'Relationship between smoking and age of natural menopause', *Lancet,* 1, pp. 1354–5.

   Linquist, O. and Begtsson, C. (1979) 'Menopausal age in relation to smoking', *Acta Med Scan,* 205, pp. 73–7.

10 Wynn, M. and Wynn, A. (1981) *The Prevention of Handicap in Early Pregnancy Origin,* Foundation for Education and Research in Childbearing, pp. 28–33.

11 Ibid.

Fielding, J.E. and Rosso, P. K. (1978) 'Smoking during pregnancy', *New England Journal of Medicine*, 298, pp. 337–9.

Naeye, R. (1979) 'The duration of maternal cigarette smoking and placental disorders', *Early Human Development*, 3, pp. 229–37.

12 Evans, H.J., Fletcher, J, Torrance, M. and Hardgreave, T.B. (1981) 'Sperm abnormalities and cigarette smoking', *Lancet*, 1, pp. 627–9.

Viczian, M. (1969) Ergebnisse von Spermautersuchungen bei Zigarrettenrauchen', *Z. Haut Geschlectskr*, 44, pp. 183–7.

Hemsworth, B.N. (1981) 'Deformation of the mouse foetus after ingestion of nicotine by the male', *IRCS Medical Science*, 9, pp. 728–9.

13 Smith, D.W. (1979) *Mothering your Unborn Baby*, W.B. Saunders Co.

Tittmar, H.G. (1978) 'Some effects of alcohol in reproduction' *British Journal of Alcohol and Alcoholism*, 13, p. 3.

14 Van Thiel, D.H., Gavaler, J.S. and Goodman, Lester R. (1975) 'Alcohol induced testicular atrophy. An experimental model for hypergonadism occurring in chronic alcoholic men', *Gastroenterology*, 69, pp. 326–32.

Bennet, H.S., Baggenstgors, A.H. and Butt, H.R. (1950) 'The testes, breast and prostate of men who die in cirrhosis of liver', *American Journal of Clinical Pathology*, 20, pp. 814–28.

15 Wichman, L (1992) 'The value of semen analysis in predicting pregnancy', *Acta Universitatis Tamperensis*, ser A, 346, p. 5.

16 Referred to by Northrup, Christiane in (2002) *Women's Bodies, Women's Wisdom*, Bantam Books.

17 Referred to by Kittel, Mary (2004) *Stay Fertile Longer*, Rodale, pp. 247–8.

18 Phipps, W.R., Martini, M.C., Lampe, J.W., et al. (1993) 'Effect of flax seed ingestion on the menstrual cycle', *Journal of Endocrinal Metabolism*, 77, pp. 1215–19.

19 Goldhaber, M.K., et al. (1988) 'The risk of miscarriage and birth defects among women who use VDU terminals during pregnancy', *American Journal of Industrial Medicine*, 13, pp. 695–706.

20 Kittel, Mary (2004) *Stay Fertile Longer*, Rodale, p. 129.

21 Ibid.

22 Lee Vliet, Elizabeth (2003) *It's my Ovaries, Stupid!*, Scribner.

23 Clark, A.M., et al. (1998) 'Weight loss in obese infertile women results in improvement in reproductive outcome for all forms of fertility treatment', *Human Reproduction*, 13, (6), pp. 1502–5.

24 Martin, D.H., et al. (1982) 'Prematurity and perinatal mortality in pregnancies complicated by maternal chlamydia trachomatis infections', *JAMA*, 247, pp. 1585–8.

Thompson, S, et al. (1982) 'A prospective study of chlamydia and mycoplasm infections during pregnancy: relation to pregnant outcome and maternal morbidity', referred to in (1982) *Chlamydial Infections*, Elsevier Biomedical Press, pp. 155–8.

25 Quinn, P. A., et al. (1983) 'Serologic evidence of Ureaplasma urealyticum infection in women with spontaneous pregnancy loss', *American Journal of Obstetrics and Gynecolology*, 145, pp. 245–9.

26 Williams, Christopher (2001) *The Fastest Way to Get Pregnant Naturally*, Hyperion.

27 Barbierei, Robert, Domar, Alice and Loughlin Kevon (2000) *6 Steps to Increased Fertility*, Simon & Schuster, p. 81.

28 Referred to on the website www.westonrpice.org.

29 Research of Dr Carl Javert of Cornell University, referred to in Salaman, Maureen Kennedy (1998) *Your Health Questions Answered Naturally*, MKS, Inc, p. 759.

30 Research of Dr Robert Greenblatt of the Medical College of Georgia, referred to in Salaman, Maureen Kennedy (1998) *Your Health Questions Answered Naturally*, MKS, Inc, p. 759.

31 Ibid., p. 762.

32 Ibid., p. 763.

33 Ibid.

34 Ozgunes, H., et al. (1994) 'Ceruplasmin activity, copper and zinc determinations in predicting the prognosis of threatened abortion', *Trace Elements and Electrolytes*, 11 (3), pp. 139–42.

Chapter 27

1 Thatcher, S., (2000) *PCOS, The Hidden Epidemic*, Perspective Press, p. 222.

2 (1988) *Lancet*, 1, pp. 870–2.

3 Harris, C. and Cheung, T. (2002) *The PCOS Diet*, Thorsons.

4 Harris, C. and Cheung, T (2004) *PCOS and Your Fertility*, Hay House, Inc.

5 Marshall, K., et al. (2001) 'Polycystic ovary syndrome: clinical considerations', *Alternative Medical Review*, 6 (3), pp. 272–92.
Richardson, M.R., et al. (2003) 'Current perspectives in polycystic ovary syndrome', *Am Fam Physician*, 68 (4), pp. 697–704.

6 Resnick, L.M. (1992) 'Cellular ions in hypertension, insulin resistance, obesity and diabetes: a unifying theme', *Journal of the American Socity of Nephrology*, 3, pp. S78–S85.

7 Franks, S., et al. (1997) 'The genetic basis of polycystic ovary syndrome', *Human Reproduction*, 12, pp. 2641–8.

8 Pasquali, R., et al. (2003) 'Obesity and reproductive disorders in women', *Humam Reproduction Update*, 9 (4), pp. 360–70.
Hartz, A., et al. (1979) 'The association of obesity with infertility and related menstrual abnormalities in women', *International Journal of Obesity*, 3, pp. 57–73.

Alieva, E.A., et al. (1993) 'The effect of a decrease in body weight in patients with the polycystic ovary syndrome', *Akush Ginekol (Mosk)*, 3, pp. 33–6.

9   Williams MD, Christopher (2001) *The Fastest Way to get Pregnant Naturally*, Hyperion.

Clark, A.M., et al. (1995) 'Weight loss results in significant improvements in pregnancy and ovulatory rates in anovulatory obese women', *Hum Reprod*, p. 10.

10 Reference to research by PCOS expert Dr Adam Balen, at Harris, Colette (2004) *PCOS and your Fertility*, Hay House, Inc., p. 86.

11 Tennant., Forrest (1995) *Carbohydrate Dependence, is this why I can't lose weight?*, Veract Handbook series.

12 Kenton, Leslie (2002) *The X Factor Diet*, Vermillion.

13 Referred to by in ibid., p. 156.

14 Evans, G.W. and Pouchnik, D.J. (1993) 'Composition and biological activity of chromium-pyridine carbosylate complexes', *Journal of Inorganic Biochemistry*, 49, pp. 177–87.

15 Fulghesu, A.M., Ciampelli, M., Muzj, G., et al. (2002) 'N-acetyl-cysteine treatment improves insulin sensitivity in women with Polycystic ovary syndrome', *Fertility and Sterility*, 77 (6), pp. 1128–35.

16 Cam, C.M., Brownsey, R.W. and McNeill, J.H. (2000) 'Mechanisms of vanadium action, Insulin mimetic or insulin enhancing agent?', *Canadian Journal of Physiology and Pharmacology*, 78 (10), pp. 829–47.

Cusi, K., Cukier, S., De Fronzo, R.A., et al. (2001) 'Vanadyl sulfate improves hepatic muscle insulin sensitivity in type 2 diabetes', *Journal of Clinical Endocrinology and Metabolism*, 86 (3), pp. 1410–17.

17 Yaginuma, T., Izumi, R., Yaui, H., et al. (1982) *Nippon Sanka Fujinka Gakkai Zasshi*, 34 (7), pp. 939–44.

Takahashi, K. and Kitao, M. (1994) *International Journal of Fertiltiy and Menopausal Studies*, 39 (2), pp. 69–76.

Bass, A., Dalla Paola, L., Erle, G., et al. (1994) *Diabetes Care*, 17 (11), p. 1356.

18 Madar, Abel, Sarnish and Arad (1998) 'Glucose lowering effect of fenugreek in non-insulin dependent diabetics', *European Journal of Clinical Nutrition*, 42, pp. 51–4.

Al-Habari and Rahan (1998) 'Antidiabetic and hypocholesterolemic effects of fenugreek', *Phytotherapy Research*, 12, pp. 233–42.

19 Ushiroyama, T., et al. (2001) 'Effects of Unikei-to an herbal medicine on endocrine function and ovulation in women with high basal levels of luteinizing hormone secretion', *Journal of Reproductive Medicine*, 46 (5), pp. 451–6.

Sakai, A., et al. (1999) 'Induction or ovulation by Sairei-to for PCOS patients', *Journal of Endicronology*, 46 (1), pp. 217–20.

Takahashi, K., et al. (1994) 'Effect of TJ-68 (shakuyaku-kanzo-to) on polycystic ovarian disease', *International Journal of Fertility and Menopausal Studies,* 39 (2), pp. 69–76.

Chapter 28

1 Sampson, J.A. (1927) 'Peritoneal endometriosis due to menstrual dissemination of endometrial tissue into the peritoneal cavity', *American Journal of Obstetrics and Gynecology,* 14, p. 422.

2 Filer, R.B. and Wu, C.H. (1989) 'Coitus during the menses. Its effect on endometriosis and pelvic inflammatory disease', *Journal of Reproductive Medicine,* 34 (11), pp. 87–90.

3 Trickey, Ruth (1998) *Women's Hormones and the Menstrual Cycle,* Allen & Unwin, Australia, p. 307.

4 Darrow, S.L., et al. 'Menstrual cycle characteristics and risk of endometriosis', *Epidemiology,* 4 (2), pp. 135–42.

5 Trickey, Ruth (1998) *Women's Hormones and the Menstrual Cycle,* Allen & Unwin, p. 3.

6 Oliker, A.J. and Harris, A.E. (1971) 'Endometriosis of the bladder in a male patient', *Journal of Urology,* 106, p. 858.

O' Connor, D.T. (1987) *Endometriosis: Current Review in Obstetrics and Gynaecology,* 12, Churchill Livingstone, p. 20.

7 Nakamaya, K., et al. 'Immunohistochemical analysis of the peritoneum adjacent to endometriotic lesions using antibodies for Ber-EP4, antigen, oestrogen receptors and progesterone receptors: implication of peritoneal metaplasia in the pathogenesis of endometriosis', *International Journal Gynecology and Pathology,* 13 (4), pp. 348–58.

8 Rier, S.E. (2002) 'The potential role of exposure to environmental toxicants in the pathophysiology of endometriosis', *New York Academy of Sciences,* 955, pp. 201–12 and 230–2.

Foster, W.G. and Agarwak, S.K. (2002) 'Environmental contaminants and dietary factors in endometriosis', *New York Academy of Sciences,* 955, pp. 213–29 and 230–2.

Zhao, D., et al., 'Dioxin stimulates RANTES expression in an in-vitro model of endometriosis', *Molecular Human Reproduction,* 8 (9), pp. 849–54.

9 Campbell, J.S., et al. (1985) 'Is Simian Endometriosis an effect of immunotoxicity?' Paper presented at the Ontario Association of Pathologists, 48th annual meeting, October, London, Ontario, Canada.

Campbell, J (1988) 'Is reproductive wastage and failure related to environmental pollution? Considerations of human data and findings from a rhesus model.' Paper presented at the Toxicological Pathology Symposium, September, Ottawa, Canada.

10 Rier, S.E., et al. (1993) 'Endometriosis in rhesus monkeys (Macaca mulatta) following chronic exposure to 2, 3, 7,8 -Tetra-chllorodibenzo-p-dioxin', *Fundamental and Applied Toxicology,* 21, pp. 433–41.

11 (2003) Scribner, p. 208.

12 Mayani, A., et al. (1997) 'Dioxin concentrations in women with endometriosis', *Human Reproduction,* 12, pp. 373–5.

13 Perper, M.M., et al. (1993) 'MAST scores, alcohol consumption and gynecological symptoms in endometriosis patients', *Alcohol Clinical and Experimental Research,* 17 (2), pp. 272–8.

14 Grodstein, F. (1994) 'Infertility in women and moderate alcohol use', *American Journal of Public Health,* 84 (9), pp. 1429–32.

15 Grodstein, F., et al. (1993) 'Relationship of female infertility to consumption of caffeinated beverages', *American Journal of Epidemiology,* 137 (12), pp. 1353–60.

16 Referred to in Kittel, Mary (2004) *Stay Fertile Longer,* Rodale.

17 Research of Daniel W. Cramer of Brigham and Women's Hospital and Harvard Medical School, referred to in Balch, Phyllis and Balch, James (2000) *Prescription for Nutritional Healing,* Avery.

18 Referred to in Kittel, Mary (2004) *Stay Fertile Longer,* Rodale.

19 Barbieri, R.L. (1990) 'Etiology and epidemiology of endometriosis', *American Journal of Obstetrics and Gynecology,* 162 (2), pp. 565–7.

Chapter 29

1 Warshowsky, Allan and Oumano, Ellen (2002) *Healing Fibroids, a Doctor's Guide to a Natural Cure,* Simon & Schuster, p. 7.

2 Ibid.

3 Ibid., p3.

4 Hutchins Jr., Francis (1990) 'Uterine fibroids: current concepts in management', *Female Patient,* October, 15, p. 29.

5 Referred to by Salaman, Maureen Kennedy (1998) *All Your Health Questions Answered Naturally,* MKS, Inc., p. 1054.

6 Quoted in Northrup, Christiane (2002) *Women's Bodies, Women's Wisdom,* Bantam Books, p. 184.

7 Ibid., p. 185.

8 Warshowsky and Oumano, *Healing Fibroids,* p. 143.

9 See www.westonprice.org/women/menorrhagia.html.

10 Referred to by Salaman, Maureen Kennedy (1998) *All Your Health Questions Answered Naturally,* MKS, Inc., p. 1058.

11 Referred to by Warshowsky and Oumano, *Healing Fibroids,* p. 131.

12 Cousens, Gabriel (2000) *Conscious Eating,* North Atlantic Books, p. 546.

13 Research of Wolfgang Sheef (Bonn) and Professor Dittmar (Starnberg), quoted by Cousens, *Conscious Eating*, p. 546.

14 Northrup, *Women's Bodies, Women's Wisdom*.

15 Referred to by Salaman, *All Your Health Questions Answered Naturally*, p. 1058.

Chapter 30

1 Reference to UK research of Dr Williams in Vliet, Elizabeth Lee (2003) *It's My Ovaries, Stupid!*, Scribner.

2 Ibid., p. 171.

3 Ibid., p. 177.

4 Cattanach, J.F. and Milne, B.J. (1988) 'Post-tubal sterilization problems correlated with ovarian steroidgenesis', *Contraception*, 38 (5), pp. 541–50. Quoted in Vliet, *It's My Ovaries, Stupid!*, p. 172.

5 Warshowsky, Allan (2002) *Healing Fibroids*, Simon & Schuster.

Chapter 31

1 Carlsten, E, et al. (1992) 'Evidence for decreasing quality of semen during the past 50 years' *British Medical Journal*, 305, pp. 609–13.

2 Swan, S.H. and Elkin, E.P. (1999) 'Declining semen quality: can the past inform the present?' *BioEssays*, 21 (7), pp. 614–21.

3 Carlsen, E., et al. (1992) 'Evidence for the decreasing quality of semen during the past 50 years'.

   Van Waeleghem, K., et al. (1994) 'Deterioration of sperm quality in young Belgian men during recent decades', *Human Reproduction*, 9 (4), p. 73.

   Auger, J., et al. (1995) 'Decline in semen quality among fertile men in Paris during the past 20 years', *New England Journal of Medicine*, 332 (5), pp. 281–5.

   Irvine, D.S. (1994) 'Failing sperm quality', *British Medical Journal*, 309, p. 476.

4 Ji, B.T., et al. (1997) 'Paternal cigarette smoking and the risk of childhood cancer among offspring of non-smoking mothers', *Journal of the National Cancer Institute*, 89 (3), pp. 238–44.

5 Pacifici, R.., et al. (1993) 'Nicotine, cotinine, and trans-3-hydroxycotionine levels in seminal plasma of smokers: effects on semen parameters', *Therapeutic Drug Monitoring*, 15, (5), pp. 358–63.

   Vine, M.F. (1996) 'Smoking and male reproduction', *International Journal of Andrology*, 19 (6), pp. 323–37.

   Vine, M.F., et al. (1996), 'Cigarette smoking and semen quality', *Fertility and Sterility*, 65 (4), pp. 835–42.

6 Bennet, H..S., et al. (1950) 'Breast and prostate in men who die of cirrhosis of the liver', *American Journal of Clinical Pathology*, 20, pp. 814–28.

7 Mendelson, J.M. (1978) 'Effects of alcohol on plasma testosterone and luteinising hormone levels', *Alcoholism Clinical & Experimental Research*, 2, pp. 225–58.

8 van Thiel, D.M. (1974) 'Hypogonadism in alcoholic liver disease: evidence for a double effect', *Gastoenterology*, 67, pp. 1188–99.

9 Wynn, M. and Wynn, A., *The Case for Preconception Care for Men and Women*, Ab Academic publishers.

10 Parazzani, F., et al. (1993) 'Risk factors for unexplained dyspermia in infertile men: a case control study', *Archive of Andrology*, 31 (2), pp. 105–13.

11 Kamen, Betty (1982) 'Nutrition dialogue, let's live', November, pp. 96–7.

12 Giblin, P. T., et al. (1988) 'Effects of stress and characteristic adaptability on semen quality in healthy men', *Fertility and Sterility*, 49, pp. 127–32.
Lenzi, A., et al. (2003) 'Stress, sexual dysfunctions and male infertility', *Journal of Endocrinological Investigation*, 26 (3), pp. 72-6.

13 Laino, Charlene (1994) 'Stress due to loss of a loved one tied to male infertility', *Medical Tribune*, 1 December, p. 16.

14 Clarke, R.N., et al. (1991) 'Relationship between psychological stress and semen quality among in-vitro fertilization patients', *Human Reproductions*, 6, (8), pp. 1170–5.

15 Howards, Stuart (1995) *New England Journal of Medicine*, 332 (5), pp. 312–17.

16 Holt Jr, L.E. and Albanese, A..A.. (1944) 'Observations on amino acid deficiencies in man', *Transactions of the Association of American Physicians*, 58, p. 143.

17 De Aloysio, D., et al. (1982) 'The clinical use of Arginine aspartate in male infertility', *Alta Europaca Fertlitatis*, 13, pp. 133–67.

18 Schater, A., et al. (1973) 'Treatment of ligospermia with the amino acid arginine', *Journal of Urology*, 110, pp. 311–13.

19 Gaby, A.R. (1996) *Townsend Letters for Doctors and Patients*, April, p. 20.

20 Costa, M.., et al. (1994) 'L-Carnitine in idiopathic asthozoospermis: a multicentre study' *Andrologia*, 26, pp. 155–9; Vitali, G., et al. (1995) 'Carnitine supplementation in human idiopathic asthenospermia. Clinical results', *Drugs under Experimental and Clinical Research*, 21, pp. 157–9.

21 Scott, R., et al. (1997) 'Selenium supplementation in sub-fertile human males', *British Journal of Urology*, 82, pp. 625–9.
Scott, R., et al. (1998) 'The effect of oral selenium supplementation on human sperm motility', *British Journal of Urology*, 82 (1), pp. 76–80.

22 Krznjavi, H., et al. (1992) 'Selenium and fertility in men', *Trace Elements in Medicine*, 9 (2), pp. 107–8.

23 Geva, E., et al. (1996) 'The effect of anti-oxidant treatment on human spermatozoa and fertilization rate in an in vitro program', *Fertility and Sterility*, 66, (3), pp. 430–4.

24 Bayer, R (1960) 'Treatment of infertility with vitamin E', *International Journal of Infertility*, 5, pp. 70–8.

25 Hunt, C.D., et al. (1992) 'Effect of dietary zinc depletion on seminal volume and zinc loss, serum testosterone concentration and sperm morphology in young men', *American Journal of Clinical Nutrition*, 56, pp. 148–57.

26 Quoted in by Brezny, Rob (2005) *Pronoia*, North Atlantic Books.

Also suggested by herbalist James Green in his book (2000) *The Male Herbal*, The Crossing Press, section entitled 'sperm trek', p. 132.

Chapter 32

1 Massachusetts Male Ageing Study as at 1998.

2 Kahn, Jason (1995) 'Smoking may increase risk of impotence', *Medical Tribune*, 19 January, p. 5.

3 Quoted by Salaman, Maureen Kennedy (1998) *All Your Health Questions Answered Naturally*, MKS, Inc., p. 599.

4 Quoted in ibid., p. 602.

5 Pennington, Jean and Young, Barbara (1991) 'Total diet study of nutritional elements', *1982–1989 Journal of the American Dietetic Association*, February, 91, pp. 179–83.

Elin, R (1995) 'Magnesium, the forgotten nutrient', *The Nutrition Report*, February.

Touyz, R.M. (1991) 'Magnesium supplementation as an adjuvant to synthetic calcium channel antoganism in the treatment of hypertension', *Medical Hypothesis*, 36, pp. 140–1.

6 Faelton, Sharon (1981) *The Complete Book of Minerals for Health*, Rodale Press, pp. 432–3.

Chapter 33

1 Vliet, Elizabeth Lee (2003) *It's My Ovaries, Stupid!*, Scribner.

2 Ross, Julia (2000) *The Diet Cure*, Penguin.

3 Buhner, Stephen Harrod (2003) *The Fasting Path*, Avery, Appendix 2, p. 174.

Chapter 34

1 A full copy of this study can be downloaded free from the website www.biolreprod.org. The reference is (2003) 'Characterization of ovarian follicular wave dynamics in women', *Biology of Reproduction*, 69, pp. 1023–31.

2 Quoted on website 25 Saskatchewan Science Achievements – medical research: www.sk25.ca.

3 Harris, Collette (2004) *PCOS and Your Fertility*, Hay House, Inc.

4 Harris, *PCOS and Your Fertility*,., p. 67.

Chapter 35

1 Cossom, J., et al. (2003) 'How spermatozoa come to be confined to surfaces', *Cell motil cytoskelton*, 54 (1), pp. 56–63.

2 Williams, Christopher (2001) *The Fastest Way to get Pregnant Naturally*, Hyperion.

3 Ibid.

4 Research of British biologists Robin Baker and Mark Bellis, referred to in Harris, Collette (2004) *PCOS and Your Fertility*, Hay House, Inc.

5 Ibid.

6 Report in (1996) *Psychology Today*, January/February.

7 Cutler, W.B., et al. (1985) 'Sexual behaviour frequency and biphasic ovulatory type menstual cycles', *Physiological Behavior*, 34 (5), pp. 805–10.

8 Ibid.

9 Harris, *PCOS and Your Fertility*

Bibliography

Balch, Phyllis and Balch James, *Nutritional Healing* (New York: Avery, 2000)

Barbierei, Robert, Domar, Alice and Loughlin Kevon, *6 Steps to Increased Fertility* (New York: Simon & Schuster, 2000)

Beck, Leslie, *The Ultimate Nutrition Guide for Women* (Hoboken, NJ: John Wiley & Sons, 2001)

Berkson, Lindsey D., *Hormone Deception* (New York: McGraw-Hill, 2000)

Bonk, Melinda, *It's Not in Your Head, It's in Your Hormones* (Gloucester, MA: Fair Winds Press, 2001)

Bradstreet, Karen, *Overcoming Infertility Naturally* (Orem, UT: Woodland Books, 1995)

Braverman, Eric, *The Healing Nutrients Within* (Laguna Beach, CA: Basic Health Publications, 2003)

Carter, Jean, *Food, Your Miracle Medicine* (New York: HarperPerennial, 1993)

Cherniske, Stephen, *The Metabolic Anti-Aging Plan* (London: Piatkus, 2003)

Chichoke, Anthony, *Enzymes & Enzyme Therapy* (Chicago: Keats Publishing, 2000)

Clarke, Adrienne, et al., *Organic Living* (Naperville, IL: Sourcebooks Inc., 2001)

Cousens, Gabriel, *Conscious Eating*, (Berkeley: North Atlantic Books, 2000)

Day Phillip, *Food for Thought* (New York: M. Evans & Co, 2001)

Domar, Alice, *Conquering Infertility* (New York: Viking Books, 2002)

Engel, Cindy, *Wild Health* (Boston: Houghton Mifflin Company, 2002)

Erasmus, Udo, *Fats that Heal, Fats that Kill* (Vancouver: Alive Books, 1993)

Glenville, Marilyn, *Natural Solutions to Infertility* (New York: M. Evans & Co., 2000)

Harris, Collete, *The PCOS Diet Book* (London: Thorsons, 2002)

Holwell, Edward, *Enzyme Nutrition* (New York: Avery, 1985)

Indichova, Julia, *Inconceivable* (New York: Broadway Books, 1997)

Jensen, Bernard, *Dr Jensen's Guide to Body Chemistry & Nutrition* (Chicago: Keats Publishing, 2000)

Klapper, Michael, *Pregnancy, Children and the Vegan Diet* (Hawaii: Gentle World Inc., 1997)

Klatz, Ronald, *Grow Young with HGH* (New York: HarperPerennial, 1997)

Magnacca, Kristen, *Girlfriend to Girlfriend, A Fertility Companion* (Bloomington, IN: 1st Books Library, 2000)

Malesky, Gale and Kittel Mary, *The Hormone Connection* (Emmaus, Pennsylvania: Rodale, 2001)

Mars, Brigitte *'Rawsome'* (Laguna Beach, CA: Basic Health Publications Inc., 2004)

McKeith, Gillian, *Living Food for Health* (London: Piatkus, 2000)

——, *You Are What You Eat* (London: Michael Joseph, 2004)

Murray, Michael, *5 HTP* (New York: Bantam Books, 1999)

Northrup, Christiane, *Women's Bodies, Women's Wisdom* (Carlsbad, California: Hay House Inc., 2006)

Null, Gary, *Power Aging* (New York: New American Library, 2003)

Ogle, Amy and Mazzullo, Lisa, *Before Your Pregnancy* (New York: Random House Publishing Group, 2002)

Payne, Niravi, *The Whole Person Fertility Program* (New York: Three Rivers Press, 1997)

Reid, Daniel P, *The Tao of Health, Sex and Longevity* (London: Simon & Schuster, 1989)

Reiss, Fern, *The Infertility Diet* (Newton, MA: Peanut Butter & Jelly Press 1999)

Richardson, Jack, *The Little Herb Encyclopedia* (Woodland Health Books, 1995)

Ross, Julia, *The Mood Cure* (London: Thorsons, 2002)

Santillo, Humbart, *Food Enzymes* (Arizona: Hohm Press, 1993)

Schmid, Ronald, F., *Traditional Foods Are Your Best Medicine* (Rochester, Vermont: Healing Arts Press, 1997)

Schmidt, Michael, *Smart Fats* (Berkeley, CA: Frog Ltd./North Atlantic Books, 1997)

Shannon, Marilyn, *Fertility Cycles & Nutrition* (Cincinnati, OH: Couple to Couple League International Inc., 1990)

Somers, Suzanne, *The Sexy Years* (New York: Crown Publishers, 2004)

Starck, Marcia, *Handbook of Natural Therapies* (Berkeley, CA: The Crossing Press/Ten Speed Press, 1998)

Trickey, Ruth, *Women, Hormones and the Menstrual Cycle* (Sydney: Allen & Unwin, 2003)

Van Stratton, Michael, *The Good Health Directory* (New York: Barrons, 2000)

Vliet, Elizabeth Lee, *Women, Weight, and Hormones* (New York: M. Evans and Company Inc., 2001)

——, *It's my Ovaries, Stupid* (New York: Scribner, 2003)

Weeson, Nicky, *Enhancing Fertility Naturally* (Rochester, VT: Healing Arts Press, 1999)

Weschler, Toni, *Taking Charge of Your Fertility* (HarperCollins: Quil, 2002)

Williams, Christopher, MD, *The Fastest Way to Get Pregnant Naturally* (New York: Hyperion, 2001)

Wolfe, David, *The Sunfood Diet Success System* (New York: Maul Brothers Publishing, 2000)

Woollams, Chris, *Oestrogen, The Killer in Our Midst* (Bath: Bath Press Ltd, 2004)

Index